PROGRESS IN PEDIATRIC NEUROLOGY II

PROGRESS IN PEDIATRIC NEUROLOGY II

Editor

J. GORDON MILLICHAP, M.D., F.R.C.P.

Professor Emeritus of Pediatrics and Neurology.
Northwestern University Medical School,
and
Children's Memorial Hospital,
Chicago, Illinois

Formerly, Pediatric Neurologist,
Mayo Clinic

P N B • Publishers
Chicago

Published and Distributed Throughout the World by

PNB • Publishers

P.O.Box 11391

Chicago, Illinois 60611, U.S.A.

Printed in the U.S.A.

ISBN 0-9629115-8-5
Library of Congress Catalog Card Number: 94-66683
ISSN 1076-2728

To

NANCY

PREFACE

The material included in this book is based on a review of the literature published during the three year period, January 1991 through December 1993. The abstracts and editorial comments have appeared in monthly issues of *Pediatric Neurology Briefs* ©, Volumes V, VI and VII. They have been compiled under subject heading and in chronological order of appearance in order to provide an update and overview of current PROGRESS IN PEDIATRIC NEUROLOGY. A comprehensive index is supplied so that the reader may have ready access to the material reviewed and the subject matter included in the editorial comments.

PROGRESS IN PEDIATRIC NEUROLOGY 1994 is the second book compiled from *Pediatric Neurology Briefs*©. The first compendium in this series was published in 1991 and included articles from the literature of 1987 through December 1990. In the current volume, I have invited colleagues who are authorities in the subject to join me in providing an introduction to chapters with their opinion and overview of the most important advances. Their most valued contributions and assistance are gratefully acknowledged.

Epilepsy, headache, attention deficit and learning disorders, neuromuscular disorders, neurocutaneous syndromes, brain neoplasms, congenital and degenerative diseases, including Rett syndrome, are some of the topics covered. The impact of advances in chromosomal and molecular genetics on our understanding of the pathogenesis, prevention, and treatment of the epilepsies and other neurological disorders is emphasized.

The specialty of pediatric neurology bridges not only pediatrics and neurology but also psychology and the education of learning disabled children. Environmental toxins, especially lead and pesticides, have received increased attention from our colleagues in public health and pharmacology, and the literature on neurotoxicology, nutrition, and diet-related illness has been reviewed. Original articles have been selected from the medical world literature and journals of pediatrics, neurology, developmental medicine, neurosurgery, psychology, psychiatry, epilepsy and other specialties. The editorial comments draw on both recent and past publications on each subject. The institutions and country of origin of the reports are provided in addition to full references.

PROGRESS IN PEDIATRIC NEUROLOGY is intended to provide pediatric neurologists, pediatricians, neurologists, neurosurgeons, psychiatrists, psychologists, geneticists, educators and other interested professionals with an update of the diagnosis, etiology, pathology, treatment and prognosis of nervous diseases of infants, children and adolescents.

J. GORDON MILLICHAP, M.D., F.R.C.P.

CONTRIBUTORS

ANITA L. BELMAN, M.D.

Professor of Neurology and Pediatrics, School of Medicine, State University of New York at Stony Brook, N.Y.

JOHN B. BODENSTEINER, M.D.

Professor of Pediatrics and Neurology, Chief, Child Neurology, West Virginia University School of Medicine, Morgantown, WV.

J. KEITH BROWN, M.D., F.R.C.P.

Paediatric Neurology Department, Royal Hospital for Sick Children, Edinburgh, Scotland, U.K.

MICHAEL E. COHEN, M.D.

Professor and Chairman, Department of Neurology, State University of New York at Buffalo School of Medicine & Biomedical Sciences.

MARTHA BRIDGE DENCKLA, M.D.

Professor of Neurology & Pediatrics, Johns Hopkins University School of Medicine; Director, Developmental Cognitive Neurology,and Learning Disabilities Research Center, Kennedy-Krieger Institute, Baltimore, MD.

PATRICIA K. DUFFNER, M.D.

Professor of Neurology and Pediatrics, Department of Neurology, State University of New York at Buffalo School of Medicine & Biomedical Sciences.

PAUL RICHARD DYKEN, M.D.

Professor and Chairman, Department of Neurology, University of South Alabama, Mobile, AL.

MANUEL R. GOMEZ, M.D.

Professor of Pediatric Neurology, Consultant Pediatric Neurologist, Mayo Clinic, Rochester, MN.

CONTRIBUTORS (continued)

GREGORY L. HOLMES, M.D.
Director, Epilepsy Program & Clinical Neurophysiology Laboratory, Children's Hospital; Associate Professor of Neurology, Harvard Medical School, Boston, MA.

JOHN H. MENKES, M.D.
Professor Emeritus of Neurology and Pediatrics, University of California, Los Angeles.

RUTH D. NASS, M.D.
Professor of Pediatrics and Neurology, Department of Neurology, New York University Medical Center, New York.

MICHAEL J. RIVKIN, M.D.
Assistant in Neurology (with Joseph J.Volpe, M.D.), Children's Hospital, Harvard Medical School, Boston, MA.

E. S. ROACH, M.D.
Director, Division of Pediatric Neurology, Professor, Department of Neurology, University of Texas Southwestern Medical School, Dallas, TX.

HARVEY B. SARNAT, M.D., F.R.C.P. (C)
Professor of Pediatrics (Neurology) and Pathology (Neuropathology), University of Washington; Head, Division of Pediatric Neurology, Children's Hospital and Medical Center, Seattle, WA.

HARVEY S. SINGER, M.D.
Professor and Chairman, Department of Pediatric Neurology, Johns Hopkins University and Hospital, Baltimore, MD.

JOHN WILSON, Ph.D., F.R.C.P.
Consultant Neurologist, Great Ormond Street Hospital for Children, and the Institute of Child Health, London.

TABLE OF CONTENTS

Progress in Pediatric Neurology II

CHAPTER 1

EPILEPSY AND RELATED DISORDERS

INTRODUCTION

Scientific articles on pediatric epilepsy selected for review and commentary in Volume II of **Progress in Pediatric Neurology**, and published in the years 1991 through 1993, totalled 145, an increase of 30 (12%) compared to the number included in Volume I of the series, which covered the years 1987 through 1990. Adverse effects of antiepileptic drugs (AEDs), chiefly carbamazepine and valproic acid, accounted for 16% of these articles in both Volumes I and Volume II of this series.

In addition to the well documented cognitive, teratogenic, and hepatotoxic effects, an apparent increase in incidence of skin rash with carbamazepine and valproate-induced reproductive endocrine disorders in girls and young women with epilepsy are cause for concern. The Editor's plea for research and development of novel AEDs based on recent advances in cellular mechanisms of epilepsy, noted in Volume I of Progress in Pediatric Neurology 1991, has been answered. The recent introduction of new AEDs, notably gabapentin and felbamate, may lead to improved seizure control without serious side effects. *Gabapentin*, a GABA analogue designed to readily penetrate the blood-brain barrier, differs from conventional AEDs although its exact mode of action is unclear. It is not metabolized by the liver and is free of interactions with other drugs. Gabapentin has been found effective for the treatment of partial and secondarily generalized seizures in children older than 12 years and in adults. Adverse effects have been minor and psychometric testing revealed no cognitive impairments.

Unlike gabapentin, *felbamate*, a dicarbamate related to meprobamate, increases the concentrations of phenytoin and valproate and is itself affected by other drugs. It is available as add on therapy for Lennox-Gastaut syndrome in children and partial seizures in adults. Reports of significant insomnia and weight loss may limit the usefulness of felbamate, however, especially as a monotherapy. Until these newer agents have passed the test of time as adjuvant therapies, the monotherapists may have to yield to polytherapists for optimal seizure control to be attained. Further research into drug interactions, synergisms and antagonisms, and the scientific management of multiple drug therapy might mitigate the bias against polytherapy and lead to improvements in control of drug resistant epilepsies.

Major advances in chromosomal and molecular genetics have identified genes for several of the childhood epilepsies, including benign familial neonatal convulsions, juvenile myoclonic epilepsy, and progressive myoclonus epilepsy. Technological developments in electroencephalography and neuroimaging have led to the identification of a variety of childhood epilepsy syndromes and pathologies, previously recognized only by biopsy or at the time of surgery or autopsy. Surgical resection of focal cortical heterotopias for the relief of infantile seizures, corpus callosotomy for the control of drop seizures, temporal lobectomy for complex partial seizures, and hemispherectomy for seizures associated with infantile hemiplegia have resulted in an improved prognosis for children with medically refractory epilepsies.

Progress in pediatric neurology and epilepsy in the future will depend on advances in molecular biology and our understanding of seizure mechanisms. The development of anticonvulsants will focus on drugs that interfere with neurotransmitter receptors and specific ion channels involved in the mechanism of epileptogenesis. The introduction of new, more effective and less toxic antiepileptic medications should be complemented by an emphasis on seizure etiology and prevention, and the earlier implementation of surgical techniques for the removal of discrete epileptogenic foci.-*J. Gordon Millichap, M.D., F.R.C.P.*

OVERVIEW OF RECENT ADVANCES

Gregory L. Holmes, M.D.
Clinical Director, Epilepsy Program
Children's Hospital, Harvard University, Boston

Clearly the evaluation and treatment of childhood epilepsy has changed dramatically during the past three years. While there have been many noteworthy articles published, I feel the most significant changes have occurred in three areas: initiation of antiepileptic drugs, surgical management of intractable epilepsy, and the release of new antiepileptic drugs.

In the not too distant past it was not unusual for children or adults to be placed on both phenytoin and phenobarbital for their partial or generalized seizure. We now know that many children presenting with their first unprovoked seizure will not have a recurrence. In a prospective study of 238 children with a first unprovoked seizure closely followed by Shinnar and colleagues seizures recurred in only about a third (Pediatrics 1990;85:1076-85). Patients with static encephalopathies and abnormal EEGs had higher risk factors for recurrence than children with idiopathic seizures and normal EEGs. Because we have also learned that AEDs in some children may lead to significant cognitive and behavioral side effects, there has been an increasing emphasis on AED monotherapy using AEDs for shorter periods of time.

The pioneering work of Drs Penfield and Jasper at the Montreal Neurological Institute was the stimulus for the wide use of epilepsy surgery for medically intractable seizures in adults. The last few years have seen a marked increase in interest in surgery for epilepsy in children and infants. Unlike adults in whom most surgical resections are performed on mesial temporal lobe structures, children frequently have extra-temporal epileptic foci(Ped Neur Briefs Feb 1991). Localization of the epileptic focus or zone has been aided by improved MRI scanning, use of subdural electrode monitoring, ictal and interictal single positron emission tomography (SPECT), and positron emission tomography (PET) scans.

The MRI is now the neurimaging test of choice in the evaluation of intractable epilepsy in children. It is particularly valuable in detecting cortical migration defects and hippocampal sclerosis in the older child.(Ped Neur Briefs Dec 1991). Computer-assisted volume analysis of the temporal lobes may detect asymmetries that are not readily apparent on visual analysis of the scan. Central to the use of SPECT in the localization of the epileptic foci are the observations that ictal hyperfusion occurs at the site of the epileptic focus while hypoperfusion is seen on the interictal scan. There is now substantial evidence that the ictal scan is superior to the interictal scan in the localization of the epileptic focus. While SPECT studies in children have been more limited, results in children appear to be similar to adults. Like SPECT, PET scanning is a noninvasive functional imaging test that has been used to evaluate cerebral metabolic rates. While over 300 agents have been labelled with positron-emitters, 2-deoxy-2(^{18}F) fluro-D-glucose (FDG) has been the agent most commonly employed in epilepsy patients.

These new technologies have helped identify epileptic zones in children who previously were felt to have generalized or multifocal seizures. For example, infantile spasms, a condition characterized clinically by generalized flexor or extensor tonic seizures and an EEG with diffuse high-voltage, slow background with multifocal spikes and sharp waves, would at first appear unlikely to be amenable to focal ablation. However, Chugani and colleagues (Ann Neurol 1990;27:406-413; Ped Neur Briefs March 1992) have used PET scanning successfully to guide the extent of the resections in selected children with infantile spasms.

While surgery is becoming increasingly used in the treatment of childhood epilepsy, antiepileptic drug (AED) therapy remains the mainstay of treatment. Gabapentin and felbamate are the first AEDs to be released since carbamazepine in 1974 and valproate in 1977. The potential role of gabapentin in the treatment of epilepsy in children younger than 12 years of age is under investigation (Ped Neur Briefs May 1994), and felbamate has been found effective in the management of Lennox-Gastaut syndrome (Ped Neur Briefs Jan 1993).

There have been significant advances in our understanding of other paroxysmal disorders. Most noteworthy have been the investigations into the mystifying disorder of alternating hemiplegia of childhood. This syndrome is characterized by episodes of hemiplegia or quadriplegia lasting from minutes to days, motor deficits, choreoathetotic movements, and moderate to severe retardation.(Burgeois M et al. J Pediatr 1993;122:673-679; Ped Neur Briefs Jan 1993). While not totally effective, flunarazine has been widely used as treatment.

While epilepsy and other paroxysmal disorders continue to be a major health issue in children, recent advances have been substantial. In this "Decade of the Brain" we all hope the next three years will be as productive as the last three.-*Gregory L. Holmes, M.D., Department of Neurology, Children's Hospital, Harvard Medical School, Boston, MA.*

NEONATAL SEIZURES

BENIGN FAMILIAL NEONATAL CONVULSIONS

Linkage studies with the chromosome 20 markers D20S19 and D20S20 were performed in two families with benign familial neonatal convulsions at the Department of Pediatrics, The University of Texas Health Science Center, San Antonio, TX. In the first family with 14 affected, none had seizures after two months of age. In the second family with 13 affected, seizures did not remit until 6 to 24 months; febrile convulsions occurred in two, and one had refractory epilepsy until late adolescence. In family one, the odds were greater than 20,000:1 against linkage at 10% recombination; whereas the data from family two favored linkake with a maximum odds ratio of 45:1 at 6% recombination. It was concluded that this autosomal dominant primary epilepsy of infancy is clinically and genetically heterogeneous. (Ryan SG et al. Benign familial neonatal convulsions: Evidence for clinical and genetic heterogeneity. Ann Neurol May 1991;29:469-473).

COMMENT. These data based on large family pedigrees suggest two distinct genetic loci for benign familial neonatal convulsions. The subtype linked to chromosome 20q may be associated with delayed remission and a higher risk for the development of epilepsy. The authors suggest that absence and benign rolandic epilepsy might also show genetic heterogeneity.- Editor. *Ped Neur Briefs* June 1991.

EEG IN BENIGN NEONATAL CONVULSIONS

An electroencephalographic-video study of 14 benign neonatal familial convulsions (BNFCs) in 3 children from two families is reported from the Hopitaux Universitaires, Strasbourg, and the Institut de Biologie, Montpellier, France. Seizures occurred during sleep and were preceded by a short period of arousal. A brief symmetrical flattening of the EEG, associated with apnea, tachycardia, and tonic motor activity, was followed by a long (1-2 minute) bilateral discharge of spikes and sharp waves, simultaneous with vocalizations, chewing, and focal or generalized clonic activity, often asymmetrical and asynchronous. EEG and clinical symptoms varied from left to right from one seizure to the next, and a stable focus was never observed. (Hirsch E et al. Electroclinical signs of benign neonatal familial convulsions. Ann Neurol Dec 1993;34:835-841). (Respond: Dr Hirsch, Service d'Epileptologie Clinique, Clinique Neurologique, Hopitaux Universitaires de Strasbourg, 1 place de l'Hopital, 67091 Strasbourg Cedex, France).

COMMENT. BNFCs are brief seizures beginning at the second or third day after birth and occurring for several days or weeks. Less than 10% have seizures in later childhood and adulthood. The gene for this syndrome has been localized to the long arm of chromosome 20, but BNFCs may be genetically heterogeneous. The pattern of the seizures is similar to that of generalized tonic-clonic epilepsy, in which the initial tonic phase may be asymmetrical. The asymmetry of BNFCs may be explained by immaturity of the corpus callosum in the neonate. The interictal EEG is either normal or shows bursts of sharp alternating theta rhythms, a *theta pointu alternant* pattern. Frequent BNFCs have no postictal deficit or exhaustion and no adverse effect on development of the child. -Editor. *Ped Neur Briefs* Dec 1993.

SEIZURES AND PARTIAL HYPOPARATHYROIDISM

Neonatal hypocalcemia and seizures in three infants who developed recurrence of hypocalcemia later in childhood are reported from the Department of Paediatrics, The Hospital for Sick Children, Toronto, Ontario, Canada. Hypocalcemia resolved in 1 week, 3 months, and 14 months and recurrences were noted at 4, 7 and 12 years of age. Plasma parathyroid hormone concentrations were low but detectable.

One patient born full term with normal birth weight became irritable and developed tonic-clonic convulsions on the first day of life. The plasma calcium was 1.43 mmol/L; magnesium, 0.86 mmol/L; and phosphate 1.95 mmol/L. She was hospitalized again at 4 weeks of age for asymptomatic hypocalcemia. Except for generalized developmental delay first noted at 7 months of age, she had no clinically important illness until 12-1/2 years of age when she experienced difficulty bending her fingers and numbness of her hands and feet. Several months later, following a minor viral illness, she lost consciousness while watching television and developed convulsions. The plasma calcium was 1.35 mmol/L and ionized calcium 0.69 mmol/L. She has received therapy with calcitriol for the last 3 years and has maintained a normal plasma calcium concentration.

In patients 2 and 3 the childhood hypocalcemia developed gradually over several years. The authors caution that congenital hypoparathydroidism is not always transient, neonatal hypocalcemia may signal permanent partial hypoparathyroidism, and hypocalcemia in an otherwise normal neonate should be followed up with blood calcium measurements during childhood and adolescence. (Kooh SW, Binet A. Partial hypopara-thyroidism. A variant of transient congenital hypo-parathyroidism. AJDC August 1991;145:877-880).

COMMENT. The authors note that DiGeorge syndrome most closely resembles congenital partial hypoparathyroidism and includes immunologic and cardiac abnormalities. Patients with MEDAC (multiple endocrine deficiency, Addison's disease, and candidiasis) may also have partial parathyroid hormone deficiency. -Editor. *Ped Neur Briefs* Aug 1991.

BENIGN NEONATAL SLEEP MYOCLONUS

Benign neonatal sleep myoclonus was diagnosed in 10 infants at the Children's Hospital, Winnipeg, Manitoba. The neonates were referred for assessment of seizures. The myoclonus increased with gentle restraint and in 2 patients it worsened in spite of anticonvulsant therapy. None of the clinical events was associated with EEG seizure phenomena. All infants were neurodevelopmentally normal between the ages of 4 months and 5 years. The myoclonus remitted by age 6 months in all but 2 infants (Daoust-Roy J, Seshia SS. Benign neonatal sleep myoclonus. A differential diagnosis of neonatal seizures. AJDC Oct 1992; 146:1236-1241). (Reprints: Dr. Seshia, Section of Pediatric Neuro~ciences, Children's Hospital, AE208, 840 Sherbrook St., Winnipeg, Manitoba, Canada R3A lS1.)

COMMENT. *Benign neonatal sleep myoclonus* has the following characteristics: 1) neonatal onset, 2) myoclonic jerks only during sleep, 3) abrupt and consistent cessation with arousal, 4) absence of EEG seizure activity and 5) good prognosis. This entity must be distinguished from benign familial neonatal seizures and anticonvulsants should be withheld. The condition should also be differentiated from neonatal hyperekplexia which is characterized by massive jerks in response to sudden tactile and acoustic stimuli and long lasting myoclonic jerks closely resembling epileptic seizures (Pascotto A, Coppola G. Neonatal hyperekplexia: a case report. Epilepsia Sept/Oct 1992;33:817-820).

Benign myoclonic epilepsy of early childhood reported in 20 children from Riyadh, Saudi Arabia (Gascon GG et al. Pediatr Neurol Sept/Oct 1992; 8:348 (abstract)) was considered a phenotype differing only in the age of onset, but sharing the same genotype as benign infantile myoclonic epilepsy and juvenile myoclonic epilepsy.

Benign myoclonus of early infancy was reported in 6 cases from Milan, Italy (Nardoccin et al. Pediatr Neurol Sept/Oct 1992; 8:404 (abstract)). The sudden onset of myoclonic jerks mainly involving the trunk and upper limbs, normal developmental milestones, absence of EEG abnormalities, and self limited course were consistent with the diagnosis as described initially by Lombroso and Fejerman. -Editor. *Ped Neur Briefs* Dec 1992.

NEONATAL ELECTROGRAPHIC SEIZURES

Preterm and full-term neonates with electrographically confirmed seizures were compared at the University of Pittsburgh School of Medicine. The incidence of seizures for all neonates admitted to a neonatal ICU was 2.3%. Of 92 neonates with EEG-confirmed seizures seen over a 4 year period, 62 were preterm and 30 were full-term. Seizure frequency of preterm 30 wk neonates was 3.9% and significantly higher than that of older neonates. Clinical seizures were noted in 45% of preterm and 53% of full-term neonates. Seizures were subtle in 71% and 68%, respectively. Ischemic brain lesions were diagnosed in 3 9% of preterm compared to 77% of full-term neonates. Intraventricular hemorrhage occurred in 45% of preterm and only in 3% of full-term neonates. Mortality was higher in the preterm than in the term populations. (Scher MS et al. Electrographic seizures in preterm and full-term neonates: Clinical correlates, associated brain lesions, and risk for neurologic sequelae. Pediatrics lan 1993; 91: 128-134). (Reprints: Dr Mark S Scher, MageeWomens Hospital, Developmental Neurophysiology Laboratory, 300 Halket St, Pittsburgh, PA 15213).

COMMENT. More than 50% of this cohort had only electrographic expression of seizures. A later onset of seizures in preterm neonates suggests adverse medical complications after birth. One cannot always rely on simultaneous electrographic confirmation of seizures, since 16% of patients exhibit electroclinical dissociation. -Editor. *Ped Neur Briefs* Jan 1993.

EEG SEIZURES IN NEONATES

Ictal and interictal electrographic seizure durations were compared in 33 preterm(PT) and 35 full-term(FT) neonates studied retrospectively at the Magee-Womens Hospital and the Children's Hospital of Pittsburgh. Average ictal durations were five times longer in FT than in PT infants(14.2 cf 3.1 min). Status epilepticus was responsible for the longer ictal durations in 33% of FT cf only 9% of PT infants. Interictal durations were longer in the older PT(>33 wks) cf young PT(<33 wks) infants. More mature neuronal networks in FT neonates are associated with longer ictal durations and more frequent status epilepticus than in PT neonates. Inhibitory networks more dominant in older than in younger PT infants are correlated with longer interictal periods. (Scher MS, Painter MJ et al. Ictal and interictal electrographic seizure durations in preterm and term neonates. Epilepsia March/April 1993; 34: 284-288). (Reprints: Dr Mark S Scher, Developmental Neurophysiology Laboratory,

Magee-Womens Hospital, 300 Halket St, Pittsburgh, PA 15213).

COMMENT. Neonatal seizures have a high mortality; 35% of this series died soon after birth. They are often difficult to diagnose, and the EEG plays a pivotal role in management. Ideally, video monitoring is used to correlate behavioral manifestations with the EEG. The effectiveness of treatment with anticonvulsant drugs should be evaluated electrographically, in addition to reliance on clinical criteria. Two thirds of neonatal seizures are unresponsive (Painter et al. J Pediatr 1978; 92:315); only 10% are confirmed by EEG (Scher et al. Pediatr Neurol 1989; 5: 17). -Editor. *Ped Neur Briefs* May 1993.

PHENOBARBITAL IN NEONATAL SEIZURES

Phenobarbital plasma levels 24 hrs after a loading dose, and drug level variations after intravenous maintenance doses, were studied in 25 newborns with seizures admitted to a neonatal intensive care unit at the Maternity-School Hospital of Vila Nova Cachoeirinha, Sao Paulo, Brazil. With a mean loading dose of 19 mg/kg for both term and pre-term infants and a mean maintenance dose of 4 mg/kg/day, a mean plasma level of 23 mcg/ml was obtained at 24 hrs, and therapeutic levels between 15-40 mcg/ml were sustained at 4, 7, 14 and 21 days. A tendency towards drug accumulation in the first week and lower levels after 7 days requires frequent monitoring and dose adjustments. Seizure control without EEG confirmation was obtained in 64%. Phenytoin iv was required in addition in 7 infants and clonazepam in 5. Side effects were limited to infants with severe neurological impairment. (Gherpelli JLD et al. Phenobarbital in newborns with neonatal seizures. A study of plasma levels after intravenous administration. Brain Dev July/Aug 1993;15:258-262). (Respond: DrJLD Gherpelli, Sevico de Neurologia Infantil, Hospital das Clinicas da Faculdade de Medicina da USP, Sao Paulo -SP-05403, Caixa Postal 30657, Brazil).

COMMENT. For newborns and infants <3 months who require phenytoin, the recommended loading dose is 12-20 mg/kg and the maintenance dose is 2-4 mg/kg/d, with 8-12 hr dosing intervals (Leppik IE. Epilepsia 1992;33. Suppl 4:S32). Phenytoin levels may be modified by phenobarbital because of an increased metabolism during chronic therapy. Phenytoin elimination half-life varies with age: preterm neonate 75 hr; neonate 21 hr; infant and child 7 h; and adult 24 h. -Editor. *Ped Neur Briefs* Sept 1993.

TREATMENT OF NEONATAL SEIZURES

Controversies in treatment of neonatal seizures are addressed by neurologists from Stanford and Yale Universities. Seizures likely to be associated with electrographic seizure activity (eg focal clonic or multifocal clonic seizures) should be treated with antiepileptic drugs (AEDs). Bilateral tonic posturing, unaccompanied by EEG seizure activity, would not be benefited by AEDs. The presence of seizures should be determined electrographically before treatment is begun. For symptomatic seizures, AEDs are administered until clinical seizures, but not necessarily all EEG seizures, are controlled. The nature and severity of the underlying cerebral lesions are the major determinants of outcome. Conventional treatment, usually with phenobarbital, is not very effective; control is obtained in only one-third of patients. The goals are to restore a normal metabolic state, control hypertension and tachycardia, and reduce the increase in glucose utilization. (Hahn JS, Young RSK. Controversies in treatment of neonatal seizures. Pediatr Neurol July/Aug 1993;9:330-332).

COMMENT. Seizures caused by hypoxic-ischemic encephalopathy and intracranial hemorrhage are the most refractory to treatment with AEDs. Seizures due to metabolic abnormalities are usually transitory and require early recognition and specific management.

Water intoxication as a potential etiology of seizures in young infants, a previously rare condition, is increasing to epidemic proportions in US inner cities.(Keating JP, Dodge PR; and Furth S, Oski FA. AJDC Sept 1993;147:932-3). The maternal motivation for offering water remains uncertain. Improper dilution of formula and feeding large amounts of free water or glucose water, especially at times of diarrhea, are common practices, and occasionally result from improper medical advice. Infants with seizures refractory to AEDs should be tested for hyponatremia. -Editor. *Ped Neur Briefs* Oct 1993.

PROGNOSIS OF NEONATAL SEIZURES

The neurologic outcome of 40 infants with EEG documented seizures of diverse etiologies was examined retrospectively at the Division of Neurology, The Children's Hospital of Philadelphia, PA. Neurologic followup of 27 survivors performed at a mean age of 31 months (range 5 to 56 months) was favorable in 30% of the study population. The remaining 70% (28 of 40) with an unfavorable outcome included mortality in 33% and severe morbidity in 38%. Epilepsy occurred in 56% of survivors (15 of 27), development delay - 67%, and cerebral palsy - 63%. Factors influencing the outcome were the etiology of the seizures, the age at the onset of seizures, birth weight and neurologic examination results. Asphyxia, meningitis and cerebral dysgenesis carried a poor prognosis. Onset of seizures within the first day of life and a severely abnormal neurologic exam significantly predicted an unfavorable outcome. An Apgar score less than 5 at 5 minutes was not significantly related to a poor prognosis. The EEG background activity was the only EEG parameter of value in prognosis: an abnormal background carried an unfavorable outcome in 81% and a normal background was predictive of a favorable prognosis in 67%. (Legido A et al. Neurologic outcome after electroencephalographically proven neonatal seizures. Pediatrics Sept 1991; 88:583-596).

COMMENT. In this retrospective study of neonates with EEG proven seizures, the mortality rate was 33% and the morbidity rate was 56%.

The long-term outcome of an infant with *pyridoxine-dependent neonatal seizures* is reported from the British Columbia's Children's Hospital, Vancouver, BC, Canada (Connolly MB et al. Intravenous immunoglobulin and pyridoxine-dependent seizures. Neurology Sept 1991; 41:1524). Generalized clonic seizures began at 6 days of age followed by partial motor seizures becoming secondarily generalized at 1 month, and episodes of status epilepticus lasting 1 hour at 2-1/2 months. Seizures were controlled and the EEG normalized by 100 mg pyridoxine daily. The patient remained seizure free until age 20 months and then developed episodes of status epilepticus twice a week, always associated with infections. Monthly IV gamma globulin therapy 400 mg/kg infused over 6 hours resulted in prevention of infections and control of convulsions. IV Ig therapy may be helpful in the treatment of neonatal pyridoxine-dependent seizures. -Editor. *Ped Neur Briefs* Oct 1991.

FEBRILE SEIZURES

ELECTROENCEPHALOGRAM IN FEBRILE SEIZURES

The clinical value of EEG investigations in children with febrile seizures is reviewed from the Section of Child and Adolescent Psychiatry, Parke Hospital for Children, Old Road, Hedington, Oxford, England. Reports of EEG abnormalities in children with a history of febrile seizures include 1) ictal, generalized spiking, or lateralized spike wave discharge; 2) postictal, slow activity, spike wave or spikes; and 3) serial EEG's showing bisynchronous theta activity, bisynchronous spike wave at rest and during over breathing, bisynchronous spike wave on photic stimulation, focal spikes or sharp waves, and hypnagogic paroxysmal spike wave.

The author concludes that an early postictal standard EEG will not be helpful in: a) the distinction between clinically simple and atypical seizures, b) the identification of a cerebral infective etiology, and c) the prediction of later occurrence of either further febrile or later afebrile seizures. A limited-place for EEG studies is proposed in connection with febrile seizures associated with suspect cerebral pathology. If the child showed developmental delay, if the first seizure occurred below the age of 12 months, or if the seizures are partial or focal in pattern, a possible structural brain pathology is more likely. In addition, a prolonged febrile seizure, especially if followed by residual neurologic signs or developmental regression, may be evidence of structural cerebral damage and may require further investigation.

EEG can be a useful ancillary investigation suggesting a persistent brain pathology, even in the presence of a normal CT scan, if it demonstrates a slow wave abnormality with or without spike or sharp waves that is persistent. This implies the use of serial EEG recordings over a period of weeks rather than a single recording. The EEG may also be helpful in research investigations concerning genetic factors and the possible connection between febrile seizures and benign rolandic epilepsy of childhood.

Also, the possibility of defining clinically important subgroups of febrile seizures might be facilitated by the use of the EEG. It is emphasized that the EEG recordings should include natural sleep and wakefulness, drowsiness, at least stages I and II of nonrapid eye movement sleep, and arousal. Failure to standardize the procedure makes comparisons between different studies very difficult. (Stores G. When does an EEG contribute to the management of febrile seizures? Arch Dis Child April 1991; 66:554-557).

COMMENT. The author correctly emphasizes the need for standardized EEG procedures, including sleep recordings, in assessing the value of the EEG in the management of febrile seizures. The conclusion that EEG findings may lack predictive value for the later occurrence of epilepsy in children with febrile seizures has been based on longitudinal EEG investigations that were sometimes lacking in this necessary standardization and activation procedures, including sleep. Some earlier reports, omitted from the list of references cited in the present review, have demonstrated a predictive value for the EEG and later occurrence of afebrile seizures (Millichap JG. Febrile Convulsions. Macmillan New York 1967). Further research would be justified. -Editor. *Ped Neur Briefs* May 1991.

THE EEG AND FEBRILE SEIZURES

The relationship between clinical characteristics and EEG classification in 676 children with febrile seizures was examined at the University Pediatric Clinic, Skopje, Yugoslavia. The initial EEG was classified as paroxysmally abnormal (spike wave complexes, generalized or focal, or spikes) in 22 % Focal seizures and those that lasted more than 15 minutes were more often associated with abnormal EEGs. Multiple seizures in the first 24 hours were not related to risk of specific paroxysmal abnormalities. The leading predictors of initial paroxysmal EEG abnormality were 1) older age at the time of EEG and 2) the number of previous febrile seizures. Motor abnormality before the index seizure and focal seizure had less predictive value. The rate of EEG abnormality in children with no previous seizures was 18 % whereas in those with 4 or more previous seizures it was 63 %. (Sofijanov N et al. Febrile seizures: clinical characteristics and initial EEG. Epilepsia Jan/Feb 1992; 33:52-57). (Reprints: Dr. K.B. Nelson at NIH, Federal Building, Room 700, Bethesda, MD 20892, U.S.A.).

COMMENT. Age at the time of the EEG, the number of seizures experienced and a focal first febrile seizure were all predictive of a paroxysmal EEG abnormality. In children more than 4 years of age abnormal EEGs were found in 5 1%. Further follow-up of this population based sample should allow correlation of the initial EEG findings and the occurrence of subsequent afebrile seizures and epilepsy.

In a questionnaire survey of pediatricians and pediatric neurologists in the U.S.A., the EEG was used in determining the need for long-term phenobarbital prophylactic therapy for febrile seizures by 51% and 45 %, respectively. Paroxysmal EEG abnormalities were more frequent in children 5 years of age and older than in younger age groups, and the incidence of EEG abnormalities in records of patients who developed afebrile seizures was 5 times that observed in children with febrile seizures alone. Paroxysmal tracings were more frequent in patients with prolonged or focal febrile seizures than in patients with short simple seizures (Millichap JG, Clinical EEG. 1991; 22:5-12. *Idem,*

Febrile Convulsions, 1968, McMillan, New York). -Editor. *Ped Neur Briefs* March 1992.

PARENTAL REACTION TO FEBRILE CONVULSIONS

The parental reaction to a child's first febrile convulsion was investigated by telephone interview from the Department of Paediatrics, Randers Central Hospital, Denmark. Interviews were conducted in 52 cases from 3-20 months after the convulsion. Fear that the child would die during the fit was volunteered by 44% of parents and another 33% admitted the same reaction when specifically asked about it. Appropriate treatment, i.e. cooling the child and/or placing him in a side position was used in 63% of cases. The child was vigorously shaken during the seizure in 15%. Changes in the behavior of the parents following the child's first seizure included restless sleep in 60%, and dyspeptic symptoms in 29%. The frequency of parental behavioral symptoms rose dramatically if the child had more than a single fit. Many parents wished they had known more about fever and febrile convulsions in children. The general level of knowledge of febrile convulsions among parents of young children is low and the reaction of the parents to the first fit is often severe and persistent. Parents should be given written general infornation about fever and febrile convulsions, and information to parents who have witnessed a convulsion must be both verbal and written. It is concluded that parents of young children should be better informed about febrile convulsions before they occur. Well informed parents managed febrile convulsions better than those uninformed. (Balslev T. Parental reactions to a child's first febrile convulsion. A follow-up investigation. Acta Paediatr Scand April 1991; 80:466-469).

COMMENT. The controversy concerning the long-term prophylactic use of phenobarbital in the management of febrile seizures and the consequent risk of a heightened prevalence of febrile seizure recurrence emphasizes the importance of parental education in the management of fever and febrile seizures. In the absence of a safe and satisfactory alternative to phenobarbital, parental anxiety may be allayed by the prescription of intermittent prophylactic treatment with diazepam at times of fever but poor compliance minimizes its effectiveness in practice. The home use of rectal diazepam, employed more frequently in Europe than in the U.S., may offer an alternative method of parental involvement in selected cases. -Editor. *Ped Neur Briefs* May 1991.

SIBLING EEGs & GENETICS OF FEBRILE SEIZURES

Waking and sleep EEGs were recorded in 67 siblings of 52 patients with febrile seizures (FS) at the Epilepsy Centre Bethel, Bielefeld, F.R.G. Epileptic activity was recorded in at least one sibling of 54 % of patients . Epileptic discharges were noted in 50% of the 67 siblings; only in waking in 3%, in waking and sleep in 31% and in sleep only in 15%. The greatest number of epileptic discharges were noted in the waking state during hyperventilation (33%) and during sleep stage C (39%). Of nine patients with complicated febrile seizures 56 % had at least one sibling with seizure discharges and of 43 patients with simple febrile seizures 54% had a sibling with seizure discharges. Of nine patients with later onset epileptic seizures, 44% had seizure discharges in the EEG. Siblings age six to ten years had the highest rates of activation (67%). Epileptic discharges occurred in 83% of siblings with seizures, but in only 46% of those without seizures. Epileptic activity in patients and in siblings was significantly greater in those who had occipital slow wave activity in the EEG. A multifactorial inheritance of EEG abnormalities was suggested and the genetic factor was important in patients with both simple or complicated FS. Exogenous brain damage may act as an accidental event or catalytic effect leading to the activation of FS, mental retardation, neurologic deficits, behavior disturbances, focal FS, and/or a higher rate of later epileptic seizures (Degen R. et al. A contribution to the genetics of febrile seizures: waking and sleep EEG in siblings. Epilepsia July/August 1991; 32:515-522).

COMMENT. The importance of sleep EEGs and other activating procedures in the prediction of prognosis in patients with febrile seizures is demonstrated by this study. Reports minimizing the value of the EEG in prognosis and later occurrence of epilepsy are often based on EEGs in the waking state only, and without sleep recordings.

A case control study of risk factors for febrile seizures in the People's Republic of China is reported from the Neurological Institute, Sun Yat-Sen University of Medical Sciences, Guangzhou, Beijing Neurosurgical Institute, Beijing, China; National Institutes of Health, Bethesda, MD ; and the World Health Organization, Geneva, Switzerland. Information was gathered by door-to-door survey in six major cities in the People's Republic of China (Zhao F et al. Epilepsia July/August 1991;32:510-514). Family history of febrile seizures, birth and postnatal factors were assessed in 182 subjects and in an equal number of matched controls. The odds ratio for risk of FS in children with a family history of FS in a first-degree relative was 10. Apart from maternal acute respiratory infection during the first trimester of preanancy none of the other examined factors was associated with an increased risk. Birth asphyxia was not a significant risk factor. -Editor. *Ped Neur Briefs* Sept 1991.

TWIN STUDIES OF FEBRILE SEIZURES

Population based twin panels containing 14,352 twin pairs established in Norway and Virginia were used to study the occurrence of febrile seizures and epilepsy at the Departments of Human Genetics and Neurology, Medical College of Virginia, Virginia Commonwealth University, Richmond, VA- and the Institute of Medical Genetics, Oslo, Norway. There was a history of febrile seizures reported in 257 pairs and a history of epilepsy in 1 or both members of 286 pairs of twins. Virginia twins reported febrile seizures (1.98%) slightly more often than Norwegian twins (1.61%). Norwegian twin pairs reported epilepsy (2.19%) slightly more often than Virginia twin pairs (1.66%). There were no significant differences in the concordance rates between Virginian and Norwegian twins for either febrile seizures or epilepsy (for febrile seizures, 0.33 in monozygotic twins and 0.11 in dizygotic twins; for epilepsy, 0.19 monozygotic and 0.07 dizygotic). The excess of concordant monozygotic twin pairs observed for both epilepsy and febrile seizures was significant and showed a factor of almost 3 to 1. (Corey LA et al. The occurrence of epilepsy and febrile seizures in Virginian and Norwegian twins. Neurology Sept 1991;41:1433-1436). (Reprints: Dr. Linda A. Corey, Department of Human Genetics, Medical College of Virginia, Box 33 MCV Station, Richmond, VA 23298).

COMMENT. The inheritance of febrile seizures is multifactorial. Siblings have approximately an 8-12% risk of also having febrile seizures. If the index child and 1 parent are affected, the risks to siblings are 30%-40% (50% if both parents are affected) (Progress in Pediatric Neurology, Millichap JG ed, Chicago, PNB Publishers, 1991).

MMR IMMUNIZATION AND FEBRILE SEIZURES

The risk of seizures following MMR or MR immunization is evaluated in a retrospective cohort study conducted among 18,364 Tennessee children from The Department of Preventive Medicine, Vanderbilt University School of Medicine, Nashville, TN. Of 100 children (0.5%) with a confirmed seizure between the first MMR or MR and age 36 months, 77 had febrile seizures, 15 afebrile seizures and 8 acute symptomatic seizures. The incidence of febrile seizures was 4.3, 5.1, and 2.8 per 1,000 person-years in the 3 age groups, 361-540, 541-720, and 721-1,080 days, respectively. 4 children had febrile seizures in the 7-14 days following MMR or MR immunization, compared with 72 in the interval 30 or more days following MMR or MR with a relative risk of 2.1. The authors concluded that the increase in febrile seizures in the 7-14 day interval following MMR was coincident with the occurrence of fever post-immunization (Griffin MR et al. Risk of seizures after measles-mumps-rubella immunization. Pediatrics Nov 1991;88:881-885).

COMMENT. This review of seizure occurrence was confined to those patients seen at a hospital and would not include seizures treated at home ar at outpatient facilities. The authors admit that the ascertainment of seizures was incomplete but would include more serious seizures or neurologic events.

Measles was the cause of fever in 1.2% of 7,000 cases of febrile seizures reported in the world literature between 1929 and 1964 (Millichap JG, Febrile Convulsions. New York Macmillan, 1968). -Editor. *Ped Neur Briefs* Dec 1991.

RECURRENCE OF FEBRILE SEIZURES

The predictive value of multiple clinical variables for febrile seizure recurrence was assessed in a follow-up study of 155 Dutch children at the Department of Paediatrics, University Hospital and Sophia Children's Hospital, Rotterdam, The Netherlands. Children between 6 months and 5 years presenting with a first febrile seizure and a body temperature of 38.5C or higher but without intracranial infection or defined cause were included. Those with a history of nonfebrile seizures or with neurological abnormalities such as cerebral palsy and mental retardation were excluded as were those treated with continuous phenobarbitone or sodium valproate. Of these initially untreated children, 37% had 1, 30% had 2, and 17% had 3 or more recurrences. The highest risk period for recurrence was during the 6 months after a seizure and the lowest risk was after 24 months freedom from seizures. The younger the child at the 2nd and 3rd seizures, the higher the likelihood of further recurrences. A first degree relative with any type of seizure predicted multiple recurrences of febrile seizures. A body temperature of 40c at initial seizure was associated with a lower risk, as was an age of 30 months or older (Offringa M et al. Seizure recurrence after a first febrile seizure: a multivariate approach. Dev Med Child Neurol Jan 1992;34:15-24). (Respond: Dr. Offringa, Room EE 2171, Erasmus University, P.O. Box 1738, 3000 DR Rotterdam, The Netherlands.)

COMMENT. The authors conclude that the predictive value of combined risk factors (age at onset, family history, height of fever) is superior to that of single variables. The association between elevated temperature and risk of recurrence is in keeping with the theory of a threshold of febrile seizures based on the height of the body temperature (Millichap JG. Studies in febrile seizures I. Height of body temperature as a measure of the febrile seizure threshold. Pediatrics Jan 1959; 23:76-85). - Editor. *Ped Neur Briefs* March 1992.

EPILEPSY AND FEBRILE CONVULSIONS

The risk of epilepsy after febrile convulsions was determined in a national population based study in the United Kingdom and reported from the Department of Paediatrics, Addenbrooke's Hospital, Cambridge and the Institute of Child Health, University of Bristol, England. Of 16,004 neonatal survivors born during 1 week in April 1970 and enrolled in the British Birth Survey, 398 (2.7% of those followed) had at least 1 febrile convulsion by 10 years of age. The ratio of simple to complex febrile seizures was 4 to 1. Those with complex febrile convulsions had a significantly greater incidence of febrile seizure recurrences than the simple febrile seizure group. Prophylactic anticonvulsants were prescribed for longer than a month in only 14% of patients; the seizure was simple in 26 and complex in 14. Afebrile seizures developed in 13 patients (3.4%) and 9 (2.3%) had epilepsy or recurrent afebrile seizures. Complex febrile convulsions and especially focal febrile convulsions were predictive of epilepsy. Afebrile complex partial seizures occurred in 9.4% of children with prolonged febrile convulsions. Of 14,278 children in this study who had no febrile convulsions, 53 (0.4%) developed epilepsy by the age of 10 years (Verity CM, Golding J. Risk of epilepsy after febrile convulsions: a national cohort study. BMJ Nov 30, 1991;303:1373-6). (Respond: Dr. Verity, Department of Paediatrics, Addenbrooke's Hospital, Cambridge CB2 2QQ, England.)

COMMENT. Complex febrile convulsions (longer than 15 minutes, focal, or multiple) accounted for 20% of the febrile seizures in this study, an incidence identical with that reported by pediatricians in the

United States (Millichap JG. Clinical EEG. 1991;22:5-12). In contrast, complex and simple febrile seizures are seen with equal frequency in pediatric neurology practice in the U.S. (Millichap IG, Colliver JA, Pediatr Neurol. 1991;7:243-248). Compared to the United Kingdom where prophylactic anticonvulsants are used infrequently (14% of patients), in the United States long-term phenobarbital is prescribed by 89% of pediatric neurologists for the prevention of complex febrile seizures and by 43% for simple febrile seizures. Parental anxiety was a factor in the prescription of anticonvulsants by 67% of respondents to a questionnaire. Despite the publicity regarding adverse effects on behavior and cognition, phenobarbital therapy is still favored by the majority of pediatric neurologists in the U.S., particularly in the prevention of complex febrile seizures. The recent Seattle study (Farwell JR et al. N Engl J Med 1990;322:364-9) failed to convince members of the Child Neurology Society that phenobarbital has any long-term persistent adverse effects on cognition and they are skeptical of the claim that phenobarbital is ineffective in the control of febrile seizures. The viewpoint stated in an editorial (Robinson RJ, BMJ Nov 30, 1991;303:1345-6) that prophylactic anticonvulsants are rarely needed and have no long term benefit in febrile convulsions is shared by only 17% of pediatric neurologists in the United States.

Several factors might explain the transatlantic differences in the management of febrile seizures: 1) a greater availability and reliance on rectal diazepam for use by parents in the U.K., 2) geographic considerations and the greater distances to hospitals for emergency room treatment of the acute seizure in rural areas of the U.S., and 3) the apparent importance of parental anxiety and physician concern for litigation in the U.S. Therapeutic guidelines may be helpful but the decision to treat must be made on an individual basis. When further and more carefully evaluated, perhaps the EEG will prove of value and receive attention in febrile seizure management.-Editor. *Ped Neur Briefs* March 1992.

FEBRILE SEIZURE V. MENINGITIS

Among 309 children with a first seizure and fever seen in two ERs in Rotterdam, The Netherlands, 23 (7%) had meningitis. The clinical findings in the patients with meningitis were compared with a control group of 69 children with seizures and fever and no meningitis. The signs of meningitis in 21 cases identified were: petechiae, nuchal rigidity, coma, persistent drowsiness, ongoing convulsions, and paresis or paralysis. Two children who proved to have meningitis had none of these signs. The median age at presentation with the first seizure associated with fever was 18 months (range: 3-52 months); 171(65%) underwent lumbar puncture. Meningitis could be excluded on clinical grounds at reevaluation in all 138 children (45%) who did not undergo lumbar puncture. Children whose seizures showed no complex features and whose febrile illness revealed no suspicious features did not have meningitis. If all children with positive indicators were considered eligible for lumbar puncture, no meningitis cases would have been missed, and 75 of the 309 children (24%) would have been spared the puncture. The authors conclude that meningitis can be ruled out clinically in children presenting with seizures and fever, and routine investigation of cerebrospinal fluid is unnecessary. (Offringa M. Seizures and fever: can we rule out meningitis on clinical grounds alone? Clin Pediat Sept 1992;31:514-522.) (Correspondence: M. Offringa, M.D., Center for Clinical Decision Analysis, Room EE 2171, Erasmus University, P.O. Box 1738, 3000 DR, Rotterdam, The Netherlands.)

COMMENT. In a questionnaire study to determine the methods of management of febrile seizures by pediatricians and family practitioners in the State of Illinois, spinal taps were employed by 70 % of respondents in the workup of an acute febrile seizure (Millichap JG. Clin EEG 1991;22:5-12). This frequency of spinal taps was higher than that routinely ordered by private pediatric practitioners for children with first febrile seizures in the United States (Nealis JGT. In:Nelson KB, Ellenberg JH (eds) Febrile Seizures, New

York, Raven Press, 1981). It was lower than the estimate for children admitted to medical centers (Rutter N, Smales ORC. Arch Dis Child 1977;52:188-191). Routine taps have been recommended in all children with an initial febrile convulsion (Ratcliffe JC, Wolff SN. Ann Neurol 1977;1:285-286). Lorber J and Sunderland R have argued against routine lumbar punctures in children with seizures and fever, but recommend examination by a senior staff member if symptoms and signs of meningitis are absent (Lancet 1980;1:785-786).

The indications for lumbar puncture should be determined not only by the patient's clinical manifestations, but also the physician's experience and clinical acumen and the opportunity for close patient observation. A selective approach avoids many unnecessary lumbar punctures and a false sense of security engendered by a normal premature tap. A second selzure with fever is no less likely to herald a bacterial meningitis than a first seizure, and the common emphasis on routine taps for first seizures with fever may be misleading.

Another source of confusion is the determination of complex features of febrile seizures. Berg AT et al. have found disagreement among pediatric neurologists regarding the assessment of focality of the seizure (Epilepsia 1992;33:661-666). The reasons for disagreement included variation in interpretation of lateral eye deviation, staring episodes and motor asymmetries of the convulsion. -Editor. *Ped Neur Briefs* Oct 1992.

EXANTHEM SUBITUM CNS COMPLICATIONS

Central nervous system complications of exanthem subitum were analyzed in 21 infants examined at thc Departments of Pediatrics and Neurology, Fujita Health University School of Medicine, Toyoake, Japan. The primary infection with human herpesvirus 6 was confirmed by isolation of the virus from the blood and/or a rise in antibody titers, and the virus DNA was detected in the cerebrospinal fluid of 6 infants, including 3 with encephalitis/encephalopathy (E/E). Convulsive seizures (15 generalized and 6 focal) occurred during the pre-eruptive stage of the illness, and persisted for more than 45 minutes in 7 infants. Four patients with E/E had prolonged focal seizures and loss of consciousness, abnormal EEGs and CT scans; 3 had a pleocytosis and elevated protein in the CSF. One developed epilepsy and one died. Infants without E/E recovered with no sequelae. (Suga S et al. Clinical and virological analyses of 21 infants with exanthem subitum(roseola infantum) and central nervous system complications. Ann Neurol June 1993;33:597-603). (Respond: Yoshizo Asano MD, Department of Pediatrics, Fujita Health University School of Medicine, Toyoake, Aichi 470-11, Japan).

COMMENT. Exanthem subitum is a common, usually benign, infectious disease of infants, characterized by a four day fever and a rash that appears after the fever subsides. Seizures may complicate the illness during the febrile stage and before the rash erupts. Human herpesvirus 6, recently identified as the causative agent, may rarely invade the CNS and cause encephalitis.

A febrile seizure has long been recognized as the most common complication of exanthem subitum, occurring in 22 percent of 581 patients reported in 11 publications (Millichap JG. Febrile Convulsions. New York, Macmillan, 1968). Evidence for an encephalitic process and a direct involvement of the brain was lacking, and the degree of fever was considered sufficient to explain the frequent complication of convulsions. The present report demonstrates that seizures associated with exanthem subitum and fever are not always simple in type. They are occasionally prolonged and complex and a manifestation of encephalitis or encephalopathy. -Editor. *Ped Neur Briefs* June 1993.

E COLI HEMORRHAGIC COLITIS AND CONVULSIONS

The neurological manifestations of hemorrhagic colitis in seven kindergarten children with *Escherichia coli* 0157:H7 infection are reported from the Saitama Children's Medical Center, Saitama, Japan. Generalized convulsions, occurring in 5 comatose patients, were intractable in 3 and required toxic doses of anticonvulsants for their control. Two patients died aftcr 5 and 7 days of illness. Transient symptoms, delayed in onset for 2 to 6 weeks and after consciousness improved, included phrenic nerve paralysis in 1 patient, neurogenic urinary incontinence in 3, gaze nystagmus in 3, action tremor and oral dyskinesia in 1, and vertigo in 1 patient. Pyrexia and hemolytic uremic syndrome were seen only in patients with neurologic complications. Diarrhea, bloody diarrhea, and abdominal pain were more frequent and severe in this group compared to 7 patients with no neurologic symptoms who were admitted to hospital. Contaminated well water was the source of infection, and verotoxin-l (Shiga-like toxin 1) was the likely cause of neurological symptoms. (Hamano S et al. Neurological manifestations of hemorrhagic colitis in the outbreak of *Escherichia coli* 0157:H7 infection in Japan. Acta Paediatr May 1993;82: 454-458). (Respond: S Hamano MD, Division of Neurology, S Children's Medical Center, 2100 Magome, Iwatsuki, Saitama 339, Japan).

COMMENT. Fever, high white blood cell count, young or old age, and prololonged antimotility drug use are risk factors for complications of this strain of *E coli* infection. The neurologic and other complications of foodborne and waterborne infections, pollutants, and additives, are covered in Environmental Poisons in Our Food, Chicago, PNB Publishers, 1993. -Editor. *Ped Neur Briefs* June 1993.

DIAZEPAM PROPHYLAXIS OF FEBRILE SEIZURES

The results of a double-blind, randomized, placebo-controlled trial of oral diazepam administered only at the time of fever are reported from Tufts University School of Medicine and Boston University School of Public Health, Boston. Among 406 children of mean age 24 months who received diazepam, 0.33 mg/kg/body wt, or placebo orally every 8 hours during febrile illnesses, the reduction in risk of recurrence of febrile seizures in the diazepam-treated group, based on an intention-to-treat analysis, was 44% during a mean follow-up of 1.9 years. An analysis restricted to children who had seizures while actually taking the prescribed medication (45 seizures in 36 children) showed 29 seizure occurrences in the placebo group and only 7 in the diazepam group, an 82% reduction in recurrence risk. Moderate side effects, including ataxia, lethargy, or irritability, were reported in 59 (39%) of 153 children who took at least one dose of diazepam. Mild side effects occurred with the same frequency. (Rosman NP et al. A controlled trial of diazepam administered during febrile illnesses to prevent recurrence of febrile seizures. N Engl J Med July 8 1993; 329: 79-84). (Reprints: Dr Rosman, Division of Pediatric Neurology, Floating Hospital for Children, New England Medical Center, 750 Washington St, Box 330, Boston, MA 02111).

COMMENT. The authors advocate the prevention of recurrence of all febrile seizures and recommend oral diazepam, taken at the first sign of illness, as the optimal prophylactic medication. The benefit demonstrated in this zealously monitored study may not be duplicated in practice when compliance is often less than satisfactory. In a previous controlled trial, Autret and colleagues in France found the results of intermittent oral diazepam therapy disappointing, a lack of efficacy explained by poor compliance (J Pediatr 1990;117:490). An approved rectal preparation of diazepam for the home treatment of the acute febrile seizure in high risk patients may offer one alternative to the universal prophylactic intermittent regimen proposed. A survey of pediatric neurologists found only 22% in favor of diazepam (mean dose, 0.46 mg/kg/day at times of fever) in 1990 (see Millichap JG. Progress in Pediatric Neurology, Chicago, PNB Publ, 1991). A more general acceptance of diazepam by pediatricians and parents may be expected following the Boston report, and the results of this wider experience will determine the practical value and safety of this form of treatment.

A clearer understanding of the mechanism of susceptibility to febrile seizures may lead to more specific therapies. Experiments at Ehime Univ School of Medicine, Japan, demonstrate a hyperthermia-induced increase in cortical extracellular glutamate correlating with a decrease in seizure threshold temperature in rats (Morimoto T et al. Pathogenic role of glutamate in hyperthermia-induced seizures. Epilepsia May/June 1993;34:447-452). -Editor. *Ped Neur Briefs* July 1993.

PROGNOSIS OF 'LENGTHY' FEBRILE CONVULSIONS

The outcome of children with status epilepticus (afebrile seizure >30 min) or lengthy febrile convulsions (>30 min) is reported by a British population based cohort study group that followed 16004 neonatal survivors born in one week in 1970 and assessed them after 5 and 10 years. Febrile convulsions (FC) in 398 children were lengthy in 19 (4.8%). Children with lengthy FC had a greater risk of afebrile seizures than those with FC <30 min (4/19 [21%] v 13/379 [3.4%]), but the rate was lower than in the status group (14/17 [82%]) and none died. Of 84 children with afebrile seizures, 18 (21%) had status epilepticus, and 2 died: one of cerebellar tumor hemorrhage and the other as a result of encephalitis and pneumonia. Neither death was directly due to status epilepticus. In 10 of 33 survivors of lengthy FC or status, measures of IQ were abnormal but 8 had preceding developmental delay or neurologic abnormality. (Verity CM, Ross EM, Golding J. Outcome of childhood status epilepticus and lengthy febrile convulsions: findings of national cohort study. BMJ 24 July 1993;307:225-228). (Respond: Dr CM Verity, Department of Paediatrics, Addenbrooke's Hospital, Cambridge CB2 2QQ UK).

COMMENT. This population based study gives a more optimistic outcome of lengthy febrile convulsions and status epilepticus than hospital based studies. A poor outcome was determined more by the underlying cause than the seizure itself.

In a prospective study of 110 patients with febrile seizures followed for up to 2 years, the incidence of afebrile seizures and of EEG seizure discharges was significantly greater in patients with 'prolonged' febrile seizures (>20 min) than in those with short seizures (<20 min). (Millichap JG et al.

Neurology 1960;10:643). Both duration of the seizure and the EEG were predictive of outcome.

Pavone L, Galli V et al, Universities of Catania and Modena, Italy, report a follow-up study of 204 children who suffered febrile (FS) and afebrile seizures (AFS) within a 12 month period. EEG specific abnormalities found in 69 (33%) were associated with AFS recurrences in 94%. EEG seizure discharges were predictive of further AFS. (Child's Nerv Syst June 1993;9:154-156). -Editor. *Ped Neur Briefs* Aug 1993.

INFANTILE SPASMS

INFANTILE SPASMS AND PARTIAL SEIZURES The concurrence of infantile spasms and partial seizures was studied in 11 infants using time-locked video electroencephalography at the Department of Pediatrics, Children's Hospital, Ohio State University School of Medicine, Columbus, OH. Partial seizures preceded the onset of infantile spasms in 7. In some, the focal EEG ictal activity was overriding the generalized slow-wave transient and in others was visible only during the generalized decrement. Interictal EEGs showed hypsarrhythmia in 6 patients and modified hypsarrhythmia in 5. Brain malformations occurred in 3 and tuberous sclerosis in 2. Accurate clinical identification of both types of seizures was not made without resort to video EEG. (Donat JF, Wright FS. Simultaneous infantile spasms and partial seizures. J Child Neurol July 1991;6:246-250).

COMMENT: The authors refer to only one previous account in the literature of the simultaneous occurrence of the two seizure types (Hrachovy RA et al. Epilepsia 1984;25:317-325). The concurrence of these seizures might support both cortical and subcortical mechanisms in the genesis of infantile spasms. Information on the relative effect of ACTH and other forms of treatment of these seizure types would be of interest.

A long term follow-up study of 42 patients with West syndrome treated with high doses of sodium valproate is presented from the Neuropaediatric Unit, Hospital de Ctuces, Bilbao, Spain. The hypsarrhythmia EEG pattern was controlled after two weeks treatment with VPA 100 to 300mg/kg/daily in 80% of patients. Relapses occurred most often in those treated with doses lower than 200 mg/kg/day. Other types of seizures developed in 50% of patients followed beyond two years of age. Side effects included thrombocytopenia, vomiting and somnolence. Hepatic enzymes were elevated in 3 patients and returned to normal when treatment was ended (Prats JM et al. Dev Med Child Neurol August 1991;33:617-625). The authors recommend that high dose valproate requires careful monitoring and admission to hospital. Somnolence, vomiting, thrombocytopenia and coagulation defects are of concern and warrant further evaluation before general acceptance of this therapy. -Editor. *Ped Neur Briefs* Aug 1991.

SURGERY IN WEST SYNDROME

The results of surgical removal of a porencephalic cyst in an 18-month old child with infantile spasms and hypsarrhythmia are reported from the Departments of Neurology and Neurosurgery, VA Medical Center and University of Florida; the State University of Stony Brook, NY; and University of Michigan Medical School, Ann Arbor, MI. Infantile spasms were evaluated first at 4 months of age. The seizures were generalized but the neurologic examination showed a left hemiparesis and a left visual field deficit. ACTH provided a transient control of spasms for 3 months. At 18 months the seizures had become refractory to medical treatment. Postoperatively, seizures have been controlled for 12 months and the use of the paretic extremities has improved. Preoperative anti-epileptic medications were continued. (Uthman BM et al. Outcome for West Syndrome following surgical treatment. Epilepsia Sept/Oct 1991;32:668-671).

COMMENT. This report indicates that infantile

spasms and hypsarrhythmia of a diffuse pattern may be associated with a focal cerebral lesion amenable to surgery.

Infantile spasms associated with *COFS syndrome* (cerebro-oculo-facial-skeletal syndrome) in a 3-month-old child is reported from the Department of Neurology, New York Medical College, New York, NY (Harden CL et al. Pediatr Neurol July/Aug 1991;7:302-304). COFS syndrome is a rare autosomal recessive condition characterized by microcephaly, microphthalmia and/or cataracts, neurogenic arthrogryposis and multiple congenital anomalies. The infantile spasms and hypsarrhythmia resolved during ACTH therapy. -Editor. *Ped Neur Briefs* Oct 1991.

CSF TRYPTOPHAN IN INFANTILE SPASMS

The levels of tryptophan (TRP) metabolites in the CSF of 8 patients with infantile spasms are reported from the Department of Pediatrics, St. Marianna University School of Medicine, Kawasaki 213, Japan. Concentrations in patients were compared to TRP metabolites in CSF from 20 age matched controls (mean age: 5.8 months). The levels of CSF serotonin, 5-hydroxyindoleacetic acid and kynurenine were significantly lower in infantile spasm patients compared to controls, whereas the levels of CSF 3-hydroxykynurenine was significantly higher in patients. Tryptophan and 5-hydroxytryptophan were not significantly different in patients compared to controls. The CSF was collected before treatment. The findings suggest that infantile spasms are associated with a decrease in serotonergic metabolites (Yamamoto H, Studies on CSF tryptophan metabolism in infantile spasms. Pediatr Neurol Nov/Dec 1991;7:411-414). (Correspondence: Dr. Yamamoto, Neurology Service (V-151), VA Medical Center, 3350 La Jolla Village Drive, San Diego, CA 92161.)

COMMENT. Yamamoto H has also found a significant inverse correlation with aging in the CSF neurotransmitters during the neonatal period (Pediatr Neurol 1991;7:406-10). Langlais PJ, Wardlow ML, and

Yamamoto H report marked increases in 5-hydroxyindoleacetic acid and decreases in kynurenine levels in the CSF of 5 infants whose infantile spasms were eliminated or reduced following treatment with ACTH. The elimination of seizures by ACTH was accompanied by increased serotonin turnover (Pediatr Neurol 1991;7:440-5).

Treatment of infantile spasms with IV gamma-globulins (lg/kg/day, the first 2 days, every 3 weeks, for 6 months) is reported in a prospective study of 23 children from the Unite de Neuropediatrie, Centre Gui de Chauliac, 34059, Montpellier, France (Echenne B et al. Brain Dev 1991;13:313-9). Five patients responded satisfactorily and 15 received no benefit. Deficiencies of IgA in one patient, IgG2 in 3, and IgG 1 in one showed no correlation with therapeutic results . IV gamma-globulin is recommended only as an auxillary therapy and not the treatment of choice for infantile spasms. -Editor. *Ped Neur Briefs* Feb 1992.

PET STUDIES OF INFANTILE SPASMS

Positron emission tomography (PET) was used to determine local cerebral metabolic rates for glucose in 44 infants with spasms at the Departments of Neurology and Pediatrics, Division of Nuclear Medicine and Biophysics and the Brain Research Institute, University of California, Los Angeles School of Medicine, CA. Ictal events were detected in the EEG in 10 studies during PET. The most consistent abnormality on PET was the. symmetrical increase of relative cerebral metabolic rate for glucose in the lenticular nuclei and was apparent in 32 of the 44 infants. This relative hypermetabolism of the lenticular nuclei occurred with both cryptogenic or symptomatic spasms, and was not characterized by any specific EEG abnormality. Every infant with focal abnormalities on CT and/or MRI also had a focal abnormality on PET in the same location, but 17 of 28 infants with focal abnormalities on PET had no detectable focal abnormalities on CT and/or MRI (Chugani HT et al. Infantile spasms: II. Lenticular nuclei and brain stem activation on positron emission tomography. Ann Neurol Jan 1992;31:212-219).

(Correspondence: Dr. Chugani, Division of Pediatric Neurology, Room 22-464 MDCC, UCLA School of Medicine, Los Angeles, CA 90024.)

COMMENT. The lenticular nuclei may contribute to the mechanism of infantile spasms. A cortical-subcortical interaction is proposed in the pathophysiology of infantile spasms. A Commission on Pediatric Epilepsy of the International League Against Epilepsy, following a workshop on infantile spasms, has proposed that the term infantile spasms is too restrictive and the term "spasms" is preferable to designate a special type of epileptic seizure that involves the axial musculature-in flexion, extension or mixed- and that often occurs in clusters. They propose that this type of seizure should be listed in the International Classification of Epileptic Syndromes (Commission 1981 and 1989). -Editor. *Ped Neur Briefs* March 1992.

VALPROATE METABOLITES DURING TREATMENT OF INFANTILE SPASMS

Metabolite profiles were measured in serum and urine of pediatric patients treated with valproic acid for infantile spasms at the Institute of Toxicology and Embryopharmacology, Free University Berlin and Department of Pediatrics, Rittberg-Krankenhaus, Berlin, Germany. The mean age was 7 months (range 4-12 months) and all 25 patients had the hypsarrhythmia pattern in the EEG. Eighteen patients were seizure free after 3 months of VPA monotherapy in a dose of 100 mg/kg body weight/day. The main VPA metabolites in serum were the *B*-oxidation products (2-en-VPA and 3-keto-VPA) and the major diunsaturated metabolite 2,3'-dien VPA; 4-en and 3-keto-4-en, 2 potential hepatotoxins, were detected only in very low concentrations. Glucuronide conjugates and the oxidation products represent the most abundant metabolites in urine. Two children had transient abnormal metabolite profiles indicating altered *B*-oxidation and associated with hepatomegaly and increased liver enzyme activity (Fisher E et al. Valproate metabolites in serum and urine during antiepileptic therapy in children with infantile spasms: abnormal metabolite pattern associated with reversible hepatotoxicity. Epilepsia Jan/Feb 1992;33:165-171). (Reprints: Professor Dr. H Nau, Institute of Toxicology and Embryopharmacology, Free University Berlin, Garystrasse 5, D-1000 Berlin 33, Germany.)

COMMENT. The initial stages of hepatotoxicity reactions to VPA may be accompanied by characteristic changes in VPA metabolism (increased levels of 2-en, 2,3'-dien and 3-en VPA). The concentrations of unsaturated metabolites and enzyme activity became normal in 2 children on reduction of VPA dose and concomitant lowering of fever. These abnormal metabolite patterns occurred predominantly in patients treated with large doses of VPA combined with dexamethasone. The authors propose that the early detection of such abnormal metabolite patterns might decrease the risk of severe hepatic injury by the timely withdrawal of VPA or reduction of dosage. -Editor. *Ped Neur Briefs* March 1992.

CSF ACTH LEVELS IN INFANTILE SPASMS

ACTH levels in CSF of 14 infants with massive infantile spasms were significantly lower than those of controls in a study from the University of Southern California and Childrens Hospital of Los Angeles, CA. Differences in cortisol levels between patients and controls were not statistically significant. The authors postulate the involvement of the corticotropin-releasing hormone-ACTH-glucocorticoid regulatory loop in the pathophysiology of infantile spasms. (Baram TZ et al. Brain-adrenal axis hormones are altered in the CSF of infants with massive infantile spasms. Neurology June 1992;42:1171-1175.) (Reprints: Dr. Tallie Z. Baram, Division of Neurology (#82), CHLA, P.O. Box 54700, Los Angeles, CA 90054-0700.)

COMMENT. Further studies of this type should help to determine the respective merits of low dose versus high dose ACTH therapy in infantile spasms (see Progress in Pediatric Neurology, ed Millichap JG. Chicago, PNB Publ, 1991; 30-34). -Editor. *Ped Neur Briefs*

July 1992.

PATHOPHYSIOLOGY OF INFANTILE SPASMS

An age-specific endogenous-convulsant hypothesis implicating corticotropin-releasing hormone (CRH), an excitant neuropeptide suppressed by ACTH/steroids, is proposed for the pathophysiology of massive infantile spasms in a report from the University of Southern California, Los Angeles, CA. Stated briefly, abnormally increased CRH synthesis and activity results in neuronal hyperexcitability. Deranged CRH-responsive brain-stem circuits may explain the spasms. ACTH treatment controls spasms and modifies the EEG by suppressing CRH synthesis. (Baram TZ. Pathophsiology of massive infantile spasms: Perspective on the putative role of the brain adrenal axis. Ann Neurol March 1993;33 231-236). (Respond: Dr Baram, Division of Neurology (#82), Childrens Hospital Los Angeles, 4650 Sunset Blvd, Los Angeles, CA 90027).

COMMENT. The author proposes that specific receptor blockers of CRH will arrest infantile spasms and may prove safer than ACTH and of some benefit to cognitive function.

The results of ACTH treatment in 21 children with intractable seizures other than infantile spasms at the Children's Hospital, Camperdown NSW, Sydney, were disappointing. Only 24% had a good response. Hypokalemia, hypertension, and infection complicated treatment in 43%, 33%, and 19%, respectively. (Charuvanij A, Ouvrier RA et al. Brain Dev 1992;14: 102). More favorable results have been reported by some. -Editor. *Ped Neur Briefs* April 1993.

PRENATAL ETIOLOGIES OF WEST SYNDROME

The etiology of West syndrome (WS) with special reference to prenatal factors was investigated in 180 patients admitted between 1969 and 1990 to the Department of Child Neurology, Okayama University Medical School, Japan. The most common cause was *prenatal,* accounting for 77 cases (43%). The frequency of perinatal factors was 14%, and postnatal 7%. Only 18 cases (10%) were idiopathic; in 48 the etiology was uncertain. Among *prenatal* factors, tuberous sclerosis was most frequent, occurring in 23 (30%) of prenatal and 13% of the total cases. Chromosome abnormalities were found in 10 (trisomy 21 in 6), and cerebral dysgenesis in 10. Seizure remission (47% of cases) and intellectual development (IQ<25 in 65%) were significantly lower in the prenatal group compared to idiopathic cases. Pyridoxal phosphate (100-400 mg daily, orally) tried in 170 cases was followed by seizure remission in 12% of the total, 12% of prenatal cases, and 28% of idiopathic cases. ACTH (0.25 mg/d/im for 26 days) was effective in 89% of 114 cases treated, including 40 (85%) prenatal cases; seizure remission with ACTH was similar in all etiological groups. (Ohtahara S et al. Prenatal etiologies of West syndrome. Epilepsia July/Aug 1993;34:716-722). (Reprints: Prof S Ohtahara, Dept of Child Neurology, Okayama University Medical School, Shikatacho, Okayama, Japan).

COMMENT. In this issue of Epilepsia, several papers refer to West syndrome (WS), 4 from the Neuropaediatric Dept, Hopital Saint-Vincent-De-Paul, Paris: 1) Cusmai R et al, reviewing 32 patients with perinatal insults, found a better prognosis in children with periventricular leukomalacia or localized porencephalic cysts than in those with diffuse cerebral lesions or extensive cysts; 2) van Bogaert P, Dulac O et al report that the MRI in 46 patients with WS of unknown etiology was more informative than CT, demonstrating one case of delayed myelination and 4 with focal lesions; 3) Jambaque I et al found that visual inattention, an early manifestation of WS, was frequently associated with long-term cognitive defects and parieto-occipital abnormalities in SPECT studies; and 4) Plouin P et al, using 24-hour ambulatory EEG monitoring, recorded partial seizures in 31 patients with an unfavorable outcome.

Additional articles on WS in Epilepsia July/Aug 1993;34: include: 5) persisting hypsarrhythmia during a cluster of infantile spasms correlated with a favorable outcome, in a report from the Bambino Gesu Children's

Hospital, Rome, Italy (Fusco L, Vigevano F); 6) the term modified hypsarrhythmia should be discarded, and unusual features of interictal EEGs in infantile spasms should be specified, according to Watanabe K et al, Dept of Pediatrics, Nagoya University, Japan; and 7) infantile spasms, with hypsarrhythmia, retardation and a poor prognosis, occurring in one member of a family with benign familial neonatal convulsions, is a unique case report from Tokushima University, Japan (Mori K, Yano I, Hashimoto T).-Editor. *Ped Neur Briefs* Sept 1993.

PROGNOSIS OF INFANTILE SPASMS

The developmental, neurologic, and seizure outcome and prognostic factors of 57 cases of infantile spasms were evaluated in relation to etiology (cryptogenic 17 cases, symptomatic 40 cases) at the Hospital for Sick Children, Toronto, Canada. Age of onset ranged from 4 weeks to 13 months (mean, 5 months), and duration of follow-up was 12 - 60 months. Cerebral dysgenesis was the most common cause (20%) in the symptomatic group. Neurologic deficits, especially hypotonia, were present in 23% of cryptogenic cases cf 75% of symptomatic. A mean developmental score of 71 in cryptogenic cases was significantly higher than 48 in symptomatic. Additional forms of seizures were more common in symptomatic cases (57% cf 35%). Unfavorable prognostic factors, particularly cognitive deficits, were the association of other seizures, neurologic deficits, delay in treatment, poor response to ACTH, and persistent EEG abnormalities after 2 weeks of therapy. All patients in the cryptogenic group responded to ACTH (80 IU/IM/d for 2 weeks, tapered over 6 to 8 weeks). Of 30 symptomatic cases receiving ACTH, 12 (40%) were completely controlled initially, and 11 had a partial response. Response was higher in patients with developmental scores >70, both cryptogenic and symptomatic cases. (Koo B et al. Infantile spasms: Outcome and prognostic factors of cryptogenic and symptomatic groups. Neurology Nov 1993;43:2322-2327). (Reprints: Dr Betty Koo, Division of Neurology, The Hospital for Sick Children, 555 University Avenue, Toronto, ON, Canada M5G lX8).

COMMENT. With improved diagnostic techniques, particularly the MRI, the increased recognition of cerebral dysgenesis as a frequent cause for infantile spasms has resulted in a lowered percentage of cryptogenic cases compared to earlier reports. In a study involving 61 cases at the Mayo Clinic (Millichap JG, Bickford RG, Klass DW, Backus RE. Epilepsia 1962;3:188-197), 43% were of undetermined etiology and only 7% were recognized with cerebral dysgenesis. The anticonvulsant efficacy and outcome of treatment with ACTH in 21 patients was related significantly to the age at the time of diagnosis and treatment; 80% of infants less than 1 year old were benefited whereas only 22% of those over 1 year showed reduction in seizures and EEG improvement. Control of seizures and hypsarrythmia was not significantly related to the etiology, but patients of borderline or normal intelligence tended to respond more frequently than did those with developmental quotients <70. (Millichap JG, Bickford RG. JAMA 1962;182:523-527).

Posterior fossa abnormalities in children with infantile spasms were associated with a poor developmental outcome in a study of 98 children from New England Medical Center and Children's Hospital, Boston, and Hadassah University Hospital, Jerusalem (Schiffmann R et al. J Child Neurol Oct 1993;8:360-365). Brain stem dysfunction and atrophy were remarkable in a study of 10 patients with infantile spasms, employing evoked potentials and MRI, at the University of Tokushima, Japan (Miyazaki M et al. Neuropediatr June 1993;24:126-130). -Editor. *Ped Neur Briefs* Dec 1993.

EPILEPTIC SYNDROMES AND ETIOLOGY

MIRTH, LAUGHTER AND GELASTIC SEIZURES

One patient with laughter-associated seizures originating in the anterior cingulate gyrus and two patients with complex partial seizures who exhibited mirth and laughter following direct cortical stimulation of the parahippocampal and fusiform gyri are reported from the Johns Hopkins University School of Medicine, Baltimore, MD. Removal of a cavernous hemangioma and the seizure focus in the first patient resulted in freedom from seizures, except when medication was withdrawn at one year following surgery. These case reports favor the localization of the motor act of laughter in the anterior cingulate region and the emotional concomitants of laughter in the basal temporal cortex. (Arroyo S et al. Mirth, laughter and gelastic seizures. Brain Aug 1993;116:757-780). (Respond: Santiago Arroyo MD, Dept of Neurology, Meyer Building 2-147, 600 North Wolfe St, Baltimore, MD 21205).

COMMENT. The authors cite several references to gelastic seizures (seizures with laughter, from the Greek *'gelos'* for mirth). Additional reports are included in the classic epilepsy monographs of Turner WA (1907), and Lennox WG (1960). In addition to complex partial seizures, infantile spasms have often been associated with attacks of paroxysmal laughter (Lacy JR, Penry JK. Infantile Spasms. New York, Raven Press, 1976).

Hypothalamic pathology, usually hamartoma, should be suspected in infants with gelastic seizures, and precocious puberty and mental retardation are frequent sequelae. The seizures respond poorly to medication and to surgical removal of the hamartoma.- Editor. *Ped Neur Briefs* Sept 1993.

NEURONAL MIGRATION DISORDERS

Thirty patients with intractable partial epilepsy and a pathological or radiological diagnosis of neuronal migration disorders (NMD) were studied at the Montreal Neurological Institute and Hospital, Montreal, Quebec, Canada. Age at onset of epilepsy ranged from 4 months to 21 years (mean 5.7). Prenatal etiological factors in 8 patients included maternal x-ray exposure or trauma, diabetes, advanced maternal age, and uterine abnormality. All patients1 had partial epilepsy: complex partial (67%), partial motor (73%), and secondary generalized seizures (73%). 8 patients (27%) had tonic or atonic drop attacks, and 6 of these had lesions involving the central region. Status epilepticus had occurred in 30%. A below average IQ was found in 1/2 of the patients. MRI was superior to CT, but did not distinguish between pachygyria, cortical dysplasia or tuberous sclerosis. White matter subcortical abnormalities were demonstrated more frequently than cortical abnormalities. In 22 of 26 surgically treated patients, the histological diagnosis was focal cortical dysplasia (12), and forme fruste of tuberous sclerosis (10). Those with a histological picture of tuberous sclerosis had none of the classical clinical diagnostic signs, but 80% had delayed psychomotor development and all 10 patients had multilobar unilateral or bilateral EEG spiking. These findings differed from patients with focal cortical dysplasia whose developmental milestones were normal and epileptogenic discharges were confined to one lobe or area of the brain (Palmini A, Andermann F et al. Focal neuronal migration disorders and intractable partial epilepsy: a study of 30 patients. Ann Neurol Dec 1991;30:741-749).

COMMENT. The results of surgical treatment of the above 26 patients are reported in the same journal (Palmini A et al. Ann Neurol Dec 1991; 30:750-757). Good or excellent seizure control was achieved in 42% and moderate control in 25%. The extent of lesion removed was most strongly correlated with the surgical outcome; 77 % receiving complete or 50% excision of the lesion had a good prognosis. When excision of epileptogenic tissue was based on scalp EEG and electrocorticography studies there was no correlation with surgical outcome.

The lack of specificity of the MRI in the diagnosis of tuberous sclerosis in this study is also alluded to by Fryer AE, geneticist at the Royal Liverpool Hospital, England, in an editorial concerning tuberous sclerosis (J Roy Soc Med Dec 1991;84:699-701). Although MRI is more sensitive than CT, CT is more specific and potentially less confusing in interpretation. A thorough clinical examination including ophthalmoscopy and ultraviolet light examination of the skin is essential to exclude the diagnosis in anyone suspect or at risk. Prenatal diagnosis is only possible by fetal echocardiography but this examination is unreliable before 26 weeks and has a high rate of false negatives.-Editor. *Ped Neur Briefs* Dec 1991.

MRI IN TUBEROUS SCLEROSIS WITH NORMAL I.Q.

The number, size and distribution of cerebral hamartomas determined by MRI in 11 patients with tuberous sclerosis and normal intellect are reported from the Bath Unit for Research into Paediatrics, Royal United Hospital, Combe Park, Bath, Avon, England and Bristol MRI Centre, Frenchay Hospital, Bristol. Nine patients had between 2 and 9 cerebral tubers seen on MRI T2 weighted images, 7 had 1-5 subependymal nodules and 2 had normal scans. The hamartomas were at least 4 mm in size. The number of lesions found on the MRI may not be used to predict neurological outcome in tuberous sclerosis. Only 3 of the 11 patients had a history of seizures and all had normal intellect (Webb DW et al. Cranial magnetic resonance imaging in patients with tuberous sclerosis and normal intellect. Arch Dis Child; Dec 1991;66:1375-1377). (Reprints: Dr. Osborne, Royal United Hospital, Comb Park, Bath, Avon BA1 3NG, England.)

COMMENT. The authors suggest that the wrong conclusions may be drawn if the number of lesions alone on cranial MRI is used to predict neurological outcome in tuberous sclerosis. Lesions seen on both MRI and CT may become less obvious with advancing age in patients with tuberous sclerosis. In the experience of these authors, individuals who reach 5 years of age with normal development do not develop mental handicap from tuberous sclerosis. While the number of cerebral hamartomas appears to be an unreliable predictor of clinical outcome it is possible that the distribution and size of lesions may be more helpful. Patients with temporal lobe or occipital lobe hamartomas are most likely to have seizures or EEG abnormalities. Tuberous sclerosis was the cause of infantile spasms in 10% of cases treated in Finland (Ped Neurol Briefs April 1990) but in only 2% reported from China (Feng YK et al. Chinese Med J. May 1991; 104:416-421). -Editor. *Ped Neur Briefs* March 1992.

SEIZURES AND IQ IN TUBEROUS SCLEROSIS

The relationship of seizures to intellectual disability was examined in 104 patients with tuberous sclerosis ascertained from the total population of the West of Scotland and reported from the Royal Hospital for Sick Children, Yorkhill, Glasgow, Scotland. Detailed analysis of the seizures was confined to the 52 patients who were born after the 1st of July, 1966: 4 (8%) had no seizures and normal intelligence. Of the 48 patients with seizures, 18 (35%) had normal intelligence, 6 (12%) had moderate intellectual disability, and 24 (45 %) had severe intellectual disability. Seizures were significantly associated with intellectual disability. No patient who developed seizures after the age of 5 years was intellectually impaired. Most individuals with intellectual disability presented with infantile spasms or other seizures under 1 year of age, or had multiple seizure types. A higher incidence of intellectual disability was found among individuals who had more than 1 seizure type. Also, children with TS whose first seizure is febrile have a high risk of developing intellectual disability (Shepherd CW, Stephenson JBP. Seizures and intellectual disability associated with tuberous sclerosis in the West of Scotland. Dev Med Child Neurol Sept 1992;34:766-774). (Correspondence: Dr. C.W. Shepherd, Craigavon Area Hospital, Portadown, Northern Ireland BT63 5QQ.)

COMMENT. Several papers on tuberous sclerosis were presented at the 6th Congress of the International Child Neurology Association, November, 1992, Buenos Aires, Argentina. Laan LA et al. Rotterdam, found vigabatrin in therapy of resistant epilepsy with tuberous sclerosis to be effective, if given early in childhood. Calderon-Gonzalez R et al. of Monterrey, Mexico, found 7 of 27 children (26%) with TS had infantile autism evident by 3.5 years of age. Rett syndrome was associated with tuberous sclerosis in 2 patients reported by Philippart M of Pomona, California. Curatolo P et al. of Rome, Italy reported topographic spike mapping of the EEG in TS which showed that "generalized" spike-and-wave discharges were of focal origin (Pediatr Neurol Sept/Oct 1992;8:

344-411). -Editor. *Ped Neur Briefs* Nov 1992.

SEIZURES AND NEUROFIBROMATOSIS I

Twenty-two (6%) patients, ages 5 to 57 years, had developed seizures among 359 attending a neurofibromatosis clinic at the Dept of Neurology, Children's Hospital, Harvard Med School, Boston. The majority of seizures could be attributed to causes unrelated to NF1: 6 had febrile seizures and 3 had primary generalized epilepsy with onset before 5 years. Complex partial seizures in 9 (41%), infantile spasms in 1, and seizures with aqueductal stenosis in 2 may have been caused by NF1, but no specific brain lesions were detected. None of the seizures was a symptom of brain tumor, and neuroimaging failed to uncover a seizure focus. Routine EEG of all patients with NF1 was considered unproductive. (Korf BR, Carrazana E, Holmes GL. Patterns of seizures observed in association with neurofibromatosis 1. Epilepsia July/Aug 1993;34:616-620). (Reprints: Dr BR Korf, Children's Hospital, 300 Longwood Ave, Boston, MA 02115).

COMMENT. Seizures appear to be relatively uncommon in association with NF1. A possible increased frequency of infantile spasms in NF1 patients was suggested in two previous reports (Huson SM et al. Brain 1988;111:1355; see Millichap JG, Ed. Progress in Pediatric Neurology, Chicago, PNB, 1991). -Editor. *Ped Neur Briefs* Sept 1993.

SEIZURE ETIOLOGY IN DOWN SYNDROME

The etiology of seizures in 47 infants, children, and young adults with Down syndrome was examined at the Floating Hospital for Infants and Children, Boston, MA and the Institute for Basic Research in Developmental Disabilities, Staten Island, NY. Of a total of 737 patients with Down syndrome, 47 (6%) had seizures; and 24 had an identifiable etiology usually related to a complication of Down syndrome, including neonatal hypoxia-ischemia, hypoxia from congenital-heart disease, or infection. The infections were bacterial meningitis in 3, viral meningoencephalitis in 1, brain abscess 1, and febrile seizures in 2. The patterns of the seizures in those of known etiology were generalized tonic-clonic in 18, infantile spasms in 2, myoclonic 2, absence 1, simple partial 3, and complex partial 1. Mixed partial and generalized seizures occurred in 2. Of 12 patients with seizures related to cardiovascular disease 4 died of complications of acute heart failure. Neonates with hypoxic ischemic injury had relatively poor outcomes. The authors recommend that all Down syndrome patients with seizures be thoroughly evaluated to determine the etiology. (Stafstrom CE et al. Seizures in children with Down syndrome: Etiology, characteristics and outcome. Dev Med Child Neurol March 1991;33:191-200).

COMMENT. Febrile seizures occurred in only two (0.9%) of the author's patients during the susceptible age range. The relative rarity of febrile seizures in Down syndrome is contrasted with the relatively frequent occurrence of infantile spasms. Wisniewski KE, one of the authors, has previously studied the arrest of neurogenesis and synaptogenesis in brains of patients with Down syndrome. (N Engl J Med 1984; 311:1187). Long necked dendritic spines persist after birth suggesting dysgenetic process, and neuronal membranes in Down syndrome are abnormally hyperexcitable. The mechanism of increased susceptibility to seizures in children with Down syndrome may involve an interplay between hyperexcitable membranes, altered dendritic spines, and reduction of inhibitory interneurons. The present study suggests that seizures in patients with Down syndrome are frequently caused by additional factors including hypoxia and infection.

The prevalence, onset, and type of seizure disorders and seizure control were studied in 405 individuals with Down syndrome aged six months to 45 years at the Departments of Pediatrics and Neurology, Rhode Island Hospital, Providence, RI. The prevalence of seizures in this group of patients was 8.1%. The onset of seizures occurred before one year of age in 40% and in the third decade of life in another 40%. Infantile spasms and tonic-clonic seizures with myoclonus were most common in the younger age group and partial simple or partial complex seizures and tonic-clonic seizures occurred in the older patients. A bimodal distribution of seizures in patients with Down svndrome was noted. (Pueschel SM et al. Seizure disorders in Down syndrome. Arch Neurol March 1991;48:318-320) -Editor. *Ped Neur Briefs* April 1991.

BENIGN PARTIAL NONROLANDIC EPILEPSIES

The syndrome of benign partial epilepsy with particular reference to the non-rolandic types is described and the relevant literature reviewed from the Pediatric Seizure Clinic and EEG Laboratory, Beilinson Medical Center, Petah Tikva, and the Sackler Faculty of Medicine, Tel Aviv University, Tel Aviv, Israel. Benign Partial Epilepsy is defined as a primary convulsive disorder belonging within the group of age- and localization-related idiopathic epilepsies and characterized by seizures, predominantly partial and amenable to anticonvulsant therapy, that begin in childhood and remit spontaneously before adulthood. The seizures, usually short and mild, include motor and/or somatosensory symptoms and tend to generalize. They are of variable frequency and occur more frequently in sleep. EEG reveals typical focal features on a normal background that tend to normalize during adolescence. Benign epilepsy occurs in normal children having no neurological or intellectual deficits and no history of brain damage. Benign partial epilepsies other than the rolandic type include occipital epilepsy, benign frontal epilepsy, benign epilepsy with affective symptomatology, benign epilepsy with extreme somatosensory evoked potentials, benign partial epilepsy of adolescence and benign epilepsy associated with multiple spike foci. The Landau-Kleffner syndrome is sometimes included among the benign epilepsies because the seizures cease before the age of 12 and the EEG normalizes before the age of 15. Aphasia resolves completely or partially in only 50% of patients. Headache and vomiting or migrainous symptoms are common in benign occipital epilepsy. Children with benign occipital epilepsy associated with headache respond best to phenytoin which relieves both seizures and headaches. (Lerman P, Kivity S. The benign partial nonrolandic epilepsies J Clin Neurophysiol July 1991;8:275-285).

COMMENT. The recognition of the partial epilepsies of childhood is important from the point of view of treatment and prognosis. In children with infrequent seizure occurrence and a diagnosis of benign partial epilepsy the use of potentially toxic anticonvulsant medications may be deferred.-Editor. *Ped Neur Briefs* Sept 1991.

DIAGNOSIS OF JUVENILE MYOCLONIC EPILEPSY

Factors contributing to the misdiagnosis of juvenile myoclonic epilepsy (JME) in an epilepsy clinic have been examined in 70 patients at the Division of Neurology, King Khalid University Hospital, Riyadh, Saudi Arabia. More than 90% were undiagnosed on referral and 33% were not recognized initially in the epilepsy clinic. The delay in diagnosis was 8 years from onset and 17 months from the first evaluation in the clinic. Factors responsible for the delayed diagnosis include the following: myoclonic jerks rarely reported by patients; generalized tonic-clonic seizures may be nocturnal without circadian relation to awakening from sleep; unilateral jerks may suggest simple partial seizures; absence seizures may antedate jerks and GTCS seizures by 4.5 years and are frequently unrecognized. The EEG was significant in confirming the diagnosis in 63% of patients. Valproate is considered the treatment of choice and clonazepam is used as an adjunctive treatment. (Panayiotopoulos CP et al. Juvenile myoclonic epilepsy: factors of error involved in the diagnosis and treatment. Epilepsia Sept/Oct 1991;32:672-676).

COMMENT. Failure to recognize JME may result in improper choice of anticonvulsant therapy, resultant status epilepticus, and failure to provide appropriate genetic counseling. This study reemphasizes the atypical history in some cases and the frequency of occurrence of absence seizures as the initial manifestation. -Editor. *Ped Neur Briefs* Oct 1991.

JUVENILE MYOCLONIC EPILEPSY: DIAGNOSIS

The clinical and EEG features and reasons for frequent misdiagnosis of juvenile myoclonic epilepsy are reviewed by the Epilepsy Research Group, Institute of Neurology, National Hospital, and St Thomas' Hospital, London, England. The triad of absence seizures, myoclonic jerks, and GTCSs shows a characteristic age-related onset. Absence seizures begin between 5 and 16 years, myoclonic jerks follow about 4 years later, usually around age 15 years, and GTCSs appear within a few months after the myoclonic jerks. Myoclonic jerks and GTCSs occur mainly on awakening. Apart from tremor, the neurologic exam is normal. Photosensitivity is present in 50% of patients, and seizures are precipitated by sleep deprivation, fatigue, alcohol, anxiety, and hyperventilation. Treatment with valproic acid is usually effective, and may be supplemented with clonazepam at bedtime if necessary. Lifelong anticonvulsant treatment is required, and withdrawal of medication may result in status epilepticus. (Grunewald RA, Panayiotopoulos CP. Juvenile myoclonic epilepsy. A review. Arch Neurol June 1993;50: 594-598). (Reprints: Dr Grunewald, Epilepsy Research Group, Institute of Neurology, National Hospital, Queen Square, London, England WCIN 3BG).

COMMENT. A high index of suspicion for JME is indicated in young patients with early-morning seizures, especially those poorly controlled with carbamazepine or associated with sleep deprivation or alcohol consumption. Diagnosis of JME was delayed by a mean of 14 years in 15 patients identified among 180 referrals to a new epilepsy clinic at St Thomas' Hospital, London, a prevalence of 8.3%. At least 11 had been examined previously by a neurologist, and 7 had received inappropriate anticonvulsants. (Grunewald RA et al. J Neur Neurosurg & Psychiat 1992;55:497). -Editor. *Ped Neur Briefs* June 1993.

EPILEPTIC PALATAL MYOCLONUS

A 14 year old girl with epilepsia partialis continua complicated by palatal myoclonus of focal cortical origin is reported from the Comprehensive Epilepsy Center, Graduate Hospital; and University of Pennsylvania School of Medicine, Philadelphia, PA. Her seizures consisted of staring, impairment of consciousness, and left facial twitching. Later she developed intermittent stuttering speech in association with palatal and lingual movements occurring up to 70 times a day. Several episodes of epilepsia partialis continua, lasting up to two weeks, were noted in the next three years. These were characterized by left facial and pharyngeal movements. They were refractory to medications. The EEG revealed theta and delta activity in the right central region with intermixed spikes, and a SPECT showed a focal area of increased perfusion in the right centrotemporal region. The epilepsia partialis continua remitted after several weeks. (Tatum WO et al. Epileptic palatal myoclonus. Neurology August 1991;41:1305-1306).

COMMENT. The myoclonus epilepsies of childhood are divided into three major groups: (1) the progressive myoclonus epilepsies which include a number of degenerative and storage diseases; (2) the myoclonus epilepsies symptomatic of non-progressive brain damage usually of prenatal or perinatal origin; (3) the cryptogenic myoclonus epilepsies (Aicardi J. Int Pediatr 1991;6:195-200). More than 15 specific disorders may cause the progressive myoclonus epilepsy syndrome; reviewed by Berkovic SF et al. (J Clin Neurophysiol July 1991;8:261-274). The major causes of PME are the Unverricht-Lundborg type, Lafora disease, neuronal ceroid lipofuscinoses, MERRF and sialidoses. Myoclonus is best controlled by valproate and/or clonazepam. -Editor. *Ped Neur Briefs* Sept 1991.

UNVERRICHT-LUNDBORG DISEASE

The progression of clinical and neurophysiological findings in a Swedish family with 4 siblings with Unverricht-Lundborg disease is reported from the Departments of Pediatrics and Clinical Neurophysiology, University of Gothenburgh, Sweden and Department of Pediatrics, University of Bergen, Norway. Stage 1 was subclinical at the age of 9-11 years with visual blackouts and polyspike EEG activity on photic stimulation. Stage 2 at 12-15 years of age was characterized by increasing segmental, stimulus sensitive myoclonias, occasional nocturnal myoclonic "cascade" seizures, and episodic 4-6 Hz bilateral sharp waves and polyspikes on photic stimulation. Stage 3, a disabling myoclonic stage at the age of 16-18 years, showed periodic generalized myoclonias, frequent nocturnal cascade seizures, ataxia, dysarthria, mental deterioration, wheelchair dependency and continuous EEG slow waves with polyspikes and intense myoclonias on photic stimulation. Obstructive apnea was seen at the peak of the cascade seizures, but consciousness was normal and post-ictal drowsiness was absent. 1 sibling died at age 18 with no apparent cause. Other causes of progressive myoclonus epilepsy were excluded. (Kyllerman M et al. Clinical and neurophysiological development of Unverricht-Lundborg disease in four Swedish siblings. Epilepsia Nov/Dec 1991;32:900-909).

COMMENT. Unverricht-Lundborg disease is diagnosed by exclusion since no specific biochemical or pathological markers have been detected. This study provides a classification of the stages of the disease together with a description of a typical "cascade" seizure monitored by video electroencephalography.

Lafora disease, another recessively inherited progressive myoclonus epilepsy, is reported in 4 children from The Department of Neurology, University of Michigan, Ann Arbor, Michigan. Each child presented in adolescence with progressive seizures, myoclonus, dementia and ataxia, and Lafora disease was proven by biopsy. The EEG in 18 studies showed 1) an early stage at age 12 with mild background slowing and trains of 3 Hz irregular spike wave activity; 2) intermediate stage at age 16 years with faster frequency spike waves up to 12 Hz and 3) late stage 4 years after onset with slow background with overlying beta activity and fast spike waves and polyspikes (Yen C et al. Longitudinal EEG studies in a kindred with Lafora disease. Epilepsia Nov/Dec 1991;32:895-899). The EEG in Lafora disease is distinguished by an increased frequency of the spike wave complexes with disease progression. At the onset of seizures the background EEG slowing should suggest a diagnosis other than an idiopathic generalized epilepsy and the progression to prominent fast spike wave complexes appears to be unique.-Editor. *Ped Neur Briefs* Dec 1991.

GENETICS OF UNVERRICHT-LUNDBORG DISEASE

Clinical and molecular genetic data on a family from the United States in which four of five sibs were affected with progressive myoclonus epilepsy of Unverricht-Lundborg type are reported from the University of Helsinki, Finland; National Cancer Institute, Bethesda, MD; and the VA Hospital, University of Florida, Gainesville, FL. Onset was between 9 and 11 years with grand mal seizures. Progressive stimulus-sensitive myoclonus developed at 11 to 13 years of age. Generalized spike-wave and polyspike-wave paroxysms and photo-sensitivity were characteristic EEG findings. The gene (EPM1) has been mapped to chromosome 21 in Finland, and the gene in this non-Finnish American family was also linked to the EPM1 region. Crossover events refined the gene localization between loci CBS and D2 1 S 112 , leading to greater accuracy of genetic prediction based on linkage analysis. (Lehesjoki A-E et al. Progressive myoclonus epilepsy of Unverricht-Lundborg type: A clinical and molecular genetic study of a family from the United States with four affected sibs. Neurology Nov 1993;43:2384-2386). (Reprints: Dr Anna-Elina Lehesjoki, Dept Med Genetics, PO Box 2 1 (Haartmanin-katu 3), 00014 University of Helsinki, Finland).

COMMENT. Causes of progressive myoclonus epilepsy include Unverricht-Lundborg disease (ULD), Lafora's disease, MERRF, Kufs' neuronal ceroid lipofuscinosis, and sialidoses. ULD is relatively common in Finland.

Cochius JI et al, at the Montreal General Hospital, have performed linkage analysis in 8 families, including 4 of neither Baltic nor Mediterranean origin. They report that ULD diagnosed in areas remote from the Baltic maps to the same locus on chromosome 21 as the Finnish form, and suggest that all ULD, regardless of geographic origin, represent mutations of the same gene (Ann Neurol Nov 1993;34:739-741). Lafora's disease, characterized by intraneuronal inclusions, is a form of myoclonus epilepsy not linked to EPM1 and chromosome 21. The recent advances in molecular genetics of neurological disease are reviewed in two current journals: Rosenberg RN et al. Arch Neurol Nov 1993;50:1123-1265, and Martin JB. Ann Neurol Dec 1993;34:757-773.-Editor. *Ped Neur Briefs* Dec 1993.

EPILEPSY AND MENTAL RETARDATION

The cumulative risk of seizures and epilepsy was studied in a prospectively identified cohort of 221 children with mental retardation born between 1951 and 1955 in Aberdeen, Scotland and reported from the Montefiore-Einstein Epilepsy Management Center, Albert Einstein College of Medicine, Bronx, NY. Epilepsy had developed in 15% by 22 years of age. The cumulative risk of developing epilepsy varied from 5% in children with mental retardation to 75% in those with mental retardation associated with a postnatal brain injury. An apparent increased risk of epilepsy associated with severe mental retardation was attributed to the higher proportion of postnatal brain injury among this group. The cumulative risk of epilepsy at 22 years was 38% in children with mental retardation and cerebral palsy and 66% in those with postnatal injury. Of 20 children whose initial seizure was a febrile convulsion, 35% went on to develop epilepsy. The authors conclude that in the absence of associated disability or postnatal injury, the risk of epilepsy in the retarded population is low. (Goulden KJ, Shinnar S et al. Epilepsy in children with mental retardation: a cohort study. Epilepsia Sept/Oct 1991 ;32: 690-697) .

COMMENT. This study is important in counseling and management of the child with mental retardation. The incidence of various seizure patterns known to be associated with mental retardation, particularly infantile spasms and Lennox-Gastaut, in the subgroups of retarded children would be of interest. West and Lennox-Gastaut syndromes are reviewed from the Children's Hospital, Ohio State University, Columbus, OH (DonatJF, Wright FS. Epilepsia July/Aug 1991;32:504-509).-Editor. *Ped Neur Briefs* Nov 1991.

ANGELMAN SYNDROME AND EPILEPSY

Characteristic epileptic seizures and EEG abnormalities are reported in three siblings with Angelman syndrome from the Kansai University Otokoyoma Hospital, Kyoto; and the Nagasaki University School of Medicine, Japan. Seizures were generalized, and interictal EEG findings included 2- to 3-Hz high-voltage slow waves bioccipitally and sporadic slow spike wave complexes bifrontally. EEG minor epileptic status occurred in a 38 month old sib and was responsive to clonazepam. The thresholds of wave V in auditory brainstem responses were increased, and the latency of wave I was prolonged in all 3 siblings. Chromosome studies were normal, but DNA deletion of the GABA receptor subunit gene was reported (Saitoh S) in the maternal grandfather, mother, and 3 siblings. (Sugimoto T et al. Angelman syndrome in three siblings: Characteristic epileptic seizures and EEG abnormalities. Epilepsia Nov/Dec 1992;33:1078-1082). (Reprints: Dr T Sugimoto, Department of Pediatrics, Kansai Medical University Otokoyama Hospital, Izumi 19, Otokoyama, Yawata-shi, Kyoto, 614 Japan).

COMMENT. Angelman syndrome is characterized by brachycephaly, microcephaly, mental retardation, jerky puppet-like movements of extremities, inappropriate laughter, and seizures. Seizures are generalized in 90% of patients. Deafness has been reported previously, but the abnormal auditory brain stem responses recorded in this study appear to be unique.

Eight sporadic cases of Angelman syndrome associated with chromosome 15ql2 deletion are reported from the Central Hospital, and Kobato Gakuen, Aichi Prefectural Colony, Japan (Matsumoto A et al. Epilepsia 1992;33:1083). Angelman syndrome is included among the etiologies of West, Lennox-Gastaut and other infantile-onset epileptic syndromes.-Editor. *Ped Neur Briefs* Jan 1993.

AUTISM AND EPILEPSY

The prevalence and clinical manifestations of epilepsy in 302 autistic and 237 dysphasic, non-autistic children were studied at the Departments of Neurology and Pediatrics, Albert Einstein College of Medicine and Montefiorei Medical Center, Bronx, New York. Epilepsy occurred in 14% of autistic children and 8% of dysphasic children. Girls were affected more frequently than boys (24% cf 11%). The seizure types included generalized tonic-clonic, atypical absence, atonic, myoclonic, infantile spasms and partial. Infantile spasms occurred in 12% of autistic patients with epilepsy. The major risk factors for epilepsy were severe mental deficiency and the combination of mental deficiency with a motor deficit. When cognitive and motor disabilities were excluded, the risk of epilepsy in autistic children was only 6% and similar to that found in dysphasic non-autistic children (Tuchman RF, Rapin I, Shinnar S. Autistic and dysphasic children. II: epilepsy. Pediatrics Dec 1991;88:1219-1225.) (Reprints: Dr. Rapin, Rose F. Kennedy Center for Research in Mental Retardation, Room 807, 1410 Pelham Parkway South, Bronx, NY 10461.)

COMMENT. The rates of epilepsy reported in autistic children have ranged from 11% to 42%. Associated cognitive and motor deficits, a higher ratio of girls, and the complication of verbal auditory agnosia in some series might explain the higher rates of epilepsy. As a group, autistic children are more likely than dysphasic children to have language subtypes affecting central processing and a history of regression of language and behavior. Girls with autism are more likely than boys to have severe mental deficiency and a motor deficit.

Epilepsy occurred in 8 (17%) of 46 children with autism and deafness (Jure R et al. Hearing impaired autistic children. Dev Med Child Neurol Dec

1991;33:1062-1072).-Editor. *Ped Neur Briefs* Jan 1992.

EPILEPTIC ACQUIRED APHASIA

The syndrome of acquired aphasia, dementia and behavior disorder in a child with partial complex epilepsy and continuous spike and waves during sleep is reported from the Service de Pediatrie, et Service de Neurologie, CHUV, Lausanne, Switzerland. The child was observed from age three to 18 years and deterioration in behavior and language occurred between the ages of 3-1/2 and 5 years, coinciding with the period of maximal EEG activity and the presence of almost continuous spike waves during sleep (CSWS). Improvement coincided with the disappearance of CSWS, between the ages of 5-1/2 and 6-1/2 years, and the onset of a unilateral focus that persisted throughout the following years. A definite correlation between the paroxysmal EEG abnormalities and the neuro-psychological deterioration and improvement was established retrospectively. (Roulet E, Deonna T et al. Acquired aphasia, dementia, and behavior disorder with epilepsy and continuous spike and waves during sleep in a child. Epilepsia July/August 1991;32:495-503).

COMMENT. Complex partial seizures with recurrence in adolescence and the persistence of an epileptic focus on the EEG are atypical features of the Landau-Kleffner syndrome. -Editor. *Ped Neur Briefs* Sept 1991.

LANDAU-KLEFFNER SYNDROME: PROGNOSIS

The long-term follow up of 6 patients and a review of the recent literature on the Landau-Kleffner syndrome ("acquired aphasia with convulsive disorder") are reported from the Department of Neurology, University Hospital Dijkzigt-Rotterdam, The Netherlands. The age at onset was 3-5 years, with epilepsy as the first sign in 3 and comprehension deficit in 3. Seizures were absence, generalized tonic-clonic, partial and complex partial in patterns. Seizures had disappeared at follow-up in 3 and epileptic activity in the EEG was absent in 4. The course of the aphasia was linked to the appearance and disappearance of electrical status epilepticus during slow sleep (ESES) which was found in 3 patients. Lasting EEG abnormalities and persisting clinical seizures, combined with the presence and duration of ESES, may impede language recovery. The disappearance of ESES may be associated with an improvement of language functions. The course of the aphasia was variable: slow and continuous improvement in 3, rapid recovery in 1, fluctuating in 1, and deterioration followed by slow improvement in 1. The follow-up period varied from 3 to 19 years. The response of the seizures and aphasia to anticonvulsants was variable; some benefit was obtained with phenytoin and phenobarbital in 1 patient, ethosuximide and valproate were helpful in 2. Prednisone in 1 patient had a variable and inconclusive effect. (Paquier PF, Van Dongen HR, Loonen MCB. The Landau-Kleffner Syndrome or "acquired aphasia with convulsive disorder" Arch Neurol April 1992;49:354-359). (Reprints: Dr. Van Dongen, Department of Neurology, Room EE 2287, University Hospital Dijkzigt-Rotterdam, P.O. Box 1738, 3000 DR Rotterdam, the Netherlands.)

COMMENT. The correlation between ESES and acquired epileptic aphasia has been emphasized previously (Jayakar PB, Seshia SS. J Clin Neurophysiol 1991;7:299-311; Deonna TW. J Clin Neurophysiol 1991;7:288-298). See also Ped Neur Briefs Sept 1991;5:71; Jan 1991;5:45). The beneficial effects of ACTH and corticosteroids have been reported from Tel Aviv University (Lerman P et al. See Ped Neur Briefs April 1991;5:28-29). Corticosteroids administered early were more effective than delayed treatments. -Editor. *Ped Neur Briefs* May 1992.

CONGENITAL HYDROCEPHALUS AND SEIZURES

The frequency of seizures and long-term outcome in 68 children with congenital hydrocephalus not associated with myelomeningocele were examined at the Washington University School of Medicine, St. Louis, MO. Mental retardation was a risk factor for the development of seizures and was diagnosed 4 times more frequently in children with seizures (76% compared to

17%). Cortical CNS malformation diagnosed on CT, such as agenesis of the corpus callosum, was another seizure predictive factor (48% v. 17%). The absence of mental retardation, older age and non-paroxysmal EEG at seizure onset, and absence of CNS malformation correlated with seizure remission. Seizures were adequately controlled by anticonvulsants in 42 % and medication was successfully discontinued in patients of normal intelligence who had been seizure free for 3 years. (Noetzel MJ, Blake JN. Seizures in children with congenital hydrocephalus: long-term outcome. Neurology July 1992;42:1277-1281.) (Reprints: Dr. Noetzel, Department of Neurology, Washington University School of Medicine, 400 S. Kingshighway, St. Louis, MO 63110.)

COMMENT. The clinical and neuroradiologic findings in a male infant with congenital hydrocephalus due to intrauterine HTLV-1 infection are reported from the Division of Child Neurology, Institute of Neurological Sciences, Tottori University Faculty of Medicine, Yonago, Japan. A 20 day old male infant was admitted with macrocephaly. The mother developed human T-cell lymphotropic virus type I (HTLV-1)-associated myelopathy shortly after the birth of the infant. The infant's serum HTLV-1 antibody was elevated, suggesting an intrauterine route of infection. (Tohyama J et al. Neurology July 1992;42:1406-1408.)

Factors affecting the prognosis of intrauterine hydrocephalus diagnosed in the third trimester are reviewed from the Department of Neurosurgery, Kobe University, School of Medicine, Japan (Oi S, Surg Neurol 1992;37:66-68). Four patients underwent transabdominal or transvaginal cephalocentesis with measurement of intracranial pressure and intrauterine pressure. Another 4 patients had pre- and post-natal CT or MRI measurements of the head performed shortly before and after birth. The results indicated extremely high intracranial pressure in the fetal brain, whereas after birth the macrocephaly was accompanied by a relatively low intracranial pressure. Fetal hydrocephalus is extremely hypertensive, and an impairment of neuronal functional development prenatally can be irreversible. The fetal ventricular amniotic shunt was not appropriate for maintaining the decompressive effect, and a more reliable drainage system is required. -Editor. *Ped Neur Briefs* Aug 1992.

REFLEX EPILEPSY INDUCED BY "SOROBAN", A JAPANESE CALCULATOR

Three patients with reflex epilepsy and myoclonic jerks of the right arm and fingers, precipitated by calculation using a Soroban, are reported from the Department of Neuropsychiatry, Osaka University Medical School, Fukushima-ku, Osaka, Japan. The Soroban (abacus) is a Japanese traditional calculator requiring complex finger movements. Calculations are made by moving the counter beads with the fingers. The quicker the fingers move the sooner the calculation is finished. A simultaneous mental task requiring a high degree of concentration and complicated and delicate finger movements was necessary to induce the epileptic discharges consisting of a spike wave complex with left central prevalence. The reflex epilepsy in these paticnts resembled that induced by writing. Valproate was effective in the control of seizures and epileptic discharges. (Yamamoto J et al. Reflex epilepsy induced by calculation using a "Soroban," a Japanese traditional calculator. Epilepsia Jan/Feb 1991;32:39-43).

COMMENT. Both mental activity under high psychological tension and complicated and delicate movements of the fingers were necessary to induce epileptic discharges and/or a clinical seizure in these patients; stimulation without these two factors had no effect. Other reflex epilepsies induced by higher mental activity include reading epilepsy, graphogenic epilepsy induced by writing, language induced epilepsy induced by reading, writing, and speaking, epilepsia arithmetices induced by calculation, decision making epilepsy induced by cards and game playing, and drawing induced seizures induced by geometric designs. Nintendo and Rubik's cube may also cause reflex epilepsy.-Editor. *Ped Neur Briefs* April 1991.

SEIZURES INDUCED BY EYE CLOSURE

A case of a 19-year-old mentally-retarded female with an unusual form of seizures induced by eye closure is reported from the Universities of Toronto and Calgary, Canada. She developed drop attacks at age 2 years and eye fluttering seizures with altered consciousness soon afterwards. Generalized tonic-clonic seizures coincided with the introduction of valproic acid therapy at age 13 years. Clobazam controlled the grand mal, but multiple absence seizures and status persisted, despite trials with numerous antiepileptic drugs. The voluntary act of eye closure was a trigger for seizure activity, but visual input was an inhibitor. Unless visual input was prevented by allowing the eyes to close, seizures did not occur. Darkness alone was insufficient to elicit a seizure. The EEG seizure pattern consisted of generalized high-amplitude beta activity alternating with delta, and typical spike-and-wave activity was absent. (Barclay CL et al. Unusual form of seizures induced by eye closure. Epilepsia March/April 1993;34: 289-293). (Reprints: Dr CL Barclay, Toronto Hospital, Western Division MP, 11th Fl, 399 Bathurst St, Toronto, Ontario, Canada M5T 2S8).

COMMENT. Seizures induced by eye closure are of two types: 1) those related to movement of the eyelids and occurring in photosensitive patients; and 2) a non-photosensitive type with scotosensitive epilepsy triggered by darkness alone or by obstruction of central visual fixation. The above patient required a combination of these two mechanisms for seizure induction. -Editor. *Ped Neur Briefs* May 1993.

METABOLIC DISORDERS AND SEIZURES

BIOTINIDASE DEFICIENCY AND SEIZURES

The clinical features of 78 symptomatic children with biotinidase deficiency were reviewed and the response to antiepileptic drugs and biotin therapy in 43 (55%) with seizures are reported from the Medical College of Virginia, Richmond, VA. Seizures were the presenting symptom in 30 (38%) patients, with onset between 2 and 24 months (mean, 8 months). Seizure patterns were generalized tonic-clonic or clonic in 56%, infantile spasms or myoclonic in 16%, and partial in only 5%. EEGs were abnormal in 16 (76%) of 21 patients tested; spike or epileptiform discharges were reported in 9. Antiepileptic drugs controlled seizures in 22 (51%) patients, but treatment was withdrawn without relapse after biotin therapy was initiated. Biotin orally, 5 to 10 mg daily, stopped seizures within 24 hours in 12 of 16 (75%) children whose seizures were uncontrolled by AEDs. Five infants died and 3 sustained permanent brain damage before the biotinidase deficiency was diagnosed. (Salbert BA, et al. Characterization of seizures associated with biotinidase deficiency. Neurology July 1993;43:1351-1355). (Reprints: Dr Barry Wolf, Dept of Human Genetics, Medical College of Virginia, Box 33, MCV Station, Richmond, VA 23298).

COMMENT. Early diagnosis by newborn screening is recommended by the authors. Biotinidase enzyme deficiency and a trial of biotin should be considered in infants or young children with poorly controlled seizures, especially in those with hypotonia, ataxia, skin rash, alopecia, metabolic ketoacidosis, or organic aciduria. Symptoms resolve rapidly after biotin therapy, but neurologic damage may be irreversible if diagnosis is delayed. (Ped Neur Briefs, Jan 1990).-Editor. *Ped Neur Briefs* July 1993.

MOLYBDENUM-COFACTOR DEFICIENCY AND SEIZURES

The clinical, biochemical, and neuropathological findings in two neonates with molybdenum-cofactor deficiency presenting with convulsions are reported from the Academic Medical Center, Amsterdam, The Netherlands. Patient 1 was admitted at day two with feeding problems, jitteriness, an abnormal cry, apneic spells, and partial and generalized seizures. Head circumference, weight and length were above the 97th percentile. EEGs showed a burst suppression pattern. CT revealed diffuse hypodense ischemic changes. Plasma and urinary cysteine were decreased, and urine sulphite, S-sulphocysteine, taurine, and thiosulphate were increased. Purine analysis showed elevated xanthine and hypoxanthine in the urine, while uric acid was very low. Seizures were refractory, and the infant died on the 10th day. Cultured fibroblasts from a skin biopsy showed absent sulfite oxidase activity. Autopsy findings were meningeal fibrosis, loss of cortical neurons, gliosis and cystic lysis of white matter. Patient 2 was admitted at age 4 days with feeding difficulties, hypertonia, jitteriness, opisthotonus, and high-pitched cry. Generalized and partial tonic-clonic seizures were resistant to treatment. EEG was a multifocal epileptic pattern. An initial diagnosis of postanoxic encephalopathy was changed to molybdenum-cofactor deficiency at 3 years, on reexamination prompted by the revelation of parental consanguinity. Clinically deteriorated, he had spastic tetraplegia, intractable epilepsy, and characteristic metabolic changes. He died 8 months later. Diagnosis was confirmed by liver biopsy and sulfite oxidase and xanthine oxidase analyses. Lens dislocation, a frequent feature of the syndrome, was absent. (Slot HMJ et al. Molybdenum-cofactor deficiency: an easily missed cause of neonatal convulsions. Neuropediatrics June 1993;24:139-142). (Respond: Mrs HMJ Slot MD, Dept of Neonatology, Academic Medical Center, Meibergdreef 9,1105 AZ Amsterdam, The Netherlands).

COMMENT. Molybdenum-cofactor deficiency is an inborn error of metabolism that results in characteristic biochemical and clinical symptoms of sulphite oxidase and xanthine dehydrogenase deficiences. Diagnosis can be made simply with a sulphite strip test in fresh urine and by measuring uric acid excretion. Antenatal diagnosis is possible by chorionic villus sampling and sulphite oxidase assay. -Editor. *Ped Neur Briefs.* July 1993.

FOLATE DEFICIENCY, PORPHYRIA, AND SEIZURES

A 12 year old, learning-disabled boy with epilepsy was admitted to the University of Connecticut Health Center, Farmington, CT because of symptomatic folate deficiency and newly diagnosed acute intermittent porphyria. Seizures and global developmental delays were noted by 12 months of age. Seizures required multiple drug combinations, and optimal control was obtained with carbamazepine, valproate, and methsuximide. The patient was hospitalized because of abdominal pain, vomiting, anorexia, and behavioral changes. He developed hypertension, hyponatremia, and anemia. The urine became brown in color, positive for urobilinogen, and showed elevated coproporphyrins, uroporphyrins, aminolevulinic acid, and porphobilinogen (PBG). Erythrocyte and maternal PBG deaminase measurements were decreased. RBC folate levels were deficient. Oral folate, 0.5 mg/d, resulted in correction of the anemia and no recurrence of porphyric crises. (DiMario FJ Jr et al. Folate deficiency and acute intermittent porphyria in a 12-year-old boy. Neurology July 1993;43:1438-1439). (Reprints: Dr Francis J DiMario Jr, Pediatric Neurology, Bldg 12, UCONN Health Center, Farmington, CT 06030).

COMMENT. Serum folate should be determined in patients with acute intermittent porphyria requiring chronic anticonvulsant therapy. A folate deficiency induced by the AEDs may further reduce red blood cell production and precipitate a porphyric crisis. Folate supplements are beneficial as an adjunct to the carbohydrate loading in therapy for a porphyric crisis or its prevention. -Editor. *Ped Neur Briefs* July 1993. ~

PYRIDOXINE DEPENDENT EPILEPSY

Four children with pyridoxine dependent seizures beginning at 2 to 19 months are reported from the Loyola University Medical Center, Maywood, IL. Patients were identified out of 51 treated routinely with pyridoxine for refractory seizures and seen over a 6 year period. The dose of pyridoxine was 50 mg orally twice daily. The seizure types were atypical absence, myoclonic, generalized clonic and simple partial and complex partial. The authors suggest that pyridoxine should be tried in all children with seizure disorders with onset at any age who are poorly responsive to anticonvulsant drugs. (Coker SB, Postneonatal vitamin B6-dependent epilepsy. Pediatrics Aug 1992;90:221-223.)

(Reprints: S.B. Coker, M.D., Loyola University Medical Center, 2160 S. First Ave., Maywood, IL 60153.)

COMMENT. Pyridoxine dependent epilepsy may present after the neonatal period and may be manifested by many seizure types. Many of us have been discouraged by failure to uncover pyridoxine dependency in drug resistant epilepsies in children. Obviously, persistence rewards, but the relationship between pyridoxine and epilepsy is complex.

The wide range of reactivity of vitamin B6 with a number of drugs and other chemicals encountered in the environment must be considered in the diagnosis. These interactions involve a condensation between the xenobiotic and pyridoxal phosphate, and vitamin B6 absorption, coenzymes, and specific vitamin B6-dependent enzymes can also be affected. Isoniazide is probably the most extensively studied drug with respect to effects on vitamin B6 metabolism. Other drugs reported to interact with vitamin B6 include ampicillin, anticonvulsants, levodopa, oral contraceptives and ethanol. The mechanism of anticonvulsant drug and vitamin B6 interaction is not well determined. One study showed that the vitamin was decreased only in males treated with anticonvulsants. Another showed that pyridoxine supplements resulted in lower plasma phenytoin and phenobarbital concentrations. An interaction between the vitamin and dyes added to medications during manufacture have also been demonstrated (Dubick MA. Interactions of vitamin B6 (pyridoxine) and xenobibotics. In <u>Nutritional Toxicology</u>, Vol III, ed. JN Hathcock. New York, Academic Press, 1989.) -Editor. *Ped Neur Briefs* Sept 1992.

ASPARTAME AND ABSENCE SEIZURES

The effect of aspartame on epilepsy was studied in 10 children with previously untreated generalized absence seizures using a double blind challenge of 40 mg/kg aspartame as a single dose at the Children's Hospital, Halifax, Canada. Ambulatory cassette recording of the EEG and quantification of numbers and length of spike wave discharges on 2 consecutive days showed that the number of seconds spent in spike-wave discharge per hour of recording was significantly increased following aspartame compared with the control day when the children received sucrose. (Camfield PR et al. Aspartame exacerbates EEG spike-wave discharge in children with generalized absence epilepsy: a double-blind controlled study. Neurology May 1992;42:1000-1003.) (Reprints: Dr. Peter Camfield, IWK Children's Hospital, Box 3070, Halifax, Nova Scotia, Canada B3J 3G9.)

COMMENT. Anecdotal claims that aspartame may exacerbate epilepsy appear to have scientific validity based on this EEG double blind controlled study in 10 children with absence seizures.

In support of the FDA decision to clear aspartame for general consumption, excepting phenylketonuric children, a study of 126 apparently healthy children and adolescents showed that there were no clinically significant differences documented between the children taking aspartame and those taking sucrose for a 13 week period, regardless of age between 2 and 21 years. Aspartame appeared to be a safe sweetening agent for use by healthy children aged 2 or older. (Frey GH. J Toxicology Environmental Health 1976;2:401.) However, studies of aspartame in children with neuropsychiatric problems are limited, and adequate data are not available to establish its safety and freedom from adverse effects. Until more specific investigations are completed to determine the effects of aspartame on seizure control it might be advisable to limit or avoid the ingestion of aspartame products in children with seizures and particularly poorly controlled absence seizures (Camfield et al. 1992). See Millichap JG. Nutrition. Diet and Child's Behavior. Charles C. Thomas, Springfield, 1986 for a review of the effects of aspartame on diseases of the nervous system in children. -Editor. *Ped Neur Briefs* June 1992.

More recent studies of aspartame failed to demonstrate adverse effects on seizures and epileptiform discharges in children with epilepsy (Shaywitz BA et al. Aspartame has no effect on seizures or epileptiform discharges in epileptic children. Ann Neurol Jan 1994;35:98-103), or on children's behavior and cognition (Wolraich ML et al. Effects of diets high in sucrose or aspartame on the behavior and cognitive performance of children. N Engl J Med Feb 3, 1994;330:301-7). The disparity in the negative conclusions of these studies compared to positive adverse effects noted in some others of comparable scientific design is unexplained. Differences in pre-challenge diets, individual idiosyncrasies, and neurological symptomatology among subjects may explain the frequency of parental reports of adverse behavioral effects of sucrose and the occasional scientific demonstration of EEG seizure exacerbation by aspartame. Further studies, preferably supported by an unbiased govermental agency, will be needed before some parents, consumers, and physicians are fully convinced of the reputed safety of the artificial sweetener aspartame, especially in children with neuro-behavioral disorders and in adults with migraine. -Editor.

INFECTIONS AND SEIZURES

SEIZURES AND CEREBRAL CYSTICERCOSIS

The results of a long-term retrospective study of 240 patients with seizures and cysticercosis of the brain parenchyma are reported from the Instituto Nacional de Neurologio y Neurocirugia Manuel Velasco Suarez de Mexico, Mexico City. Of 118 patients who received cysticidal therapy (albendazole, prasiquantel, or both) for lesions without inflammation on imaging studies, there was an 82% reduction in the mean number of brain cysts and a 95% reduction in the mean frequency of seizures. After 3 years of follow-up, 54% of patients were seizure free. By contrast, the untreated patients averaged 11 seizures per year and none was seizure free. Of 58 patients with inflammation around cysts who did not receive cysticidal medication, there was a 74% reduction in the frequency of seizures and 31% became seizure free. After surgical treatment of unmedicated patients there was an 87 % reduction in seizure frequency and 40 % became seizure free. (Vazquez V, Sotelo J. The course of seizures after treatment for cerebral cysticercosis. N Engl J Med Sept 3, 1992;327:696-701.) (Reprints: Dr. Sotelo, National Institue of Neurology and Neurosurgery, Insurgentes sur 3877, 14269, Mexico City, Mexico.)

COMMENT. The outcome for patients with epilepsy due to neurocysticercosis was better after treatment with cysticidal agents than when the primary disease was left to follow its natural course. There were fewer seizures after medical treatment than after surgical excision of the cyst. In the patients with inflammation around cysts, spontaneous resolution of the cysts occurred frequently but the number of seizures per year in this group was 31% higher than in those who received medical treatment with cysticidal drugs. Granulomas remaining after the cysts destruction may account for the high incidence of persistent seizures. The patients in this study were adults, but most had suffered from frequent seizures for many years because of persistence of the paracystic epileptic focus. Children in endemic areas who have seizures related to cysticercosis should be considered for cysticidal therapy at the time of diagnosis. The use of these drugs in children may require further definition .

Cysticercosis of the CNS is rare in the United States, but accounts for 25 % of intracranial tumors in Mexico. Increased intracranial pressure is found in about 75 % of cases (Menkes JH. Textbook of Child Neurology 3rd Ed. Philadelphia. Lee and Febiger 1981). -Editor. *Ped Neur Briefs* Oct 1992.

RASMUSSEN'S SYNDROME AND UVEITIS

Two children with Rasmussen's syndrome complicated by asymptomatic uveitis are reported from the Royal Children's Hospital, Melbourne, Australia, and Montreal Neurological Institute, Montreal, Canada. A 10-year-old girl developed somatosensorimotor seizures affected her right leg and left sided acute uveitis.

Epilepsia partialis continua, with onset 9 months later, was associated with right hemiparesis and cortical sensory loss, and dysphasia. EEG showed epileptic discharges in the left central region. CT revealed atrophy of the left hemisphere. Left frontal corticectomy failed to control seizures. The cortex showed chronic encephalitis. The second patient, a 5-year-old girl, had complex partial status epilepticus which responded to IV gammaglobulin, left facial weakness, and right sided uveitis. Right anterior temporal lobectomy revealed leptomeningeal inflammation. Seizures became intractable, and a dense left hemiparesis developed. She died 2 years 7 months after the onset of seizures. (Harvey AS, Andermann F et al. Chronic encephalitis (Rasmussen's syndrome) and ipsilateral uveitis. Ann Neurol Dec 1992;32:826-829). (Correspondence: Dr Harvey, Dept of Neurology, Royal Children's Hospital, Flemington Rd, Parkville, Victoria 3052, Australia).

COMMENT. A viral cause seemed likely but was not confirmed by serology or tissue culture. Slit-lamp examination of the eye should be included in the evaluation of children with Rasmussen's syndrome.-Editor. *Ped Neur Briefs.* Jan 1993.

SEVERE REACTIONS TO DTP VACCINE

Severe reactions experienced by 60 children within 48 hours of DTP immunization were reported from the UCLA School of Medicine, Los Angeles, CA. These included seizures in 40 or 66% (6 with fever >40.5°C), collapse episodes in 14, and persistent crying in 6. Subjects with encephalopathy were not included in the study. Those with seizures had a high rate of personal and family histories of seizures, and 10% were afebrile. Chinese hamster ovary cell assays failed to reveal active pertussis toxin in acute sera. Long-term follow-up for possible neurologic sequelae was not performed. (Blumberg DA, Cherry JD et al. Severe reactions associated with diphtheria-tetanus-pertussis vaccine: Detailed study of children with seizures, hypotonic-hyporesponsive episodes, high fevers, and persistent crying. Pediatrics June 1993;91:1158-1165).

(Reprints: Dean A Blumberg MD, Dept of Pediatrics, UCLA School of Medicine, 10833 Le Conte Ave, Los Angeles, CA 90024).

COMMENT. Seizures induced by pertussis immunization and fever are more severe than simple febrile seizures. Cherry JD and associates report that a first febrile convulsion within 3 or 7 days of pertussis immunization is more likely to last longer than 10 minutes, to be recurrent, and to have a focal pattern when compared to first .seizures occurring more than 7 days after immunization (J Pediatr June 1993;122:900-3). They have estimated that one in a 1000 children immunized will have a seizure, and 6% of first febrile seizures are associated with pertussis immunization. The use of acellular DTP vaccines, recently approved by the FDA, may hopefully reduce the frequency and severity of neurological complications. -Editor. *Ped Neur Briefs*. June 1993.

EPILEPSY IN A MITOCHONDRIAL DISORDER

Epilepsy in 9 (22%) of 37 members of a family with maternally inherited mitochondrial disease is reported from the Department of Neurology, University Hospital, Tromso, Norway. The epilepsy began in infancy or childhood in 3 patients and during adult life in the remainder. The different clinical expressions of epilepsy in the family were myoclonus, partial epilepsy and generalized tonic-clonic seizures. The neuropsychiatric disorders included intellectual deterioration, muscle weakness, pigmental retinal degeneration, progressive hearing loss, cerebellar ataxia and in 1 patient a hemiplegia and paranoid psychosis. The CT scan showed cerebral atrophy, cerebellar atrophy and calcification in the basal ganglia. The EEG abnormalities included slowing and spikes, sometimes focal, and a bilateral paroxysmal response to photic stimulation. A muscle biopsy from the proband revealed a mild defect in the NADH-ubiquinone oxidoreductase step (complex 1) in the respiratory chain (Torbergsen T et al. Epilepsy in a mitochondrial disorder. J Neur Neurosurg & Psych Dec 1991;54:1073-1076). (Correspondence: Dr. Torbergsen,

Department of Neurology, 9038 University Hospital, Tromso, Norway)

COMMENT. The various clinical manifestations of epilepsy including partial motor and/or complex partial epilepsy in different branches of this family were remarkable and worthy of publication. The authors postulate that mitochondrial dysfunctions may be the cause of some epileptic syndromes of undetermined etiology. -Editor. *Ped Neur Briefs* Feb 1992.

SEIZURES AND THYROTOXICOSIS

Two thyrotoxic children, ages 10 and 11 years, who presented with seizures and coma are reported from the Departments of Pediatrics, Bolzano Hospital and the University of Pavia, Italy. Patient 1 was admitted with vomiting, headache, and stupor. He had dilated pupils, nuchal rigidity, and tachycardia. A goiter was palpable. A generalized seizure lasting 20 min was repeated despite diazepam intravenously. Serum thyroid hormone levels were markedly elevated. Patient 2 had a thyrotoxic crisis complicated by status epilepticus and coma. Both patients had abnormal EEGs, with slow activity in temporal regions and high voltage fast activity in frontal areas. (Radetti G et al. Thyrotoxicosis presenting with seizures and coma in two children. AJDC Sept 1993;147:925-7). (Reprints: Dr Radetti, Dept of Pediatrics, Regional Hospital of Bolzano, via L Boehler no 5, 39100 Bolzano, Italy).

COMMENT. The authors cite only one other child with these symptoms reported in the literature, and 10 adult cases. Patients with seizures and coma of undetermined cause should be tested for hyperthyroidism.-Editor. *Ped Neur Briefs.* Oct 1993.

OCCIPITAL LOBE SEIZURES AND CELIAC DISEASE

The electroclinical ictal findings of 4 epileptic patients with clinically asymptomatic celiac disease are reported from the University of Bologna, Italy. All patients had paroxysmal visual manifestations and EEG seizure discharges arising from the occipital lobe. CT in

2 patients showed occipital calcifications. A gluten-free diet was not beneficial and polytherapy with antiepileptic drugs aggravated the seizures in 3 cases. Epilepsy and evidence of steatorrhea and growth failure were present in early childhood. The diagnosis of celiac disease was made by tests for serum folate level, a d-zylose absorption test, anti-gliadin antibody test and jejunal biopsy which showed villous atrophy (Ambrosetto G et al. Occipital lobe seizures related to clinically asymptomatic celiac disease in adulthood. Epilepsia May/June 1992;33:476-481). (Reprints: Professor G. Ambrosetto, Institute of Neurology, Via Ugo Foscolo 7, 40123, Bologna, Italy.)

COMMENT. The same authors had investigated 10 patients with epilepsy and occipital cerebral calcification and had found evidence of celiac disease in 6. All patients with epilepsy and posterior cerebral calcification should be investigated for possible celiac disease. (Gobbi G, Ambrosetto P et al. Celiac disease, posterior cerebral calcifications and epilepsy. Brain Dev Jan 1992;14:23-29.).-Editor. *Ped Neur Briefs* Aug 1992.

SEIZURES, CVA AND CELIAC DISEASE

Cortical vascular abnormalities including pial angiomatosis and fibrosis of small veins are described in a 12 year old girl with celiac disease, occipital calcifications, and folate deficiency who underwent surgery for intractable complex partial seizures at the Montreal Neurological Institute, Canada. She was first diagnosed with Sturge-Weber syndrome without nevus flammeus. A right occipital resection was performed and was followed by seizure remission. Subsequently, low folic acid levels and iron deficiency anemia led to a diagnosis of celiac disease. Antigliadin antibodies were 182 arbitrary units (normal: < 25), and small bowel biopsy showed villous atrophy. A gluten-free diet with folate, vitamin E, and iron supplementation resulted in improved appetite and weight increase. (Bye AME et al. Cortical vascular abnormalities in the syndrome of celiac disease, epilepsy, bilateral occipital calcifications, and folate deficiency. Ann Neurol Sept

1993;34:399-403). (Respond: Dr Anderman, Montreal Neurological Hospital, 3801 University St, Montreal, Quebec, Canada H3A 2B4).

COMMENT. The pathological abnormalities in this case were considered similar but not identical to those in Sturge-Weber syndrome. A syndrome of celiac disease, epilepsy, and cerebral calcifications, resembling Sturge-Weber syndrome, has been reported frequently, especially in Italy (Gobbi G et al. Lancet 1992;340:439; Tiacci C et al. Epilepsia 1993;34:528; Piattella L et al. Child's Nerv Syst 1993;9:172.). Patients with occipital cerebral calcification of unknown cause and patients with celiac disease should receive an EEG, followed by an MRI if the EEG is abnormal. A new, rapid, noninvasive screening test for celiac disease, a strip-AGA (antigliadin antibody) test, performed on a drop of whole blood, is described from the Instituto per l'Infancia, Trieste, Italy (Not T et al. J Pediat Sept 1993;123:425-7).-Editor. *Ped Neur Briefs* Sept 1993.

DESMOPRESSIN AND IMIPRAMINE-INDUCED CONVULSION

A 10 year old boy with enuresis was admitted in coma to the Dumfries Royal Infirmary, Scotland. Treatment with intranasal desmopressin 40 mcg nightly for 5 months had recently been supplemented with imipramine 25 mg. A generalized tonic seizure on admission was terminated by 5 mg rectal diazepam and treatment for hyponatremia (serum sodium 113 mmol/L). (Hamed M et al. Hyponatremic convulsion associated with desmopressin and imipramine treatment. BMJ May 1 1993;306:1169).

COMMENT. Avoid drug combination and limit fluids with desmopressin.-Editor. *Ped Neur Briefs* May 1993.

MIGRAINE AND EPILEPSY

The coexistence of classical migraine, visual phenomena and seizures and occipital spike-wave complexes in the EEG are reported in 14 children from the Department of Neurological Sciences, University La Sapienza, Rome, Italy. The age of onset was 3 to 9 years (mean age 5.4 years) and the clinical and EEG follow-up ranged from 4 to 16 years (mean 11.2 years). Visual phenomena were described as bright rings, bands, red-colored disks, in both visual fields or in the visual hemifield opposite the spike-wave localization. Amaurosis followed the appearance of the phosphenes. In some patients the migraine with aura and epilepsy were chronologically related phenomena; migraine might occur immediately before or after seizures; migraine may act as a triggering factor for epilepsy. In others, visual phenomena either preceded migraine with aura or occurred as an isolated event or even preceded epileptic seizures (De Romanis F et al. Migraine and epilepsy with infantile onset and electroencephalographic findings of occipital spike-wave complexes. Headache June 1991;31:378-383).

COMMENT. In 50% of the patients in this study, migraine with aura, with phosphenes and amaurosis as prodromal symptoms, replaces epileptic seizures when they disappear or improve following antiepileptic treatment. Ergot alkaloids or pizotifen were of little or no benefit whereas migraine with aura responded to anti-epileptic treatment. Occipital epilepsy in childhood in this study was not benign and seizures were controlled by anti-epileptic treatment in only 2 subjects .

Migraine during pregnancy is reviewed by Uknis A and Silberstein SD in the same issue of Headache 1991;31:372-374. A first attack of migraine with unilateral parasthesias and blurred vision occurred in a 27-year-old woman during the first trimester and led to the diagnosis of her pregnancy. Pre-existing migraine usually improves with pregnancy, whereas relapse frequently occurs in the post-partum period. Children born to migraineurs have no increased incidence of birth defects. -Editor. *Ped Neur Briefs* Oct 1991.

EEG STUDIES

EPIDEMIOLOGY OF ABSENCE EPILEPSY

A population based electroencephalographic study of absence epilepsy in 97 children is reported from the Departments of Neurophysiology and Pediatrics, Goteborg University, Sweden. All patients had regular bilaterally synchronous and symmetrical 2-4 Hz spike-and-slow wave discharges and absences with or without generalized tonic-clonic seizures (GTCS). Patients with absence seizures not complicated by GTCS had long episodes of 2-4 Hz spike-and-slow wave discharges (> 10 seconds). Posterior delta rhythms occurred only in patients with pure uncomplicated absence whereas focal abnormalities were predictive of GTCS complication. There was no correlation between polyspike and slow wave and the developnent of GTCS. Brief episodes of 2-4 Hz spike-and-slow wave (< 10 seconds) were predictive of a two-fold increased risk of GTCS. GTCS appeared in spite of a normalized EEG in seven of 14 patients. Favorable seizure control was correlated with the normalization of EEG but a normal EEG was no guarantee that GTCS would not develop. (Hedstron A, Olsson I. Epidemiology of absence epilepsy: EEG findings and their predictive value. Pediatr Neurol March/April 1991;7:100-4).

COMMENT. This study demonstrates the predictive value of the EEG in prognosis of absence epilepsy. Posterior delta rhythm and long episodes of spike-and-wave with clinical correlates favor a good prognosis whereas brief spike-and-wave discharges without clinical correlates increase the risk of future generalized tonic-clonic seizures. Editor. *Ped Neur Briefs* June 1991.

MULTIFOCAL DISCHARGES AND EPILEPSY

Continuous EEG/video recordings on 4 children with the interictal EEG pattern of multifocal independent epileptiform discharges (MIED) are reported from the Epilepsy Center, The Johns Hopkins University School of Medicine, Baltimore, MD. The predominant seizure pattern consisted of bilateral tonic seizures with fencing postures. Most seizures arose from surgically resectable regions and epilepsy surgery performed in three patients resulted in improved seizure control. One patient had a focal resection of superior frontal-parietal cortex and two had hemidecorticectomies. Because the scalp recorded EEG data did not provide adequate localization, intracranial electrodes were placed in 2 patients prior to the resections (Burnstine TH et al. Multifocal independent epileptiform discharges in children: ictal correlates and surgical therapy. Neurology August 1991;41:1223-1228).

COMMENT. The presence of bilateral independent or generalized epileptiform discharges as in patients with MIED is not an absolute contraindication to performing a hemispherectomy, according to the experience of these authors. If the majority of seizures do not originate in one hemisphere and the patient is having frequent generalized seizures, then a corpus callosotomy should be considered.-Editor. *Ped Neur Briefs* Sept 1991.

EEG MAPPING AND BECT

Sequential topographic EEG mapping performed to differentiate "epileptic" from "non-epileptic" rolandic spikes has shown a characteristic pattern significantly related to classical BECT (benign focal epilepsy of childhood with centro-temporal spikes) in a study at the Department of Clinical Neurophysiology and Department of Child Neurology, University Hospital Utrecht, The Netherlands. There were 2 patterns: 1) stationary potential fields, and 2) non-stationary potential fields. The non-stationary patterns represented by a double spike showed a specific sequence starting with a dipolar field, with the negative pole in the frontal region and the positive pole in the centro-temporal region, and changing to a unipolar or dipolar field, with a negative potential field in the centro-temporal region and a simultaneous positive potential field in the frontal region. This characteristic pattern appeared to be significantly related to classical BECT. (Van der Meij W. et al. Sequential EEG mapping may differentiate "epileptic" from "non-epileptic" rolandic spikes. EEG and Clin Neurophysiol June 1992;82:408-414.) (Correspondence: Dr. W. Van der Meij, Department of Clinical Neurophysiology, University Hospital Utrecht, P.O. Box 85500, 3508 GA Utrecht The Netherlands).

COMMENT. The spike morphology in 40 uncontrolled childhood focal epilepsy patients was quantified by a computer-based technique and analyzed in relationship to epileptic syndromes at the Baylor College of Medicine, Houston, TX. The spikes of patients in the benign focal epilepsy category differed from those in other syndromes; they were higher in amplitude, longer in duration, less sharp, and had a higher spike parameter. (Frost JD et al. Epilepsia May/June 1992 33:531-536.)

A report of unilateral opercular macrogyria underlying benign childhood epilepsy with centrotemporal rolandic spikes in an 18 year old boy emphasizes the need for MRI in detecting neuronal migration disorders and other structural lesions in cases of apparent idiopathic partial epilepsies. (Ambrosetto G. Epilepsia May/June 1992;33:499-503.) -Editor. *Ped Neur Briefs* July 1992.

SEIZURES, FOCAL EEG ABNORMALITIES, AND CT

The prevalence and nature of abnormalities on CT associated with focal EEG abnormalities were evaluated in 964 consecutive children with epileptic and non-epileptic seizures seen over one year at the Royal Liverpool Children's Hospital, England. Of 157 (16%) children with a focus on the EEG, 83 had slow waves and 74 had spike or sharp wave foci. Of 121 with CT head scans, 26 (21%) scans were abnormal, and 81% of abnormalities were localized. Abnormal scans were uncommon in children with a single seizure, occurring in 8%. Frequency of abnormal scans in patients with delta foci (25%) was not significantly different from those with spike foci (17%). Focal neurological signs or partial seizures were predictive of abnormal scans.

Focal CT findings prompted surgery in two patients with drug resistant partial seizures but lacking focal neurological signs; one had a parietal astocytoma, the other a frontal encephalocele. (Gibbs J, Appleton RE et al. Focal electroencephalographic abnormalities and computerized tomography findings in children with seizures. J Neurol Neurosurg Psychiatry April 1993;56: 368-371). (Respond: Dr RE Appleton, Department of Paediatric Neurology, Royal Liverpool Children's Hospital, Eaton Road, Liverpool L12 2AP, England).

COMMENT. The authors advise CT in children with intractable partial seizures or lateralizing neurological findings or both, but not necessarily in all those with focal EEG abnormalities. Their findings suggest that no distinction should be made between delta and spike wave foci as criteria for CT and exclusion of neurosurgical lesion. These results confirm a study of the electroencephalogram in 50 children with intracranial tumors and seizures reported from the Mayo Clinic (Millichap JG, Bickford RG, Miller RH, Backus RE. Neurology May 1962;12:329-336). A delta pattern occurred in 57%, and spike, sharp wave, or spike-and-wave seizure discharges were recorded in 32% of children with supratentorial tumors. The EEG was of localizing value in 21(88%) of 24 patients with tumors involving the cerebral cortex, and the accuracy of EEG localization was almost equal to that of pneumography. The value of the EEG in diagnostic differentiation of a brain tumor and a scar or microgyrus was less than its localizing value. -Editor. *Ped Neur Briefs* May 1993.

TEMPORAL LOBE EPILEPSY: ELECTROCLINICAL FEATURES

Results of video-EEG, PET, MRI, and pathological findings in 14 children aged 16 months to 12 years who were seizure-free after temporal lobectomy are reported in a multicenter, international study at Cleveland, Singapore, Naples, and Helsinki. In 4 children with mesiotemporal sclerosis and in 1 with cortical dysplasia, EEG showed anterior/inferior temporal interictal sharp waves and unilateral temporal seizure onset. In 9 with low- grade temporal neoplasms, the EEG findings were complex, including multifocal interictal sharp waves or falsely lateralized EEG seizure onset. Video-EEG recording was most useful for localization of the epileptogenic zone for resection in those without tumors. In patients with tumors, video-EEG confirmed the epileptic nature of the complex partial seizures but was of less localizing value. (Wyllie E et al. Temporal lobe epilepsy in early childhood. Epilepsia Sept/Oct 1993;34 859-868). (Reprints: Dr E Wyllie, Pediatric Epilepsy Program, Cleveland Clinic Foundation, 9500 Euclid Ave, Cleveland, OH 44195).

COMMENT. Three of 4 patients in this study with mesiotemporal sclerosis had a history of infantile compex febrile seizures compared with none of 10 with tumor or cortical dysplasia. An excellent outcome after temporal surgical resection in a group of 19 patients with mesiotemporal sclerosis following prolonged febrile convulsions is reported from the Montreal Neurological Institute (Abou-Khalil B, Andermann F et al. Epilepsia Sept/Oct 1993;34 878). The response and seizure control in this group was significantly better than in those without antecedent febrile convulsions.

In 15 children with temporal lobe epilepsy, aged 7-14 years, studied at the Royal Children's Hospital, Melbourne, Australia, ictal SPECT provided reliable lateralizing information to confirm that obtained from surface EEG and MRI. In 4, ictal SPECT was superior to ictal EEG in localizing value. (Harvey AS et al. Epilepsia Sept/Oct 1993;34:869).

Anterior left temporal lobectomy and seizure control had an apparent beneficial effect on illogical thinking in a group of 7 children treated for intractable temporal lobe epilepsy at the University of California at Los Angeles (Caplan R, Shields WD et al. J Am Acad Child Adolesc Psychiatry 1993;32 604).-Editor. *Ped Neur Briefs* Nov 1993.

ATTENTION, BEHAVIOR AND EPILEPSY

LEARNING DISABILITIES IN EPILEPSY

Neurophysiological mechanisms by which epilepsy may interfere with learning ability are reviewed from the Department of Clinical Meurophysiology, Maudsley Hospital, and Department of Psychology, Middlesex Hospital, London, England. Five mechanisms are listed: 1) Disruption of ongoing processing by epileptiform activity that interferes with attention to incoming information, its storage or retrieval; 2) disruption of storage and retrieval of information by discharges temporally distant from the learning experience; 3) permanent damage to neural tissue; 4) antiepileptic drug toxicity; 5) disruption of brain function by chronic frequent discharges during sleep. Subclinical generalized spike wave discharges may be accompanied by transitory cognitive impairment demonstrable by psychological testing during EEG recording. Left-sided focal spiking produces errors on verbal tasks whereas right-sided discharges impair handling of non-verbal material. Subclinical discharges may disrupt educational skills in children and impair driving performance in motorists. Suppression of discharges by antiepileptic drugs may improve psychological functioning. Spike wave monitors may find a place in special schools to alert teachers to a child's absence attacks. (Binnie CD et al. Learning disabilities in epilepsy: Neurophysiological aspects. Epilepsia 1990;31 (Suppl 4):S2-8).

COMMENT. The above article is the first in a report of the Symposium on Epilepsy and Education at the XVIIIth International Epilepsy Congress, New Delhi, India, October 1989. Other reports in this Epilepsia supplement include references to epileptic syndromes and cognitive functioning (Dam M); effects of antiepileptic drugs (Trimble MR); the EEG in assessing cognitive function (Stores G); and the effects of discontinuing antiepileptic drugs on cognition (Blennow G et al). Community based studies in the United Kingdom have shown that up to 30% of children with epilepsy underachieved in school and many are referred for special education. -Editor. *Ped Neur Briefs* Feb 1991.

REACTION TIME AND ATTENTION IN EPILEPSY

Reaction time, attention and impulsivity in 112 children with epilepsy (4.5-13 years of age) were studied using a computerized test at the Division of Neurology, Children's Hospital Los Angeles, Los Angeles, CA. Measures included simple reaction time, forced choice reaction time, choice reaction time with distraction, variability of speed of response and errors of omission and commission. Compared to controls, children with epilepsy were significantly slower, more variable and made more omission errors but not commission or impulsive errors. Reaction times showed a negative correlation with IQ but were not related to seizure severity or duration of seizure disorder. Differences related to treatment history were small although patients with less total exposure to antiepileptic medications tended to perform better than those with greater total exposure. A small unmedicated group did not differ from patients on antiepileptic drugs on the day of the test, however. (Mitchell WG et al. Reaction time, attention, and impulsivity in epilepsy. Pediatr Neurol Jan/Feb 1992;8:19-24). (Correspondence: Dr. Mitchell, Neurology Division, Box 82, Children's Hospital Los Angeles, Los Angeles, CA 90054.)

COMMENT. The authors conclude that the slowed reaction times and inattention demonstrated by epileptic patients were not primarily a result of the seizures or treatment. The names of the specific anticonvulsants were not included. A slowed motor speed may contribute to a relatively low performance IQ score.

Absence seizures may complicate learning disabilities and the diagnosis may be overlooked when using routine EEGs. Borkowski WJ, Jr. et al. at the Alfred I. duPont Institute, Wilmington, DE have demonstrated the value of 24 hour sleep deprivation in the activation of spike and wave discharges in the EEG in 8 of 9 learning impaired children with a history of absence seizures (Clinical EEG April 1992;23:62-64).-Editor. *Ped Neur Briefs* May 1992.

ANTIEPILEPTIC DRUGS, REACTION TIME, AND IMPULSIVITY

The effects of antiepileptic drugs (AED) on reaction time, attention, and impulsivity in 111 epileptic children, aged 5 to 13 years, are reported from the Children's Hospital of Los Angeles and University of Southern California School of Medicine. Higher total serum levels of AEDs correlated significantly with more impulsive errors. Carbamazepine (CBZ) monotherapy levels in 54 children were negatively correlated with simple and complex reaction times and omission errors, and positively correlated with commission errors; higher serum levels were associated with faster responses and fewer omission errors but impulsive errors on complex reaction time tests were increased. Among 73 children receiving phenobarbital monotherapy, minimal slowing of reaction times and increased omission errors were noted with higher serum levels, but changes were not significant. A number of other AEDs were included in the total drug score analysis, but none was large enough to analyze individually as monotherapy, except for phenobarbital and CBZ. (Mitchell WG et al. Effects of antiepileptic drugs on reaction time, attention, and impulsivity in children. Pediatrics Jan 1993;91:101-105). (Reprints: Wendy G Mitchell MD, Neurology, Mail Stop 82, Children's Hospital of Los Angeles, PO Box 54700, Los Angeles, CA 90054).

COMMENT. Contrary to recent concern regarding possible adverse effects of phenobarbital on cognitive function, this study shows no significant effects on reaction time and attention. The authors do not recommend CBZ in preference to other AEDs. -Editor. *Ped Neur Briefs* Jan 1993.

COGNITIVE EFFECTS OF CARBAMAZEPINE AND PHENYTOIN: A REANALYSIS

A previous report from the Univers1ty of Washington School of Medicine, Seattle, WA that carbamazepine had fewer adverse neuropsychological effects than phenytoin has been re-evaluate. When patients with disproportionately high phenytoin levels were excluded, the neuropsychological differences originally reported could not be demonstrated by statistical analysis. (Dodrill CB, Troupin AS. Neuropsychological effects of carbamazepine and phenytoin: A reanalysis. Neurology Jan 1991;41:141-143).

COMMENT. Two additional studies have found no definite adverse cognitive effects that could be related to phenytoin (Meador KJ et al. Neurology 1990;40:391-394; Dodrill CB, Temkin NR. Epilepsia 1989,30:453-457). The authors comment that many studies reporting adverse cognitive effects of phenytoin use computerized tests heavily loaded with motor speed. When the motor speed element is factored out, the cognitive effects also disappear.

Cognitive function in relation to time-of-day variation in serum carbamazepine concentration in epileptic patients is reported from the Neuropsychology Laboratory, Department of Psychosomatic and Behavioral Medicine, Rikshospitalet, Oslo, Norway (Reinvang I et al Epilepsia Jan/Feb 1991;32:116-121) . Patients had been seizure-free for at least one month and took 2 daily CBZ doses. The test battery showed no differences between performance at times of high versus low serum concentrations. A 33% fluctuation in CBZ concentrations during the day was significant. The subjects were mainly adults and different results might be obtained in children. -Editor. *Ped Neur Briefs* Feb 1991.

PHENYTOIN AND NEUROPSYCHOLOGICAL ABILITY

A comprehensive neuropsychological assessment of young adults (mean age 32) before and after treatment with phenytoin (PHT) for a 5 year study period is reported from the Regional Epilepsy Center, University of Washington School of Medicine, Seattle, Washington. In 3 groups of 11 patients each, the following medications were not changed and the median number of seizures per subject was 2: (a) PHT monotherapy; (b) PHT and other drugs; (c) drug regimens excluding PHT. Of 20 neuropsychological variables, none showed losses and 3 showed statistically significant improvements (Trail Making Part B, WAIS Performance IQ, WAIS Full-Scale IQ). The mental abilities of the groups were similar to each other at both the beginning and the end of the study. With normal therapeutic serum levels and well controlled seizures there was no evidence for any cognitive losses in patients treated with phenytoin over extended periods. (Dodrill CB, Wilensky AJ. Neuropsychological abilities before and after 5 years of stable antiepileptic drug therapy. Epilepsia March/April 1992;33:327-334.) (Reprints: Dr. C.B. Dodrill, Regional Epilepsy Center, Harborview Medical Center, 325 Ninth Avenue, Seattle,WA 98104)

COMMENT. Chronic use of phenytoin did not result in cognitive deterioration in young adults with well controlled seizures with onset after 16 years of age. Previous reports suggesting PHT-related cognitive deterioration were complicated by poor seizure control and were limited by less sophisticated tests than those used in the above study.

Mikati M et al. at the Department of Neurology, Children's Hospital, Harvard Medical School, have found significant differences in potency and plasma concentrations of brand name PHT and generic PHT monotherapy (Epilepsia March/April 1992;33:359-365). Variability in capsule content may be an important factor to be considered in trials of medications such as PHT that manifest nonlinear pharmacokinetics. -Editor. *Ped Neur Briefs* May 1992.

BEHAVIOR DISORDERS AND EPILEPSY

A longitudinal study of 127 children with epilepsy aged 8-12 years and their mothers, designed to identify factors contributing to behavior problems, is reported from the Indiana University School of Nursing, Indianapolis; the Minnesota Comprehensive Epilepsy Program, Minneapolis; and the Harvard School of Public Health, Boston. Variables that accounted for 30% of the variation in child behavior problems included female gender, seizure frequency, family stress, and family social support. Family stress and seizure frequency were positively related whereas family social support was negatively associated with behavior problems. Children experiencing behavior problems had poorer seizure control and came from troubled families with mothers receiving inadequate support from relatives. (Austin JK et al. Correlates of behavior problems in children with epilepsy. Epilepsia Nov/Dec 1992;33:1115-1122). (Reprints: Dr JK Austin, Indiana University School of Nursing, 1111 Middle Dr, Indianapolis, IN).

COMMENT. Family variables and seizure frequency are important correlates of behavior problems in children with epilepsy. Neurological dysfunction may predispose children to both epilepsy and psychiatric disturbance, but family stress may have a stronger influence on child adjustment than seizure severity. In addition to treatment with antiepileptic drugs, attention to family relationships is important in clinical management of childhood epilepsy. -Editor. *Ped Neur Briefs* Jan 1993.

STATUS EPILEPTICUS

TREATMENT OF STATUS EPILEPTICUS

The drugs used in status epilepticus, primary care in the community, secondary hospital care, and tertiary or intensive care are reviewed from the Royal Hospital for Sick Children, Edinburgh. The two preferred drugs recommended for first line care are rectal diazepam and intramuscular paraldehyde. In second line care at a hospital emergency room, intravenous diazepam is preferred in a dosage of 0.25 to 0.3 mg/kg with a glass syringe. Third line management in intensive care includes 20% mannitol given over 20 minutes in a dose of 7 ml/kg for cerebral edema. EEG monitoring is essential to demonstrate seizure activity, paradoxical reactions to drugs such as diazepam, and overdosage with drugs, eg barbiturates causing burst suppression. The authors stress the need to consider hemophilus influenzae and pneumococcal meningitis as an underlying cause of status epilepticus and caution that lumbar puncture must never be done in an unconscious child without a CT scan to exclude signs of brain swelling or edema. The need for tertiary intensive care is usually a sign of failure of early control resulting from inappropriate anticonvulsant medication rather than drug resistance. (Brown JK, Hussain IHMI. Status epilepticus II: Treatment. Dev Med Child Neurol Feb 1991;33:97-109).

COMMENT. The primary care of seizures is all important so that status epilepticus of prolonged duration may be avoided. Mortality from status epilepticus is usually the result of the underlying disease, with an 8% incidence at the above institution. A paradoxical convulsant response to the anticonvulsant diazepam should be considered in children whose seizures are not rapidly controlled, and an alternative anticonvulsant should be used (Livingston and Brown, 1988).

The home use of rectal diazepam for cluster and prolonged seizures is reported from the Department of Neurology, Hennepin County Medical Center; Department of Pharmacy Practice, University of Minnesota, Minneapolis; and the Department of Pediatric Neurology, Gillette Children's Hospital St. Paul, MN (Kriel RL, Cloyd JC et al. Pediatr Neurol Jan/Feb 1991;7:13-17). Rectal diazepam was effective in controlling seizures in 85% of patients. Adverse reactions were mild and consisted of drowsiness and/or behavioral changes. Improvements in quality of life associated with the availability of rectal diazepam were observed by 58% of users and 27% of nonusers. In addition to improved management of seizures there was increased flexibility in family activities and less parental anxiety. The diazepam injectable solution in a dose ranging fron 0.3 to 0.5 mg/kg was used for rectal administration. It was administered with a needleless lubricated 3 ml plastic syringe inserted 2 to 4 cm into the rectal cavity. Effective serum concentrations are usually reached within ten minutes. -Editor. *Ped Neur Briefs* March 1991.

RECURRENT STATUS EPILEPTICUS

The risk of recurrent status epilepticus in 95 children followed prospectively for a mean of 29 months was determined at the Montefiore Medical Center and affiliated hospitals of Albert Einstein College of Medicine, Bronx, New York. Ages ranged from 1 month to 18 years (mean 4 years). The cause was idiopathic in 24, remote symptomatic in 18, febrile in 29, acute asymptomatic in 18 or a progressive neurologic disorder in 6. Neurologically abnormal children (34% of the study population) accounted for 88% of the recurrent status group and for all 5 children with multiple episodes of status epilepticus. The risk was related to the severity of the neurological abnormality, the multiply handicapped children being at highest risk. Fifteen of 16 children with recurrent status epilepticus were being treated with antiepileptic drugs at the time of recurrence. The morbidity and mortality of status epilepticus were low. (Shinnar S et al. Recurrent status epilepticus in children. Ann Neurol June 1992;31:598-604.) (Correspondence: Dr. Shinnar, Division of Pediatric Neurology, VCP-207, Montefiore Medical Center, 111 E. 210th St., Bronx, NY 10467.)

COMMENT. The authors indicate that status epilepticus in neurologically normal children is by and large an isolated event that should not unduly influence decisions regarding further therapy. The high risk subgroup of neurologically abnormal children with recurrent status epilepticus underscored the need for better treatment strategies.

The more frequent use of neurosurgical treatment of refractory status epilepticus is suggested by Gorman DG et al. in a report from the UCLA Pediatric Epilepsy Research Program, Los Angeles, CA. (Epilepsia May/June 1992;33:546-549.) The resection of a right frontal focus in a 9 year old boy with left focal motor seizures and status epilepticus was followed by immediate control of the seizures and no seizures for more than 1 year post-operatively while using carbamazepine monotherapy.-Editor. *Ped Neur Briefs* July 1992.

TONIC CLONIC STATUS EPILEPTICUS

The phases of status epilepticus and management with anticonvulsant drugs are reviewed from the Institute of Neurology, National Hospital, Queen Square, London. In phase I, seizure activity greatly increases cerebral metabolism, but physiological mechanisms, including increased cerebral blood flow and maintenance of glucose supply to the brain, are compensatory. In phase 2, the compensatory mechanisms begin to fail. Cerebral blood flow becomes dependent on systemic blood pressure which falls due to autonomic and cardiorespiratory changes and drug treatment. The high metabolic demands of the epileptic cerebral tissue cannot be met and ischemic or metabolic damage ensues. Drug treatment, administered parenterally, is also divided into stages: 1) and 2) premonitory and early status; diazepam or other lipid-soluble, rapidly-acting, but short-duration anticonvulsant; 3) established status; phenytoin is a drug of first choice, highly effective, and long acting, often administered with diazepam. Phenobarbitone is also a drug of choice, but should not be used in a solution containing other drugs, as precipitation may occur. Numerous second-line treatment options are discussed; 4) refractory status; thiopentone is traditional in Europe; propofol, a non-barbiturate, is widely used but its safety in children has not been established. Reasons for drug treatment failure include inadequate initial dosage and maintenance, undiscovered cause or complication, and misdiagnosis.(Shorvon S. Tonic clonic status epilepticus. J Neurol Neurosurg Psychiatry Feb 1993;56: 125-134). (Respond: Dr Shorvon, Institute of Neurology, Queen Square, London WC1N 3BG, UK).

COMMENT. The annual incidence of new cases of tonic clonic status in the USA is estimated at 45,000 -70,000. It occurs in 10 - 25% of children with epilepsy.

Mortality is 5 - 10%, and morbidity increases with the duration of the status episode. Successful treatment of this medical emergency depends on the balance of a rapid control of seizures and the avoidance of complications of therapy. (Shorvon SD. Status epilepticus: its clinical features and treatment in children and adults. Cambridge, Cambridge University Press, 1993).

Phenytoin monitoring in status epilepticus in infants and children is reported from the Service de Neuropediatrie, Hopital Saint-Vincent de Paul, Paris, and Hopital du Bocage, Dijon, France. (Richard MO et al. Epilepsia Jan/Feb 1993;34:144150). A loading dose of 15 mg/kg was followed by three injections in the first 24 hours. Monitoring with nine plasma samples during the first day allowed for dosage adjustment with increased efficacy and reduced toxicity. Older children responded better than younger children who had lower plasma levels. -Editor. *Ped Neur Briefs* March 1993.

SERUM CORTISOL AND PROGNOSIS OF STATUS EPILEPTICUS

The relation of serum cortisol and CSF *B*-endorphin levels to the prognosis of status epilepticus was evaluated in 27 adults treated in the Comprehensive Epilepsy Program of the Medical College of Virginia, Richmond, VA. Poor prognosis was defined as death or severe neurologic or medical complications during or within one week after status epilepticus of more than 30 minutes. Blood cortisol levels were significantly elevated in patients with a poor outcome. CSF *B*-endorphins were significantly increased but did not correlate with prognosis. (Calabrese VP et al. Serum cortisol and cerebrospinal fluid *B*-endorphins in status epilepticus. Their possible relation to prognosis. Arch Neurol July 1993;50:689-693). (Reprints: Dr Calabrese, Dept of Neurology, MCV Station-Box 599, Richmond, VA 23298).

COMMENT. Serum cortisol determinations within 12 hours after control of status epilepticus may predict prognosis. The authors also propose that the rise in cortisol levels may contribute to the pathology of status epilepticus. -Editor. *Ped Neur Briefs* July 1993.

OCCULT CORTICAL DYSPLASLIA AND FOCAL STATUS

Four patients, ages 4, 6, 13, and 21 years, with life-threatening focal motor status epilepticus, normal pre-operative MRI, and focal cortical dysplasia defined only in the surgical specimens obtained by corticectomies, are reported from the Montreal Neurological Institute; Austin Hospital, Heidelberg, Australia; University of California, San Francisco; and Royal Children's Hospital, Melbourne, Australia. Seizures began between 3 months and 18 years of age, and therapy-resistant focal status developed after 18 months to 3 years, resulting in persistent motor deficits. A total of 12 MRIs failed to reveal abnormalities. Ictal SPECT was positive in 2 patients. Seizures were controlled after surgery, and 2 patients were seizure-free. (Desbiens R et al. Life-threatening focal status epilepticus due to occult cortical dysplasia. Arch Neurol July 1993;50:695-700). (Reprints: Dr Frederick Andermann, Montreal Neurological Hosp and Institute, 3801 University St, Montreal, Quebec, Canada H3A 2B4).

COMMENT. Neuronal migration disorder as a cause of focal motor status epilepticus or epilepsia partialis continua in a child may not be excluded by the MRI and may require surgical intervention for diagnosis and treatment. -Editor. *Ped Neur Briefs* July 1993.

TREATMENT OF CONVULSIVE STATUS

Definition, etiology, treatment, and outcome of convulsive status epilepticus in children and adults are outlined by a group of experts and sponsored by the Epilepsy Foundation of America. Common to all patients, recommendations include a clear predetermined plan of action, prompt administration of appropriate drugs in adequate doses, and attention to the possibility of apnea, hypoventilation, or other metabolic abnormalities. The major drugs include diazepam, lorazepam, phenytoin, and phenobarbital, administered intravenously. If diazepam is used, phenytoin is also necessary to prevent recurrence. After 20-60 min, if status persists, 15-20 mg/kg phenytoin no faster than 50 mg/min in adults and 1 mg/kg/min in children by IV; monitor ECG and blood pressure; purge IV with normal saline before phenytoin infusion - phenytoin is incompatible with glucose-containing solutions. If phenobarbital is used after a benzodiazepine, apnea often occurs and assisted ventilation is required. Compared to sedative drugs, phenytoin is less likely to depress consciousness. (Dodson WE et al. Treatment of convulsive status epilepticus. Recommendations of the Epilepsy Foundation of America's working group on status epilepticus. JAMA Aug 18 1993;270:854-859). (Reprints: Dr Dodson, Epilepsy Foundation of America, 4351 Garden City Dr, Landover, MD 20785).

COMMENTS. The details of this action plan will become a fixture in many hospital ERs. The authors are to be commended for a thorough review of this medical emergency. Although prognosis is closely related to the etiology of the status, appropriate and timely therapy reduces the risk of mortality and morbidity.

Barry E and Hauser WA discuss the interaction of epilepsy and acute brain disease in 217 patients with status epilepticus (Neurology Aug 1993;43:1473-1478). The 6-month mortality in this series (37%) was higher than most other reports, and reflected a high percentage of organic brain disease. In patients with a previous history of epilepsy the mortality was 16%, and in those with no epilepsy but a high proportion of acute brain insults, the mortality rate was 54%. In children, the mortality from status has been reported in the range of 3 - 8%, and much lower than in the elderly. -Editor. *Ped Neur Briefs* Aug 1993.

DIAGNOSIS AND TREATMENT

CAPILLARY PROLACTIN AND SEIZURE DIAGNOSIS

The validity of prolactin measurements using capillary blood in the diagnosis of epilepsy was tested in the Departments of Neurology, Neurosurgery, and Pathology, The Johns Hopkins University School of Medicine, Baltimore, MD. Venous and capillary prolactin levels were determined 10 to 20 minutes after seizure-like episodes in 20 patients studied in an epilepsy monitoring unit. All patients had documentation of their seizure type by simultaneous video-EEG monitoring. Using the low crlterion of elevation (18 ng/ml), capillary prolactin values were predictive of seizures versus pseudoseizures in 9 (100%) of 9 patients with generalized tonic-clonic patterns, in 5 (71%) of 7 patients with complex partial seizures, and 4 (100%) of 4 patients with pseudoseizures. Venous and capillary prolactin values correlated and were unaffected by leaving filter paper samples at room temperature for up to one week. (Fisher RS et al. Capillary prolactin measurement for diagnosis of seizures. Ann Neurol Feb 1991;29:187-190).

COMMENT Capillary blood collection for prolactin measurement may assist in the diagnosis of epilepsy in an outpatient clinic. Prolactin serum levels are elevated in children after tonic-clonic and complex partial seizures but determinations must be interpreted with reference to the complete clinical findings. -Editor. *Ped Neur Briefs* Feb 1991.

TREATMENT ONSET AND EPILEPSY PROGNOSIS

The efficacy of treatment in relation to the lost time "tiempo perdido" in a group of 3529 epileptic patients was evaluated in the Division of Neurology and Clinical Neurophysiology, Hospital General du Cataluna, Barcelona, Spain. The mean follow-up period was ten years. The "lost time" is the period elapsed from the onset of symptoms and the beginning of long-term anticonvulsant treatment. In 970 patients with a lost time of less than a year, 86% were seizure-free whereas in 922 patients whose treatment was delayed greater than 11 years, 64% were seizure-free. Delay in starting anticonvulsant medication influenced the success of drug withdrawal. Of 710 patients who discontinued treatment, 315 (44%) had treatment initiated within one year of onset of seizures whereas drug withdrawal was possible in only 106 (15%) of the group in which treatment was delayed over 11 years. A total of 144 (20%) patients had seizure recurrences after drug withdrawal and of this number, 14% occurred in the group treated early and 41% in the group with the longest period of delay in treatment. (Oller-Daurella L, Oller L F-V. Influence of the "lost time" on the outcome of epilepsy. Eur Neurol May/June 1991;31:175-177).

COMMENT. The sooner the correct diagnosis of epilepsy is made and treatment is begun, the fewer seizures a patient will suffer, and the greater the likelihood of successful antiepileptic control and subsequent withdrawal of antiepileptic drugs. Gowers, in 1881, pointed out that seizures beget seizures, and the greater the number of epileptic seizures the greater the likelihood of their continued reoccurrence. The results of this study should caution those who advocate delays in the initiation of anticonvulsant therapy and should encourage a more vigorous attempt to prevent seizure recurrences after the first epileptic seizure. -Editor. *Ped Neur Briefs* May 1991.

POLYTHERAPY IN INSTITUTIONALIZED EPILEPTIC CHILDREN

An attempt to minimize polypharmacotherapy, to discontinue the use of phenobarbital, and to assess the relation between drug levels and antiepileptic effect in institutionalized severely retarded children is reported from the Department of Pediatrics, St. Goran's Hospital, Stockholm, and the Division of Clinical Pharmacology, University Hospital, Uppsala, Sweden. Nine severely mentally retarded patients with severe epilepsy were studied during a three year period by a multidisciplinary team. Combination therapy with two or three drugs gave the best antiepileptic effect and monotherapy was possible in only two patients. Phenobarbital withdrawal was possible in two of four patients. Regular phenytoin serum monitoring was necessary to avoid high levels that could be unnoticed for long periods and possibly result in chronic long-term side effects. (Ferngren H et al. Mono- or polypharmacotherapy in institutionalized epileptic children with severe mental retardation? A team approach for optimizing antiepileptic therapy. Acta Paediatr Scand April 1991;80:458-465).

COMMENT. The tendency among neurologists to attempt conversion from polytherapy to monotherapy in severely retarded institutionalized patients may be hazardous and inadvisable. This study has demonstrated that polytherapy is frequently required. The recognition of anticonvulsant side effects may be more difficult in retarded patients compared to clinic patients and frequent serum drug monitoring is important. -Editor. *Ped Neur Briefs* May 1991.

TREATMENT OF BENIGN ROLANDIC EPILEPSY

The outcome of ten untreated and 20 treated patients with benign childhood epilepsy with Rolandic spikes was studied retrospectively after recovery at the Institute of Neurology, University of Bologna, Italy. The patients had been seizure free for at least five years. The mean period of active epilepsy was 16 months for patients and 28 months for controls. All patients and controls had Rolandic and/or centrotemporal spikes on their awake EEG recording during the active epilepsy period. Seizure frequencies, seizure occurrence and duration of active epilepsy were similar in both the treated and untreated groups. No differences were found in social adjustment of the patients. The authors conclude that antiepileptic treatment may be unnecessary in most cases of benign epilepsy with Rolandic spikes (Ambrosetto, G, Tassinari CA Antiepileptic drug treatment of benign childhood epilepsy with Rolandic spikes: is it necessary? Epilepsia Nov/Dec 1990;31:802-805).

COMMENT. The authors comment that the results should be interpreted with caution because the study was retrospective. If the data are confirmed by prospective studies, antiepileptic drugs should be withheld unless seizures are frequently recurrent. Since the seizures are generally nocturnal and usually involve the oropharynx, parental anxiety and dangers of suffocation are factors that may dictate the need for treatment. -Editor. *Ped Neur Briefs* March 1991.

DISCONTINUING MEDICATION: RECURRENCE RISK FACTORS

The results of discontinuation of antiepileptic drugs in epileptic children who were seizure free for at least 2 years are reported from the Services of Child Neurology and Psychology, Department of Neurology, Clinics Hospital University of Sao Paulo Medical School, Sao Paulo, Brazil. Twenty children (28%) had a recurrence, 75% during, or less than 6 months after, discontinuation of AED. The risk factors related to seizure recurrence were 1) more than 10 seizures before seizure control, 2) abnormal EEG in the year before discontinuation, 3) focal neurologic signs and/or mental retardation, and 4) a mixed seizure pattern. Two or more risk factors were associated with recurrence of seizures in 14 children (70%), whereas patients with none or only 1 risk factor had no recurrence (72%). (Gherpelli JLD et al. Discontinuing medication in epileptic children: a study of risk factors related to recurrence. Epilepsia July/Aug 1992;33:681-686.) (Reprints: Dr. J.L.D. Gherpelli, Service of Child Neurology, Department of Neurology, Hospital das Clinicas da F.M.U.S.P., Sao Paulo 01000, P.O. Box 8091, Brazil.)

COMMENT. Risk factors may be of help in determining the safety of discontinuing antiepileptic medications in children who are seizure free for a period of at least 2 years. There was no correlation between age at seizure onset and recurrence in this study, which is at variance with some other reports.

The finding of a higher sleep tendency in children with epilepsy than in controls, even 4-5 months after drug discontinuation, was unexpected in a study from the University of Lund, Sweden (Palm L et al. Epilepsia July/Aug 1992;33:687-691). The patients had been free of seizures for some time, and the EEG showed no epileptiform activity, so that the sleepiness could not be a direct effect of epileptic seizures.-Editor. *Ped Neur Briefs* Sept 1992.

OUTCOME OF CHILDHOOD EPILEPSY

Factors predictive of remission of epilepsy were evaluated in 504 patients followed for an average of 7 years at the Departments of Pediatrics and Mathematics, Dalhousie University and Children's Hospital, Halifax, Nova Scotia, Canada. At the end of follow-up, 55% of the total cohort were off medication and in remission. Approximately 70% of those stopping medication remained seizure free. At the time of diagnosis, the best predictors of remission, determined by a multivariate analysis scoring system, were 1) age <12 years at onset, 2) normal intelligence, 3) no prior neonatal seizures, and 4) fewer than 21 seizures before treatment. Prediction was improved after 12 months follow-up, when a score for the seizure frequency between 6 and 12 months was included. Patients with absence and minor motor seizures were excluded from the study. Seizure type and the EEG were not of predictive value. (Camfield C, Camfield P et al. Outcome of childhood epilepsy: A population-based study with a simple predictive scoring system for those treated with medication. J Pediatr June 1993;122:861-868). (Reprints: Carol Camfield MD, IWK Children's Hospital, BOX 3070, Halifax, Nova Scotia B3H 3G9, Canada).

COMMENT. During the study period, 1977-1985, the number of seizure-free years required before attempting mediction withdrawal changed from 4 to 2 years. The authors endorse the stopping of medication after 2 seizure-free years, regardless of the predicted prognosis.

A social outcome of epilepsy study in 337 intellectually normal children included in this Nova Scotia population found school failure in 34%, mental health consultation in 22%, psychotropic medication used in 5%, unemployment 20%, and criminal conviction in 2%. Learning disorders and more than 21 seizures before treatment were predictive of an unfavorable social outcome; seizure control and EEG were non-predictive. (Camfield C, Camfield P et al. J Pediatr June 1993;122:869-873) -Editor. *Ped Neur Briefs* June 1993.

ANTIEPILEPTIC DRUGS

AED LEVELS: USE BY PEDIATRIC NEUROLOGISTS

Replies from 56 of 60 pediatric neurologists surveyed regarding the use and value of antiepileptic drug (AED) levels were evaluated in the Departments of Pediatrics and Toxicology, Dalhousie University and The IWK Children's Hospital, Halifax, Canada. The majority of respondents were in academic practice. Drug concentrations were measured frequently or always at the following times: 1) pre-dose (trough) by 63%, 2) at the expected peak by 18%, 3) at time of clinic visit by 60%, 4) at each office visit by 38%, 5) when a second AED was introduced by 77%, 6) on high doses by 96%, 7) for possible toxicity by 96%, 8) when compliance in doubt by 95%, 9) routinely once or twice a year by 60%, and 10) more than twice a year by 18% of respondents. AED monitoring was generally perceived as valuable and results frequently (75%) influenced clinical decisions. Therapeutic ranges in laboratories varied; they were most consistent for phenytoin (10-20 mcg/ml) and most variable for carbamazepine, with lower limits from 3 - 9 and upper limits from 8 - 12 mcg/ml. (Dooley JM et al. The use of antiepileptic drug levels in children: a survey of Canadian pediatric neurologists. Can J Neurol Sci Aug 1993;20:217-221). (Reprints: Dr JM Dooley, Neurology Division, The IWK Children's Hospital, University Ave, Halifax, Nova Scotia, Canada B3J 3G9).

COMMENT. The interpretation of AED levels may be misleading because trough level specimens are often impractical and therapeutic ranges used by laboratories are variable. The authors question the value of carbamazepine levels in children in particular, based on the findings in their survey. Their conclusions and concerns are confirmed by a report from the Poison Centers of Philadelphia and Pittsburgh (Spiller HA, Krenzelok EP. Carbamazepine overdose: serum concentration less predictive in children. Clin Toxicol Sept 1993;31:459-460). A group of 29 children ages 1 - 12 years were at risk of serious morbidity (seizures, coma, and mechanical ventilator) from CBZ overdose at lower serum concentrations (27 mg/L) than a group of 33 adult patients whose mean toxic CBZ levels for coma were 41-44 mg/L. Serum levels were not accurate predictors of risk of toxic overdosage from carbamazepine in children. A report of massive poisoning with CBZ in 28 adults in Sweden showed that CBZ levels are more predictive of severe toxicity and morbidity in adults. Serum levels at or above 40 mg/L were associated with increased risk of serious complications. (Hojer J et al. Clinical features in 28 consecutive cases of laboratory confirmed massive poisoning with carbamazepine alone. Clin Toxicol Sept 1993;31:449-458).-Editor. *Ped Neur Briefs* Sept 1993.

CHEWABLE VERSUS REGULAR CARBAMAZEPINE

A comparison of chewable and regular carbamazepine (CBZ tablets) in 44 children receiving chronic CBZ monotherapy is reported from the IWK Children's Hospital, Halifax, Nova Scotia. Weekly levels showed no consistent differences between the 1 month on chewable CBZ and on regular CBZ. Seizure control and rates of reported side effects were similar in the 2 periods. Chewable CBZ produced higher peak CBZ levels in 5 patients and a similar number had higher peaks with regular CBZ. (Camfield P et al. The pharmacology of chewable versus regular carbamazepine in chronically treated children with epilepsy. Can J Neurol Sci May 1992;19:204-207.)

COMMENT. Chewable and regular CBZ appear to have similar pharmacokinetics but individual patients may show some differences. Those with peak level side effects using one form of CBZ should receive the alternative form of tablet.

A therapeutic bioequivalency study of brand name versus generic carbamazepine in 40 epileptic patients studied at the Bowman Gray School of Medicine, Winston-Salem, NC showed that both performed equally well in clinical efficacy and bioequivalency. (Oles KS et al. Neurology June 1992;42:1147-1153.).-Editor. *Ped Neur*

Briefs July 1992.

UNBOUND PHENYTOIN AND VALPROATE MONITORING

All antiepileptic drug blood level determinations at the University of Virginia Medical Center were analyzed over a 13 month period. Those values with unbound fractions outside the expected range and discordance between unbound and total levels were compared to seizure control and occurrence of side effects. Unbound phenytoin (PHT) levels were clinically significant (outside the expected range, a discordant ratio of unbound to total level, and seizures or side effects necessitating dosage change) in 61 of 254 determinations (24%) and 44 of 155 patients (28%). The clinical significance involved current seizures for 52 values and side effects for 24 (both for 15). The frequency of clinically significant values was similar with PHT monotherapy (20%) and polytherapy (27%). The rates of current seizures and side effects were also similar in these 2 subgroups. For valproate (VPA), 15% of unbound values from 18% of patients were clinically significant with regard to current seizures and side effects and the rate was similar for monotherapy and polytherapy. There were no clinically significant unbound levels for carbamazepine (Lenn NJ, Robertson M. Clinical utility of unbound antiepileptic drug blood levels in the management of epilepsy. Neurology May 1992;42:988-990). (Reprints: Dr. Nicholas J. Lenn, Department of Neurology, Health Sciences Center T12-020, SUNY, Stony Brook, NY 11794-8121.)

COMMENT. These data suggest that some patients receiving phenytoin or valproate have unbound drug levels and ratios that may add information of importance to improvement of seizure control and reduction of side effects. The authors suggest that patients receiving PHT as mono- or polytherapy be monitored with either unbound blood level measurements only or have unbound blood levels regardless of the total level if there is an unresolved clinical problem. The expected unbound fraction of PHT is 8-12%.

In a 17-year-old girl with thrombotic thrombocytopenic purpura who was treated by plasmapheresis the free and total concentrations of phenytoin used for the treatment of a coincident seizure disorder were examined in the patient's serum and in the plasma removed by plasmapheresis. The free concentration was similar in both the plasma removed and in the patient's serum. Plasmapheresis did not significantly alter the serum concentration of phenytoin. Dosage adjustments of phenytoin are therefore unnecessary when single volume exchanges are performed. (Tobias JD et al. Removal of phenytoin by plasmapheresis in a patient with thrombotic thrombocytopenia purpura. Clin Pediatrics Feb 1992; 31:105-108.) These authors question the value of plasmapheresis and single volume exchange as an appropriate therapeutic intervention for phenytoin overdose. (Correspondence: Dr. Tobias, Vanderbilt University, Department of Pediatrics, Division of Pediatric Critical Care, Medical Center North T-0118, Nashville, TN 37232.) -Editor. *Ped Neur Briefs* June 1992.

PHENYTOIN AND FOLIC ACID

The pharmacokinetics of phenytoin (PHT) before and after administration of 1 and 5 mg of folic acid is reported from the Colleges of Pharmacy and Medicine, University of Iowa, Iowa City and University of Health Sciences/The Chicago Medical School, Chicago, IL. The measured total serum PHT concentration was always greater than the calculated concentration and the days to the steady state concentration were always longer than the number calculated before folic acid was given. All subjects showed decreased serum folic acid following PHT. Since folate is assumed to be a co-factor in PHT metabolism, these results were expected because depletion of the vitamin would result in reduced metabolism of PHT and higher total serum PHT and longer time to reach steady state. When folic acid was added the same results were obtained. The depletion of folic acid had to be corrected first before its role as a co-factor in PHT metabolism could be used. (Berg MJ et al. Phenytoin pharmacokinetics: before and after folic acid administration. Epilepsia July/Aug 1992;33:712-20.) (Reprints: Dr. M.J. Berg, College of Pharmacy, University of Iowa, Iowa City, IA 52242.)

COMMENT. The authors suggest that folic acid should be prescribed when phenytoin therapy is initiated. Further studies may be indicated. -Editor. *Ped Neur Briefs* Sept 1992.

ACTH FOR LANDAU-KLEFFNER SYNDROME

Four children between 5 and 9 years of age with Landau-Kleffner syndrome were treated with ACTH or corticosteroids at the Department of Pediatrics, Beilinson Medical Centre, and Sackler Faculty of Medicine, Tel Aviv University, Israel. ACTH in one patient was given for three months starting with 80 units/day followed by a gradual reduction of the dose. An EEG three weeks after the start of the treatment showed complete disappearance of epileptic activity but the aphasia was initially unchanged. Complete remission of the aphasia occurred eight months after the completion of the ACTH course. Two years later the aphasia recurred with the concomitant appearance of multiple spike discharges on the EEG. Prompt prescription of ACTH therapy led to a recovery of speech and a normal EEG within a few weeks. Prednisone 60 mg/day for two to three months in two patients caused a prompt improvement in the EEG followed by normal speech. Dexamethasone 4 mg/day resulted in full recovery of speech and a completely normal EEG within two weeks of starting treatment in a 9 year old child. Three to six years after discontinuing therapy the children are off anticonvulsant medication and free from seizures and language disability. (Lerman P et al. Effect of early corticosteroid therapy for Landau-Kleffner syndrome. Dev Med Child Neurol March 1991;33:257-266).

COMMENT. These results are encouraging and warrant further trials of hormone therapy in children with the aphasic epilepsy syndrome. As in the treatment of West syndrome, corticosteroids administered early are more effective than delayed treatments.

Hypsarrhythmia is not a sine qua non for ACTH therapy. Tho children, aged 3 years and 2 years 8 months with status absence and generalized tonic-clonic seizures refractory to anticonvulsant medication were benefitted by ACTH 10 units intramuscular daily. Control of seizures, improvement in the EEG, and a dramatic recovery of mental and motor abilities occurred within two hours of the first injection in one patient, and seizure control and EEG improvement occurred in the second after a three week course of therapy. Further trials of ACTH in children with seizures other than infantile spasms are recommended. (Millichap JG. Neurology March 1991; 41 (Suppl 1):201).-Editor. *Ped Neur Briefs* April 1991.

VALPROATE FOR INTRACTABLE EPILEPSY

The efficacy and side effects of high dose valproic acid (VPA) therapy in 46 children with refractory epilepsy were studied at the Department of Child Neurology, Okayama University Medical School, Okayama, Japan. Serum VPA concentrations ranged from 105.1 to 198.4 mcg/ml. Seizures were completely controlled in 15 (32.6%) and improved in 12 (26.1%). This degree of control was sustained at 6 months or more follow-up. VPA therapy was especially effective for West syndrome and for epilepsy with continuous spike waves during slow wave sleep. Symptomatic generalized epilepsy and symptomatic partial epilepsy were benefited equally. No significant difference in efficacy was noted between the monotherapy and bipharmacy groups, but adverse side effects appeared more frequently and higher serum levels of VPA were difficult to obtain in the bipharmacy group. Liver enzymes were transiently increased in 50%, and elevated serum amylase occurred in 10% of patients. Hyperammonemia in 6.5% of patients necessitated withdrawal of the drug. Thrombocytopenia less than 100,000/mm^3 occurred in 21.7% and hypofibrinogenemia was detected in 65% of patients. These side effects were reversible with reduction of dosage (Ohtsuka Y, Ohtahara S et al. Treatment of intractable childhood epilepsy with high-dose valproate. Epilepsia Jan/Feb 1992;33:158-164). (Reprints: Dr. Y. Ohtsuka, Department of Child Neurology, Okayama University Medical School, 2-5-1, Shikata-cho, Okayama 700, Japan.)

COMMENT. The authors recommend high dose VPA therapy for intractable childhood epilepsy of generalized and partial types and particularly for patients with West syndrome. The monitoring of platelet counts and fibrinogen levels in addition to liver function tests is advised.

Kreuz W et al. from Frankfort, Germany report the induction of von Willebrand disease type I in 67 % of 30 children receiving VPA therapy (Epilepsia Jan/Feb 1991;33:178-184). The decrease in coagulation parameters were not dependent on either VPA dose or the period of drug administration. This increased tendency to hemorrhage in patients receiving VPA must be considered, especially during surgical intervention and after traumatic events.

Kondo T et al. from Hirosaki University, Japan, report that 3 risk factors (young age, polypharmacy, and high VPA serum level) enhance the susceptibility to VPA hepatotoxicity by altering the metabolism of VPA and by increasing the conversion of VPA to 4-en, the most toxic VPA metabolite (Epilepsia Jan/Feb 1992; 33:172-177). -Editor. *Ped Neur Briefs* March 1992.

METHSUXIMIDE FOR INTRACTABLE SEIZURES

The use of methsuximide in 25 children with intractable epilepsy is reported from the Department of Neurology and School of Pharmacy, University of North Carolina, Chapel Hill. In 15 patients methsuximide was well tolerated and resulted in a 50% or greater reduction in seizure frequency. The predominant seizure types were tonic, complex partial, secondary generalized and astatic/myoclonic. The EEG showed generalized slow spike and wave in 14 and focal spikes in three. Two developed hypersensitivity rashes, two had intractable hiccups and four reported nausea. Patients had failed therapy with phenobarbital, primidone, phenytoin, carbamazepine and valproic acid alone or in various combinations. Decreases in carbamazepine serum concentrations occurred after starting methsuximide as an adjunctive anti-epileptic. (Tennison MB et al Methsuximide for intractable childhood seizures Pediatrics Feb 1991;87:186-189).

COMMENT. Methsuximide has been reported of benefit in the treatment of petit mal, partial myoclonic, atonic and tonic seizures. As monotherapy methsuximide is not well established, but as an adjunct therapy further trials should be considered. The occurrence of skin rash is not uncommon, and methsuximide may be contraindicated in patients with a history of hypersensitivity reactions to other anticonvulsants -Editor. *Ped Neur Briefs* March 1991.

VIGABATRIN AND INTRACTABLE EPILEPSY

The relatlonship between vigabatrin dosage and plasma concentrations, platelet GABA-transaminase inhibition and seizure reduction in 16 children with refractory epilepsy was studied at the University of Cantabria, Santander, Spain. Vigabatrin dosages of 57 mg/kg/day and plasma concentrations of 8 mg/L reduced the GABA-T activity from 13.9 to 5.1 and seizures were reduced from 51 to 22 per month. Seizure reduction was correlated with the dosage but not with the plasma concentration or with platelet GABA inhibition. The initial dose of vigabatrin recommended was 50 mg/kg/day and was increased to 75 or 100 mg/kg/day (Arteaga R et al. Vinyl GABA (vigabatrin): Relationship between dosage, plasma concentrations, platelet GABA-transaminase inhibition, and seizure reduction in epileptic children. Epilepsia Sept/Oct; 33:923-931). (Reprints: Dr. J.A. Armijo at Farmacologia Clinica, Hospital ~M. de Valdecilla," E-39008 Santander, Spain.)

COMMENT. A study of vigabatrin in 43 children with intractable epilepsy is reported from the Royal Liverpool Children's Hospital, England. The results showed that complex partial seizures, with or without secondary generalization, responded best with more than 1/2 achieving a greater than 50% reduction.

Generalized tonic-clonic seizures also improved. Absence or myoclonic seizures were not benefited. Only 4 patients (10%) were seizure free on monotherapy with vigabatrin (Gibbs JM et al. Vigabatrin in intractable childhood epilepsy: a retrospective study. Pediatr Neurol Sept/Oct 1992;8:338-40).

In a study of 45 patients ages 2-21 years treated with vigabatrin in Paris, France, 20 (44%) showed no benefit and 24% were well controlled. Partial seizures were most responsive. -Editor. *Ped Neur Briefs* Nov 1992.

AMANTADINE IN ABSENCE EPILEPSY

Refractory absence epilepsy in 4 children was treated with amantadine as an add-on drug at the Tel Aviv University Sackler School of Medicine, Israel. The patients responded within 1 week and remained free of symptoms for 27-36 months without adverse effects. The dosage was 5-7 mg/kg per day given twice a day up to a maximum of 200 mg daily (Shahar EM, Brand N. Effect of add-on amantadine therapy for refractory absence epilepsy. Pediatr Neurol Nov 1992;121:819-821). (Reprints: Eli M. Shahar, M.D., Child Neurology Unit, Chaim Sheba Medical Center, Tel Hashomer 52621, Israel.)

COMMENT. Amantadine was initially used by Shields et al. in the treatment of 10 children with minor motor seizures refractory to medications. Myoclonic seizures and atypical absence seizures responded well. (Neurology 1985;35:579). -Editor. *Ped Neur Briefs* Dec 1992.

FELBAMATE IN LENNOX-GASTAUT SYNDROME

The Felbamate Study Group report results in 73 patients ages 4 to 36 years with the Lennox-Gastaut syndrome, using a double-blind, placebo-controlled, add-on trial design. A maximum dosage of 45 mg/kg/body wt or 3600 mg/day was titrated within 14 days. Felbamate-treated patients had a 34% decrease in frequency of atonic seizures, as compared with a 9% decrease in those receiving placebo. The total frequency of seizures was decreased by 19% in felbamate-treated patients, as compared with a 4% increase in the placebo group. Side-effects were similar in the two groups. Anorexia, vomiting, and somnolence occurred more frequently in the felbamate group, whereas diarrhea occurred more frequently in the placebo group. (Ritter FJ et al. Efficacy of felbamate in childhood epileptic encephalopathy (Lennox-Gastaut syndrome). N Engl J Med Jan 7 1993;328:29-33). (Reprints: Dr Frank J Ritter, Minnesota Epilepsy Group, 310 N Smith Ave, Ste 300, St Paul, MN 55102).

COMMENT. Felbamate (2-phenyl-1,3-propanediol dicarbamate) appears to be effective in the treatment of various types of seizures associated with the Lennox-Gastaut syndrome. Side effects are typically mild or moderate in severity and require no change in dosage. According to parental observations, the overall quality of life is also improved by increased alertness and verbal responsiveness. -Editor. *Ped Neur Briefs* Jan 1993.

KETOGENIC DIET FOR INTRACTABLE SEIZURES

The efficacy of the ketogenic diet in 58 children with multiple seizure types resistant to antiepileptic drugs has been evaluated at the Johns Hopkins University School of Medicine, Baltimore. All patients had severe neurologic handicaps: mental retardation (84%), cerebral palsy (45%), and microcephaly (15%). Mean age at diet initiation was 60 months (range 12-235 months). EEGs showed Lennox-Gastaut pattern (33%), hypsarrhythmia (19%), and focal activity (14%). Antiepileptic drugs, including valproate, showed no adverse interaction. Seizures were completely controlled in 29%, and reduced by half in 38%. Diet was continued for an average of 24 months in those controlled and for 4 months in the unimproved group. Dietary benefit was not determined by seizure type. Renal stones required withdrawal of the diet in 2 patients. (Kinsman SL et al. Efficacy of the ketogenic diet for intractable seizure disorders: Review of 58 cases. Epilepsia Nov/Dec 1992;33:1132-1136). (Reprints: Dr SL Kinsman, Kennedy Krieger Institute, 707 N Broadway, Baltimore, MD 21205).

COMMENT. Despite further demonstration of its efficacy and relative safety, the ketogenic diet is not a popular method of therapy among neurologists generally. Apart from the Mayo Clinic and Johns Hopkins, the diet is not frequently promoted in the training of pediatric neurologists and dieticians. Furthermore, the bias against fat in the diet in today's society adds to the difficulty in convincing mothers to become enthusiastic partners in the treatment program. Millichap JG at the Mayo Clinic (Epilepsia 1964;5:239) and Schwartz RM at the John Radcliffe Hospital, Oxford (Dev Med Child Neurol 1989;31:145) studied the metabolic effects of the diet and were unable to document any significant changes in blood lipid profiles using the classical diet. For an account of the mechanism of action of the diet, see Millichap JG. Progress in Pediatric Neurology, Chicago, PNB Publ, 1991, p 87-88. -Editor. *Ped Neur Briefs* Jan 1993.

COMBINATION PHENOBARBITAL/ANTIBIOTIC DRUG REACTIONS

Undesirable drug reactions during simultaneous administration of high dosage phenobarbital and beta lactam antibiotics, mainly Cefotaxim, are reported in 24 of 49 children admitted to intensive care at the Klinikum der J W Goethe Universitat, Frankfort, Germany. The reactions were mainly exanthematous skin rashes which in some cases progressed to Stevens-Johnson syndrome. (Harder S et al. Unerwunschte Arzneimittelreaktionen bei gleichzeitiger Gabe von hochdosiertem Phenobarbital und Betalaktam-Antibiotika. Klin Padiatr Nov/Dez 1990;202:404-407) .

COMMENT. The incidence of skin reaction with phenobarbital is relatively rare compared to the anticonvulsants phenytoin and carbamazepine but the risk of serious skin reactions may be increased by the simultaneous administration of the antibiotic Cefotaxim. -Editor. *Ped Neur Briefs* May 1991.

CARBAMAZEPINE RASH AND PREDNISONE

The use of prednisone in the treatment of

carbamazepine-induced rash in 20 patients is reported from the Divisions of Neurology and Allergy and Immunology, Danbury Hospital, Danbury, CT. Fifteen were female and 5 were male. Their ages ranged from 4 to 73. In 16 patients the rash was suppressed and carbamazepine was continued; the drug had to be discontinued in four patients, 2 of whom had developed fever. (Murphy JM et al. Suppression of carbamazepine-induced rash with prednisone. Neurology Jan 1991;41:144-145).

COMMENT. Fifty cases of serious skin reaction related to carbamazepine have been reported to CIBA-GEIGY in an eight year period, 1982-89 (personal communication), with an estimated incidence of 1 in 70-180,000 patients treated. Stevens-Johnson syndrome occurred in 30, erythema multiforme in 8, exfoliative dermatitis in 7, and toxic epidermal necrolysis (Lyell's syndrome) in 5.

A 12 year old girl developed Stevens-Johnson syndrome after two weeks' treatment with carbamazepine which was substituted for valproate therapy found ineffective in the control of generalized tonic-clonic seizures. Despite immediate withdrawal of both anticonvulsant drugs within 6 hours of the appearance of the rash the patient developed fever and a generalized rash with extensive blistering which was not prevented by the early introduction of oral prednisone treatment. (Millichap JG. Ped Neur Briefs Feb 1991;5:11)). Seizures of an absence pattern with generalized atypical spike wave in the EEG developed when prednisone was withdrawn, and both tonic-clonic and absence attacks were completely controlled by clonazepam without adverse effects or skin rash recurrence. The value of steroids in the treatment of Stevens-Johnson syndrome is debated; most dermatologists advocate steroid use in early cases when caused by adverse drug reaction. The increased risk of superimposed infection might contraindicate the use of steroids in some cases. -Editor. *Ped Neur Briefs* Feb 1991.

CARBAMAZEPINE-INDUCED SKIN RASH

Of 335 children who were treated with carbamazepine at the Department of Paediatrics, Toyama Medical University, Japan, 33 (10%) developed a skin rash. Five had exfoliative dermatitis and 2 had Stevens-Johnson syndrome. The eleventh day of therapy was the most frequent day of onset; 88% developed the rash between 8 and 15 days. Children over 6 years of age were more susceptible to skin rash than younger patients, with frequencies of 20% and 5%, respectively. Leucopenia in 9 patients (27%), thrombocytopenia in 6 (18%), and hepatic dysfunction manifested by elevated transaminases in 9 (27%) occurred concomitantly with the skin rash. (Konishi T et al. Carbamazepine-induced skin rash in children with epilepsy. Eur J Pediatr July 1993;152:605-608). (Respond: Dr T Konishi, Dept of Paediatrics, Toyama Medical and Pharmaceutical University, 2630, Sugitani, Toyama City, Japan).

COMMENT. The frequency of skin rash with carbamazepine in this study is disturbingly high, particularly in children over 6 years of age. For additional reports, see Ped Neur Briefs Feb 1991. The introduction of dyes in the carbamazepine tablet in recent years may explain an apparent increase in reports of allergic skin reactions.

In a report from The Liverpool Hospital, New South Wales, Australia, the substitution of oxcarbazepine, a keto derivative thought to be less toxic than CBZ, caused a cross-reactive skin eruption in 3 adult patients who had previously developed exfoliative dermatitis with CBZ. (Beran RG. Epilepsia Jan/Feb 1993;34:163). -Editor. *Ped Neur Briefs* July 1993.

SPINA BIFIDA AND CARBAMAZEPINE

The records of all pregnant Medicaid recipients in Michigan who were taking anti-epileptic agents during pregnancy were studied at the Center for Drug Evaluation and Research, Food and Drug Administration, Rockville, Maryland. Four cases of spina bifida were identified in infants born to 1,490 women who took anticonvulsants during pregnancy. Among 107 women taking carbamazepine three gave birth with spina bifida; one was taking valproic acid in addition and two were taking phenytoin, barbiturates or primidone in combination with carbamazepine. Among 1,018 infants of mothers taking barbiturates alone only one had spina bifida. Anong 444 women taking phenytoin and 50 taking primidone alone, none gave birth to an infant with spina bifida. When the data from approximately 20 published studies were pooled, nine cases of spina bifida occurred among a total of 984 in utero exposures to carbamazepine, and the relative risk was 13.7 times the expected rate (approximately one in 1,500 births). Five cases of spina bifida occurred in infants whose mothers took carbamazepine alone during pregnancy. While exposure to carbamazepine in utero carried a 1% risk of spina bifida the risk with valproic acid was close to 2% but the difference was not significant. The risks with other anticonvulsant drugs was only 0.14% or one in 748 cases. (Rosa E.W. Spina bifida in infants of women treated with carbamazepine during pregnancy. N Engl J Med March 7, 1991;324:674-677).

COMMENT. The incidence of meningomyelocele has declined steadily from 12 per 10, 000 in 1970 to 6 to 8 per 10, 000 in 1980 among babies born in the United States. The neural tube closes between 22 and 29 days after conception and exposure to anti-epileptic agents such as valproic acid and carbamazepine may interfere with closure. Meningomyelocele may be diagnosed in the fetus with 75 to 80% accuracy by measurements of serum alpha-fetoprotein levels, and ultrasonography can identify the extent and location of these defects. (Hobbins, J.C., Diagnosis and management of neural tube defects today. N Engl J Med, March 7 1991;324:690-691).

The outcome of a neural tube defect may be improved by cesarean section before labor begins (Luthy, D A et al. Cesarean section before the onset of labor and subsequent motor function in infants with meningomyelocele diagnosed antenatally, N Engl J Med

March 7, 1991;324:662-666). Infants who had been exposed to labor were 2.2 times more likely to have severe paralysis than those delivered by cesarean section without labor. The mean functional motor level was at the second lumbar vertebra in fetuses exposed to labor and at the fourth lumbar vertebra in those delivered before labor began. Cesarean section before onset of labor may result in better subsequent motor function and the ability to walk with minimal mechanical assistance.-Editor. *Ped Neur Briefs* March 1991.

TERATOGENICITY OF ANTICONVULSANTS (AEDs)

The risks of teratogenic effects of AEDs are reported from Erasmus University, Rotterdam, The Netherlands. These consist of major malformations, minor anomalies, intrauterine or postnatal growth failure, and psychomotor retardation. The absolute risk of 7-10% is about 3-5% higher than that in the general population. None of the currently available AEDs is free of possible adverse effects on the fetus. Valproate and carbamazepine are associated predominately with spina bifida and hypospadias. Barbiturates and phenytoin are associated with congenital heart malformations and facial clefts. Risk factors include a high daily AED dosage, high maternal serum AED levels, low folate levels, or polytherapy. Genetic predisposition plays a role but no tests are available for identifying parents or fetuses at high risk. Prenatal diagnosis consists of fetal ultrasound during week 18-20, and *a*-fetoprotein analysis of amniotic fluid in week 16 in mothers receiving VPA or CBZ (Lindhout D, Omtzigt JGC. Pregnancy and the risk of teratogenicity. Epilepsia 1992;33 (Suppl 4):S41-S48). (Reprints: Dr. Dick Lindhout, Department of Clinical Genetics, Erasmus University, P.O Box 1738, 3000 DR Rotterdam, The Netherlands .)

COMMENT. Prevention of teratogenetic AED side effects should include the evaluation of the patient before conception, the need for AED therapy, monotherapy with the lowest possible dosage, avoidance of high peak levels by dividing daily dosage into 2 or 3 doses, folic acid supplement in cases of obvious deficiency and exclusion of vitamin B_{12} deficiency. Minor anomalies tend to lessen or disappear with age (e.g. nail hypoplasia). Pregnancy and teratogenesis in epilepsy was the subject of a Neurology supplement 5, April 1992. The effects of prenatal exposure to anticonvulsants on intellectual functioning of 4-8 year olds are reported by Vanoverloop D et al. from the Department of Pediatrics, Harvard Medical School, Boston (Neurotox Teratol Sept/Oct 1992;14:329-335). None of the children was mentally retarded, but scores for performance IQ and full scale IQ were lowered.-Editor. *Ped Neur Briefs* Dec 1992.

COGNITIVE IMPAIRMENT AND CARBAMAZEPINE

The effects on cognition of carbamazepine, phenytoin and sodium valproate were compared in 64 new cases of childhood epilepsy treated at the Leeds General Infirmary, England. The children age 5-14 years had no neurological deficit and were allocated randomly and assessed prospectively over a 12 month period. They were seizure-free throughout the 12 months. Psychological tests included visual recall, auditory recall (memory), visual scanning (vigilance), Stroop test (concentration), speed of information processing, and standard scales of intellectual functioning and reading. Serum levels of carbamazepine (CBZ) showed a significant negative correlation with changes in scores on the sum of five memory tests from before medication to 6 months and a year later. No significant correlations with memory scores were found for children treated with phenytoin (PHT). Only 10 of 126 serum level estimations of CBZ gave a value greater than 8.2 mcg/L. In the sodium valproate (SV) group significant positive correlations were found between serum levels and the sum of five memory tests at 1 month and at 6 months after starting treatment. The memory test clearly showed that there was impaired recent recall on CBZ apparent by 6 months of treatment and even more definite after a year. Reading scores were also lower in the CBZ compared with the PHT group after a year on drug treatment. Doses of CBZ were usually in the lower half of the accepted therapeutic range of 5-15 mcg/L

(Forsythe I et al. Cognitive impairment in new cases of epilepsy randomly assigned to carbamazepine, phenytoin and sodium valproate. Dev Med Child Neurol June 1991;33:524-534).

COMMENT . In this study involving children with epilepsy previously untreated, carbamazepine in moderate dosage adversely affected memory but sodium valproate and phenytoin did not. The tendency to favor carbamazepine in preference to phenytoin on the basis of reported cognitive deficits seems questionable and unfounded. A phenytoin-induced improvement in auditory memory has been demonstrated in children with EEG dysrhythmias (Millichap J G et al. Auditory perceptual deficit correlated with EEG dysrhythmias. Response to diphenylhydantoin sodium. Neurology 1969;19:870-872). Editor. *Ped Neur Briefs* July 1991.

CARBAMAZEPINE-INDUCED DIARRHEA

Intractable diarrhea induced by carbamazepine (CBZ) in 3 patients and necessitating discontinuation of the drug is reported from the Departments of Neurology and Medicine, University of Louisville School of Medicine, Kentucky. A 3 year old boy with generalized tonic-clonic seizures received CBZ 125 mg/day, increasing to 125 mg 3 times daily. The CBZ serum level was 7.4 mcg/ml. Frequent diarrhea was associated with negative stool examination and cultures. Liver function studies showed minimal LDH elevation. The gradual withdrawal of CBZ and substitution of phenytoin were followed promptly by recovery. The 2 other patients were adults, both of whom recovered after CBZ was withdrawn and phenytoin or primidone was substituted (Iyer V, Holmes JW, Richardson RL. Intractable diarrhea from carbamazepine. Epilepsia Jan/Feb 1992;33:185-187). (Reprints: Dr. V. Iyer, Department of Neurology, University of Louisville, Louisville, KY 40292.)

COMMENT. The authors note that diarrhea is described as a complication of CBZ in the package insert but gastrointestinal adverse effects of CBZ have received little attention in the literature. Other GI complications include anorexia, nausea, vomiting and constipation. Hepatic toxicity has been reported in 5%-10% of patients.

Carbamazepine-induced eosinophilic colitis with severe watery diarrhea is reported in an adult from Helsinki, Finland (Anttila VI, Valtonen M. Epilepsia Jan/Feb 1992;33:119-121). With 2 reports of CBZ-induced diarrhea appearing in the same issue of Epilepsia, the gastrointestinal side effects of CBZ need to be taken seriously and treated by prompt discontinuation of CBZ. -Editor. *Ped Neur Briefs* March 1992.

CARBAMAZEPINE ACUTE TOXICITY

The clinical toxic effects and serum concentrations after ingestion of carbamazepine are reported in 82 pediatric patients from the Intensive Care Unit, Royal Children's Hospital, Melbourne, Australia. Two died, 1 of cardiac failure and 1 of aspiration pneumonitis with septicemia. In 10 patients in deep coma with a Glasgow Coma Scale (GCS) of 3-4, the mean serum level was 213 *u*mol/L. The serum carbamazepine level was related to the depth of coma, convulsions, hypotension caused by myocardial failure and conduction defects, and to the requirement for mechanical ventilation. In 27 patients with moderate coma (GCS 5-8) the mean serum level of carbamazepine was 112 *u*mol/L; convulsions occurred in 2 patients in this group. In 45 patients with mildly depressed consciousness (GCS 9-15) the serum level was 73 *u*mol/L and symptoms included drowsiness (80%), ataxia (53%), nystagmus (38%), vomiting (17%), and dystonia (7%). Patients with carbamazepine serum levels greater than 150 *u*mol/L may require intensive life support. (Tibballs J. Acute toxic reaction to carbamazepine: clinical effects and serum concentrations. J Pediatr Aug 1992;121:295-299.) (Reprints: James Tibballs, MBBS, Intensive Care Unit, Royal Children's Hospital, Flemington Road., Parkville, Victoria, Australia 3052.)

COMMENT. In a study from the University of Cincinnati, Ohio, the administration of activated charcoal resulted in a statistically significant reduction in carbamazepine half-life but the time to complete recovery from overdose was not affected. (Wason S et al. Carbamazepine overdose - the effects of multiple dose activated charcoal. Clin Toxicol March 1992;30:39-48.) The authors recommend no more than 2 to 3 doses (1 g/kg) of activated charcoal to prevent formation of concretions and continued absorption of the drug. Prolonged repeated use of activated charcoal after carbamazepine overdose in comatose patients is not beneficial and carries a hazard of aspiration. -Editor. *Ped Neur Briefs* Sept 1992.

MASSIVE CARBAMAZEPINE POISONING

The clinical features in 2 8 consecutive adult cases of laboratory confirmed massive overdosage with CBZ alone treated in an intensive care unit during the period 1981-1991 are reported from Southern Hospital, Karolinska Institute, Stockholm, Sweden. Serum levels at or above 40 mg/L were significantly associated with an increased risk of serious complications including coma, seizures, respiratory failure and cardiac conduction defects. Two patients died. In 61% CBZ had been used therapeutically for the treatment of epilepsy. Five patients with repeated generalized seizures despite CBZ concentrations above 40 mg/L were controlled with diazepam or clonazepam intravenously. Ataxia, vertigo, nystagmus, diplopia, dysarthria, and/or dyskinesia were recorded in 11 cases (39%). Multiple dose activated charcoal was administered routinely. (Hojer J et al. Clinical features in 28 consecutive cases of laboratory confirmed massive poisoning with carbamazepine alone. Clin Toxicol Sept 1993;31:449-458). (Reprints: Dr Jonas Hojer, Medical Intensive Care Unit, Sodersjukhuset (Southern Hospital), S-118 83, Stockholm, Sweden).

COMMENT. An increased risk of seizures was a sign of CBZ overdose in this study, but in at least six previous reports, one involving 26 well documented cases in children, carbamazepine induced exacerbation of seizures at therapeutic dose levels. (Ped Neur Briefs June 1987; Progress in Pediatric Neurology, 1991, pp 108-9). The epileptic syndromes worsened by CBZ include childhood absence, Lennox Gastaut, myoclonic epilepsy, focal frontal lobe, and generalized tonic clonic epilepsy. A slow withdrawal of the CBZ results in improved seizure control. -Editor. *Ped Neur Briefs* Sept 1993.

ANTICONVULSANTS AND SERUM CHOLESTEROL

The effect of antiepileptic drugs (AED) on total cholesterol, high density lipoprotein (HDL) cholesterol and triglycerides was studied in 208 epileptic children compared with 175 normal children at the University of Bologna, Italy. In epileptic patients the mean total cholesterol plasma level was higher (195 mg/dl) than that of controls (184 mg/dl). HDL cholesterol and triglyceride levels were not different in the two groups. Carbamazepine- and phenobarbital-treated patients had significant elevations of mean cholesterol values and valproate treated patients had a significant lowering of cholesterol. An increase in cholesterol in the primidone and phenytoin treated patients was not significant. In a group of 32 patients studied before and during AED therapy the total cholesterol level before therapy was 168 mg/dl and after therapy 203 mg/dl. The highest level (313 mg/dl) of total cholesterol was observed in a boy receiving carbamazepine therapy (Franzoni E et al. Total cholesterol, high-density lipoprotein cholesterol, and triglycerides in children receiving antiepileptic drugs. Epilepsia Sept/Oct 1992;33:932-935). (Reprints: Professor E. Franzoni, Centro di Neurologia Pediatrica, Universita di Bologna, Via Massarenti 11, 4013B Bologna, Italy.)

COMMENT. Carbamazepine treated patients with a family history of hypercholesterolemia or cardiac infarction should be followed carefully for elevated levels of total cholesterol. The effect of antiepileptic drugs on cholesterol levels during treatment with the ketogenic diet should be carefully monitored, especially when treatment is combined with carbamazepine or phenobarbital.

Carbamazepine appeared to be responsible for a nonconvulsive status epilepticus in a 12 year old epileptic girl, in a report from Washington University School of Medicine, St. Louis, MO (Callahan DJ, Noetzel

MJ. Neurology Nov 1992;42:2198). CBZ level was 7.1 mcg/ml on admission. The absence status was resistant to multiple AEDs and was associated with increased intracranial pressure and transient MRI abnormalities. CBZ should be avoided in patients with generalized, synchronous, spike-and-wave EEG patterns. -Editor. *Ped Neur Briefs* Nov 1992.

CARBAMAZEPINE-INDUCED ACUTE PANCREATITIS

A 5-year-old mentally retarded child who developed pancreatitis during accidental acute carbamazepine (CBZ) intoxication is reported from the Department of Pediatrics, Ohio State University, Columbus, Ohio. He presented with vomiting and lethargy, but no abdominal pain. Serum amylase and lipase levels were increased for several days, and they returned to normal on recovery. (Tsao CY, Wright FS. Acute chemical pancreatitis associated with carbamazepine intoxication. Epilepsia Jan/Feb 1993;34: 174-176). (Reprints: Dr CY Tsao, Department of Pediatrics, Ohio State University, Children's Hospital, 700 Children's Dr, Columbus, OH 43205).

COMMENT. Among antiepileptic drugs, valproate is the most likely to be associated with pancreatitis. In a study at the Bowman Gray School of Medicine, Winston Salem, North Carolina, and the University of Virginia, Charlottesville, 14.5% of 366 physicians treating epilepsy reported a case of valproate-associated pancreatitis. Thirty nine cases were available for review from the physicians surveyed, the authors' patient population, and from the medical literature. Pancreatitis was more common in young persons (mean age 16 years) and during the early months of treatment. Three deaths were reported. Asymptomatic elevation of serum amylase was observed by 40 (11%) of the physicians using valproate. (Asconape JJ, Penry JK, Dreifuss FE et al. Valproate-associated pancreatitis. Epilepsia Jan/Feb 1993;34: 177-183). -Editor. *Ped Neur Briefs* March 1993.

CARBAMAZEPINE AND SERUM LIPID LEVELS

The effects of carbamazepine on serum lipid

levels in 36 previously untreated patients with recently diagnosed idiopathic epilepsy were evaluated in a 1 to 5-year follow-up study at the Departments of Neurology and Clinical Chemistry, University of Oulu, Finland. Serum cholesterol, high-density lipoprotein (HDL) cholesterol, and *g*-glutamyltransferase (GGT) levels increased after 2 months' carbamazepine treatment and remained high after 1 and 5 years follow-up. Cholesterol/HDL cholesterol ratios remained unchanged. Serum low-density lipoprotein (LDL) cholesterol and triglycerides (TG) increased during the first year but were normal after 5 years on medication. The change in lipid metabolism may be associated with induction of liver enzymes during carbamazepine treatment for epilepsy, and may also have clinical relevance to the increased incidence of atherosclerosis and coronary heart disease in patients with epilepsy. (Isojarvi JIT et al. Serum lipid levels during carbamazepine medication. A prospective study. Arch Neurol. June 1993;50:590-593). (Reprints: Dr Isojarvi, Department of Neurology, University of Oulo, SF-90220 Oulo, Finland).

COMMENT. The data support the hypothesis that the increase in serum cholesterol levels during carbamazepine therapy for epilepsy may be associated with liver enzyme induction. The changes in serum lipids may also be a consequence of hormonal effects, notably a decrease in free thyroxine, observed with carbamazepine. Patients receiving carbamazepine should have base line lipid profiles and serum lipid monitoring. Carbamazepine may not be an adjunct drug of choice in children receiving the ketogenic diet for refractory epilepsy. An elevation of very long chain fatty acids found in 13 of 22 plasma samples from patients on a standard ketogenic diet for uncontrolled seizures may lead to diagnostic confusion with peroxisomal disorders. Valproic acid was taken by 5 of the patients tested. (Theda C et al. J Pediatr May 1993;122:724-6). -Editor. *Ped Neur Briefs* June 1993.

CARBAMAZEPINE CARDIOTOXICITY

A 13-month-old boy with complex partial

seizures complicating tuberous sclerosis developed a cardiac conduction abnormality and heart block during treatment with carbamazepine in a report from the University of Massachusetts Medical School, Worcester, MA. The CBZ serum level was 6 mcg/ml and CBZ-10,11-epoxide level, 1 mcg/ml. After CBZ was discontinued a repeat EKG was normal. The echocardiogram, at first thought to show a small rhabdomyoma, was normal on repeat study 2 years later. (Weig SG, Pollack P. Carbamazepine-induced heart block in a child with tuberous sclerosis and cardiac rhabdomyoma: Implications for evaluation and follow-up. Ann Neurol Oct 1993;34:617-619). (Respond: Dr Weig, Department of Pediatrics, University of Massachusetts Medical Center, Worcester, MA 01655).

COMMENT. The authors cite one previous report of heart block secondary to erythromycin-induced CBZ toxicity in a 10-year-old boy. This child had no evidence of underlying cardiac disease. Additional cases in adults have been reported. Although CBZ cardiotoxicity is rare, an echocardiogram is recommended in patients with tuberous sclerosis treated with carbamazepine, and cardiac rhythm should be carefully monitored. -Editor. *Ped Neur Briefs* Oct 1993.

VALPROIC ACID AND CARNITINE METABOLISM

Plasma total, free, and acyl carnitine levels were determined in children treated with valproic acid at the Valley Children's Hospital and University of California, San Francisco, Fresno, CA. The mean total carnitine level was significantly lower in patients given valproic acid polytherapy compared with normal subjects and with those receiving valproic acid monotherapy. The levels in both the valproic acid monotherapy and polytherapy groups were significantly lower than those treated with other antiepileptic drugs. The mean free carnitine level was significantly lower in both the valproic acid monotherapy and polytherapy groups compared to normal subjects and the other antiepileptic drug group. Acylcarnitine levels were also lower in the polytherapy valproic acid group compared to the monotherapy valproic acid group and those receiving other antiepileptic drugs. The study indicates that a general decrease in the carnitine pool should be anticipated in patients taking valproic acid polytherapy and to a lesser degree, monotherapy. (Opala G, et al. The effect of valproic acid on plasma carnitine levels. AJDC Sept 1991;145:999-1001).

COMMENT. Plasma and erythrocyte carnitine was significantly lower in 37 children on sodium valproate alone or in combination with other drugs compared to levels in 22 children on drugs other than sodium valproate in a study from the Royal Aberdeen Children's Hospital, University of Aberdeen, Scotland (Thom H et al. Ammonia and carnitine concentrations in children treated with sodium valproate compared with other anticonvulsant drugs. Dev Med Child Neurol Sept 1991;33:795-802). Plasma ammonia was also elevated in the valproate group. Urinary free carnitine was reduced in valproate treated children with a significant increase in the ratio of bound to free carnitine. Carnitine supplementation is recommended.

Alterations of renal carnitine metabolism by valproic acid were studied in mice at the University of Santiago de Compostela, Spain (Camina MF et al. Neurology Sept 1991;41:1444-1448). Valproic acid induced a significant increase in renal clearance of acylcarnitine without affecting that of free carnitine, whereas other anticonvulsants increased clearance of free carnitine but not that of acylcarnitine. -Editor. *Ped Neur Briefs* Nov 1991.

VPA METABOLITES AND HYPERAMMONEMIA

The association between valproate metabolism (VPA) and VPA-induced hyperammonemia was studied at Hirosaki University Hospital, Japan. In 53 monopharmacy patients, plasma ammonia levels did not depend on age, VPA dosage or serum levels and showed a negative correlation with the 4-en metabolite of VPA. In polypharmacy patients, plasma ammonia levels were significantly higher, while 2-en VPA serum level and bilirubin were lower than in monopharmacy patients. (Kondo T et al. Is 2-propyl-4-pentonoic acid (4-en), a hepatotoxic metabolite of valproate, responsible for valproate-induced hyperammonemia? Epilepsia May/June 1992;33:550-554.) (Reprints: Dr. S. Kaneko, Department of Neuropsychiatry, Hirosaki 036, Japan.)

COMMENT. This study indicates that young age and high VPA serum levels are not risk factors for hyperammonemia induced by VPA and 4-en metabolite is not causally related to this adverse effect. These authors had previously reported that young age, polypharmacy, and high VPA serum level enhance the susceptibility to VPA hepatotoxicity by altering the metabolism of VPA and by increasing the conversion of VPA to 4-en, the most toxic VPA metabolite (Ped Neur Briefs March 1992, 6 :21) .

In 43 children with epilepsy who were treated with VPA monotherapy or polytherapy, serum levels of copper were significantly lower than in normal control patients, whereas serum zinc levels were not altered. (Kaji M et al. Epilepsia May/June 1992;33:555-557.)

Valproate and carbamazepine, and in a lesser frequency, phenytoin and phenobarbital, were the most common causes of red blood cell macrocytosis in children in a study from the Children's Medical Center, Dallas, TX (Pappo AS et al. Pediatrics June 1992;89:1063-1067). Macrocytosis and pancytopenia may be the first manifestation of bone marrow failure and aplastic anemia. An MCV of more than 90 fL in a patient taking antiepileptic medications deserves careful monitoring. -Editor. *Ped Neur Briefs* July 1992.

VALPROATE-INDUCED PUBERTAL ARREST

A 12-year-old girl with complex partial seizures who had pubertal arrest of both growth and secondary sexual development while receiving VPA is reported from the Department of Pediatrics, Wright State University, Dayton, OH and the University of Iowa, Iowa City, IA. She had received Depakote from 10 years 7 months of age in doses ranging from 750 mg/day (17 mg/kg/day) to 1,500 mg/day (36 mg/kg/day) and a maximum VPA level of 135.5 mcg/dL. Her growth rate during treatment decreased to 1.9 cm/yr compared to 4.9 cm/yr prior to treatment. When treatment was discontinued, normal-pubertal growth and maturation resumed with a growth rate of 10 cm/yr. Cranial MRI with gadolinium and CT were normal (Cook JS et al. Pubertal arrest associated with valproic acid therapy. Pediatr Neurol May/June 1992;8:229-231). (Respond: Dr. Cook, Department of Pediatrics, Wright State University, Dayton, OH 45402.)

COMMENT. The authors recommend that children and adolescents on VPA therapy should have height, weight and Tanner staging of genitalia and pubic hair assessed at each clinic visit to detect arrest of growth and development.

A causal association between maternal use of VPA and fetal spina bifida has been reported (Omtzigt JGC et al. The risk of spina bifida aperta after first trimester exposure to valproate in a prenatal cohort. Neurology 1992; 42(suppl 5):119-125.) Of 261 pregnant women receiving antiepileptic drugs, 6.3% of fetuses with VPA exposure had spina bifida aperta, whereas other antiepileptic drugs were not implicated in this developmental abnormality. High serum levels of VPA in the mother may have increased the risk which might be diminished by reduction of the daily dose. Editor. *Ped Neur Briefs* Aug 1992.

VALPROATE-INDUCED REPRODUCTIVE DISORDERS

The relation of antiepileptic therapy to the occurrence of reproductive endocrine disorders in 238 women with epilepsy has been studied at the University Hospital, Oulu, Finland. Age ranged from 18 to 45 years (mean, 33 yrs); the mean duration of therapy was 9 years. Menstrual disturbances occurring in 20% of patients were unrelated to the type of epilepsy but were significantly more frequent in those treated with valproate alone than in patients receiving other AEDs. Polycystic ovaries and elevated serum testosterone concentrations were found in the majority of women who were taking valproate and especially in those beginning treatment in adolescence; 80% receiving valproate before age 20 years were affected, compared to 27% of women treated with other AEDs. (Isojarvi JIT et al. Polycystic ovaries and hyperandrogenism in women taking valproate for epilepsy. N Engl T Med Nov 4 1993;329:1383-8). (Reprints: Dr Isojarvi, Dept of Neurology, University of Oulu, SF-90220 Oulu, Finland).

COMMENT. Polycystic ovaries, hyperandrogenism, obesity, menstrual disturbances, and hirsutism, characteristic findings of the polycystic ovary syndrome, may be secondary to valproate therapy for epilepsy. Women who begin treatment in adolescence are especially at risk. The authors voice concern regarding the use of valproate in adolescent and young women with epilepsy, and alternative antiepileptic medications should be selected for female patients in these age groups when possible.

Impaired fatty acid oxidation in 12 children taking valproic acid and at low risk for hepatotoxicity (>2 years of age and monotherapy) is reported from the University of Chicago (Kossak BD et al. Neurology Nov 1993;43:2362-8). The valproate-induced metabolic abnormalities resembled those found in inborn errors of mitochondrial *B*-oxidation and were not corrected by L-carnitine supplementation. These findings refute the hypothesis of "carnitine insufficiency" as the cause of valproate hepatotoxicity, and the routine supplements of carnitine in patients taking valproate are not advised. -Editor. *Ped Neur Briefs* Dec 1993.

VALPROATE-INDUCED CEREBRAL EDEMA

A case of cerebral edema resulting from acute sodium valproate poisoning in a 19 year old male is reported from Northwick Park and East Birmingham Hospitals, UK. On admission the patient was unconscious and the plasma valproate concentration was 900 mg/L. He had taken 1200 mg of sodium valproate along with 1500 mg of aspirin. The salicylate blood level was 70 mg/L. CT showed gross cerebral edema with slit-like ventricles and absence of cortical sulci and basal cisterns. Gastric lavage, fluid restriction and IV dexamethasone resulted in slow recovery. Acute complications included liver and renal dysfunction, hypocalcaemia and generalized muscle spasms. (Khoo SH, Leyland MJ. Cerebral edema following acute sodium valproate overdose. Clin Toxicol June 1992;30:209-214.) (Reprints: Dr. S.H. Khoo, Monsall Hospital, Newton Heath, Manchester, M108WR, UK.)

COMMENT. External leakage from feeding gastrostomies was reported in 4 of 8 children who received valproate sprinkle at the Hennepin County Medical Center, Minneapolis, MN (Jones-Saete C et al. Epilepsia July/Aug 1992;33:692-695). Adherence of undissolved valproate particles to the exterior of the tube appeared to prevent the close approximation of the tube to the gastrostomies stoma. The problem was reduced by changing the tube more frequently or using a larger size tube -Editor. *Ped Neur Briefs* Sept 1992.

VALPROATE AND EEG ABNORMALITIES

The effect of valproate on EEG epileptic abnormalities was investigated at the Institute of Neurophysiology, Genoa, Italy. Sixteen patients aged 14 to 44 years were administered a single (14-37 mg/kg) oral dose of magnesium valproate. At peak serum concentrations of 65-139 mcg/ml of valproate, there were increases in spike wave frequency at 2, 3, 4 and 5 hours. The peak concentrations of ammonia ranged from 15-72 mcg/l, with values exceeding normal in 13 determinations. The VPA and ammonia concentrations varied independently. The frequency of EEG epileptic abnormalities was not correlated with either the ammonemia level or the amount of variation in ammonemia concentration (Sannita WG. Valproate acute administration, EEG epileptic abnormalities, and ammonemia. Neurology Oct 1992;42:2003-2005). (Reprints: Professor Walter G. Sannita, Centro Farmaci Neuroattivi, Dipartimento di Scienze Motorie, Universita, Ospedale San Martino, viale Benedetto XV, I-16132 Genova, Italy.).

COMMENT. A direct CNS drug action has been

proposed to explain the quantitative EEG abnormalities in response to acute VPA administration and the stupor states in some patients. The stupor was not necessarily related to the increased ammonia concentration in the blood.-Editor. *Ped Neur Briefs* Dec 1993.

HEPATOCEREBRAL DEGENERATION OR VALPROATE TOXICITY

Six children with refractory seizures and focal neuronal damage who died of liver failure are reported from the Washington University School of Medicine, St Louis, MO. Four were treated with valproic acid (VPA) and developed liver failure within 30 - 68 days. Two of these children each had one sibling who was not exposed to VPA and developed the same clinical picture, but liver failure was delayed. Siblings receiving VPA survived only 3 and 5 months after onset of seizures, whereas those not treated with VPA lived for 7 to 16 months. (Bicknese AR et al. Early childhood hepatocerebral degeneration misdiagnosed as valproate hepatotoxicity. Ann Neurol Dec 1992;32:767-775). (Correspondence: Dr WE Dodson, St Louis Children's Hospital, 400 S Kingshighway Blvd, St Louis, MO 63110).

COMMENT. The authors propose that many of the reported patients with VPA-associated hepatotoxicity represent undiagnosed hepatocerebral degeneration, the Huttenlocher variant of Alpers' syndrome. Their experience suggests that liver failure is accelerated by exposure to VPA, and an alternative antiepileptic treatment should be employed in young children with resistant seizures and mental and motor regression, indicative of cerebral degeneration. Recurrence of this syndrome in family members suggests an autosomal recessive inheritance, but the biochemical basis remains undetermined. Of 13 similar cases reported from the Hospital for Sick Children, London (Egger J et al. Clin Pediatrics 1987;26:167), only 4 had received VPA and 2 may have died from VPA-hepatotoxicity.(Ped Neur Briefs July 1987). -Editor. *Ped Neur Briefs* Jan 1993.

VALPROATE (VPA)-ASSOCIATED HEPATOTOXICITY

The metabolic pattern of VPA in 170 epileptic

patients without symptoms or signs of hepatic side effects was compared to that in 11 patients with early symptoms and signs of hepatotoxicity and in 5 children with fulminant liver failure. A cohort of 470 patients in whom VPA serum metabolites had been measured were examined at several pediatric epilepsy clinics between 1986 and 1991 and results were evaluated at the Departments of Pediatrics, Rittberg-Krankenhaus; and Free University, Berlin, Germany; and University Hospital, Bern, Switzerland. In the reference group, infants receiving VPA monotherapy and comedication with other AEDs showed lower concentrations of the potential hepatotoxin 4-ene-VPA than did older children. Three of 4 children who died had massive lactic acidosis. In all children with probable VPA-associated hepatotoxicity, VPA metabolic patterns were different from the reference group, but were not specific or distinct, even in those who died. Increased values of 4-ene-VPA were found in only 1 of the 5 children with fulminant liver failure. The pattern of VPA metabolites did not distinguish between benign and life-threatening hepatic toxicities. (Siemes H et al. Valproate (VPA) metabolites in various clinical conditions of probable VPA-associated hepatotoxicity. Epilepsia March/April 1993;34:332-346). (Reprints: Professor Dr Med Harmut Siemes, Rittberg-Kinderklinik, CarstennstraBe 58, D-1000 Berlin 45, Germany).

COMMENT. This most extensive study of VPA liver toxicity has shown that the primary toxic agent is most likely VPA itself and not the VPA metabolite, 4-ene-VPA. An inherited or acquired defect in the B-oxidation of VPA may be contributory, and VPA may unmask an underlying metabolic disorder leading to mitochondrial dysfunction. (Appleton et al. Can J Neurol Sci 1990;17:145). The initial symptoms and pattern of metabolites do not distinguish between those patients with a benign reversible liver dysfunction and those who may develop a fulminant and fatal liver failure. Young age, polypharmacy, status epilepticus, and febrile illness are factors associated with VPA toxicity.- Editor. *Ped Neur Briefs* May 1993.

VALPROATE-INDUCED FATAL HEPATOTOXICITY

An 18 month old infant with fatal VPA-related hepatic toxicity is reported from Children's Mercy Hospital, Kansas City, MO, and the Mayo Clinic, Rochester, MN. The infant had received L-carnitine supplements and did not have Alpers disease. The child presented at 15 months with developmental delay, periodic vomiting, ataxia, chorea, hypotonia, areflexia, and nocturnal myoclonus. VPA, 15 mg/kg per day, supplemented with L-carnitine, 200 mg 4xdaily, resulted in initial partial control of the chorea and myoclonus. Relapse after 9 weeks therapy was accompanied by lethargy, vomiting, and hepatic dysfunction, resulting in death in 6 weeks. The liver was small, atrophic, and yellow at autopsy, and the brain showed neuronal loss and gliosis in the brain stem, cerebellar nuclei, and spinal cord. (Murphy JV, Groover RV, Hodge C. Hepatotoxic effects in a child receiving valproate and carnitine. J Pediatr Aug 1993;123:318-320). (Reprints: Jerome V Murphy MD, Children's Mercy Hospital, 2401 Gillham Rd, Kansas City, MO 64108).

COMMENT. The authors contend that the clinical features and pathological findings ruled out Alpers disease, but an undiscovered explanation for the neurological disorder and some contributory metabolic cause could not be definitely excluded. Nonetheless, this experience demonstrates the potential hazard of valproic acid therapy, particularly in young and neurologically impaired children, and carnitine supplements are not a prophylactic panacea against VPA liver toxicity.

Fanconi syndrome associated with valproate therapy for seizures in two developmentally delayed children, aged 4 and 9 years, is reported from Harvard Medical School, and Northampton Area Pediatrics, MA (Lande MB et al. Reversible Fanconi syndrome associated with valproate therapy. J Pediatr Aug 1993;123:320-322).-Editor. *Ped Neur Briefs* Aug 1993.

FETAL VALPROATE SYNDROME

The high frequency of minor abnormalities and major malformations, the withdrawal manifestations, and hypoglycemia in infants born to mothers who received sodium valproate during pregnancy are reported from the Department of Paediatrics, Aalborg Hospital, Denmark. Of 17 mothers, 11 had valproate monotherapy, and 6 had valproate combined with another anticonvulsant, usually carbamazepine. Minor abnormalities (epicanthic folds, hypertelorism, low set ears, etc) affected 9 (53%) infants, of whom 5 also had major malformations, predominantly congenital heart disease, present in 4. The frequency of abnormalities was related to the valproate dosage in the first trimester. Of 6 infants born to mothers receiving >2.5 g daily, 5 had minor abnormalities, and 3 had major malformations. Withdrawal symptoms in 9 (53%) infants included irritability, jitteriness, seizures, and feeding problems; hypoglycemia occurred in 4. At 2.0 - 3.5 year follow up, 3 showed psychomotor retardation. (Thisted E, Ebbesen F. Malformations, withdrawal manifestations, and hypoglycemia after exposure to valproate in utero. Arch Dis Child Sept 1993;69:288-291). (Respond: Dr Ebbe Thisted, Department of Paediatrics, University Hospital of Hvidovre, Kettegards Alle 30, DK-2650 Denmark).

COMMENT. Fetal valproate syndrome is related to the valproate dosage in the first trimester, while withdrawal symptoms are related to the dose and free fraction plasma concentration in the third trimester. These serious complications of valproate therapy for epilepsy during pregnancy occur during monotherapy as well as polytherapy. If the use of valproate during pregnancy cannot be avoided, despite the relatively high risk of teratogenicity, and especially spina bifida, the dosage and blood levels must be meticulously monitored and maintained as low as possible. (Omtzigt JGC, Lindhout D et al. Neurology 1992;42(suppl 5):119-125) -Editor. *Ped Neur Briefs* Nov 1993. ~

SURGERY AND EPILEPSY

TEMPORAL LOBECTOMY FOR COMPLEX PARTIAL SEIZURES

The outcome of 11 children who had undergone temporal lobectomy for the treatment of intractable complex partial seizures is reported from the Royal Children's Hospital, Melbourne, Australia. The average age at the time of surgery was 5 years 6 months (range, 1 to 9 years). The interval between onset of epilepsy and surgery averaged 3 1/2 years. The cause of the epilepsy was mesial temporal sclerosis in 4, glioma in 5, dysplasia in 1, and chronic progressive encephalitis in 1. Four patients had had febrile convulsions lasting more than 15 minutes. Seven patients had behavior disorders preoperatively, including hyperactivity, rage reactions, and destructive aggressive tendencies. At 2 to 7 years follow-up after surgery eight patients were seizure-free, two had seizures reduced in frequency, and only one with encephalitis had not benefited. Behavior was significantly improved in four of seven patients evaluated. Postoperative sequelae, including visual field defects and minor hemiparesis, occurred in four. (Hopkins IJ, Klug GL. Temporal lobectomy for the treatment of intractable complex partial seizures of temporal lobe origin in early childhood. Dev Med Child Neurol Jan 1991;33:26-31).

COMMENT. These results are encouraging and should lead to more frequent referral of children with refractory epilepsies to our neurosurgical colleagues. The occurrence of febrile convulsions as antecedents of the complex partial seizures in 36% of this group of children invalidates reports that stress the benign nature of the febrile seizure and are opposed to prophylactic therapy -Editor. *Ped Neur Briefs* Feb 1991.

TEMPORAL LOBECTOMY FOR INTRACTABLE SEIZURES

The results of temporal lobectomy in 16 children under the age of 12 years who had intractable seizures of temporal lobe origin are reported from the Miami

Children's Hospital, Florida. All had seizures for at least 2 years despite multiple antiepileptic drugs. Structural lesions were demonstrated by neuroimaging in 11 patients. At follow-up from 1 to 4 years 11 children were seizure free, 3 were 90 % improved, 1 was 50 % improved and 1 was unchanged. Of 9 families contacted 7 reported substantial improvement in the child's psychosocial function. Neuropathological abnormalities identified in all children showed findings consistent with disordered neuronal migration in 7, tuberous sclerosis in 1, and mesial temporal sclerosis only in 2 children. (Duchowny M et al. Temporal lobectomy in early childhood. Epilepsia March/April 1992;33:298-303.) (Reprints: Dr. M. Duchowny, Comprehensive Epilepsy Center, Miami Children's Hospital, 3200 S.W. 60 Court, Miami, FL 33155.)

COMMENT. Anterior temporal lobectomy tailored according to the extent of the lesion and epileptogenic field may be beneficial in pre-adolescent children with medically refractory seizures. Compared to adults, children undergoing temporal lobectomy have a higher incidence of abnormalities of neurogenesis and lesions that are poorly circumscribed and often widespread. -Editor. *Ped Neur Briefs* June 1992.

TEMPORAL LOBECTOMY FOR COMPLEX PARTIAL SEIZURES

The results of anterior temporal lobectomy performed for medically intractable, complex partial seizures, with onset before 16 years of age, in 42 consecutive patients are reported from various centers. All patients underwent surgery at the Children's Hospital, Boston, between 1972 and 1987, before implanted electrodes were routine. Total or near total seizure control was achieved in 85%. (96% of 28 operated after the introduction of long-term EEG monitoring). Results were comparable to series using invasive monitoring. Post-operative follow-up was at least 2 years. The median age at operation was 17 years (range 3.9-27 years) in the seizure-free group compared to 20 years (range 12-34 years) in the group with persistent seizures after surgery. (Erba G et al.

Temporal lobectomy for complex partial seizures that began in childhood. Surg Neurol Dec 1992;38:424-432). (Reprints: Ken R Winston MD, Box B467, Children's Health Center, 1950 Ogden St, Denver, CO 80218).

COMMENT. Patients may be selected successfully for temporal resection without the risk and expense of invasive presurgical depth electrodes and subdural monitoring. Neoplasm was the cause of seizures in 57%, and surgery at an earlier age may have improved prognosis and seizure control. The outcome from anterior temporal resection in patients with localized lesions was particularly favorable.

Positron emission tomography showing temporal hypometabolism correlated with good outcome following temporal lobectomy for uncontrolled seizures in a study of 53 patients at the National Institutes of Health (Theodore WH et al. Ann Neurol Dec 1992;32:789). PET identified the seizure focus and allowed limitation of invasive electrode placements for mapping.-Editor. *Ped Neur Briefs* Jan 1993.

SURGERY FOR EXTRATEMPORAL PARTIAL EPILEPSY

The results of surgery for extratemporal partial epilepsy that began in childhood are reported from the Department of Surgery, Stanford University Medical School; Department of Neurology, University of Rochester; University of Colorado Health Sciences Center; and the Children's Hospital, Boston MA. Of 35 patients who underwent 39 operations, 63% were either seizure-free or had a significant reduction in frequency of seizures. The locations of the cortical resections were frontal, parietal, occipital, or multilobar. Tumors accounted for 31%, malformation 17%, atrophy 14%, encephalitis 5.7%, Sturge-Weber syndrome 2.9%, and vascular malformation 8.6%. The lesion was a nonspecific gliosis in 20% Patients for surgery were selected by clinical criteria, neural imaging, and EEG with long-term monitoring. Invasive preoperative investigations such as depth electrodes were not employed. The authors advocate early operation in children with intractable epilepsy even when the seizure focus is not involving the temporal lobe. (Adler J et al. Results of surgery for extratemporal partial epilepsy that began in childhood. Arch Neurol Feb 1991;48:133-140).

COMMENT. In retrospect the authors believed that surgery was delayed in most patients much longer than necessary and that years of needless suffering from epilepsy and the adverse effects of antiepileptic medications might have been avoided by surgery before adolescence. Patients with vascular malformations often had the longest delay between onset of seizures and surgery and these would have benefited greatly from earlier intervention. -Editor. *Ped Neur Briefs* Feb 1991.

VAGUS NERVE STIMULATION FOR CONTROL OF EPILEPSY

Results of intermittent stimulation of the vagus nerve in four patients with intractable partial seizures are reported from the Department of Neurology, Bowman Gray School of Medicine, Wake Forest University, Winston-Salem, NC. The criteria for implantation of the device were 1) refractory partial seizures, 2) adequate trials of antiepileptic drugs, 3) adequate trials of investigational drugs, 4) age 18 to 55, and 5) not a candidate for epilepsy brain surgery. The stimulation electrodes are placed around the vagus nerve at or above the omohyoid muscle. The leads are tunneled through to a subcutaneous pocket in the subclavicular region and connected to the pulse generator. Complex and simple partial seizures as well as secondarily generalized seizures were reduced by 100% in patients 1 and 2 and by 40% in patient 4. Side effects were transient and occurred concomitantly with stimulation; they included hoarseness and a stimulation sensation in the neck. One patient had an episode of uncontrolled hiccups. (Penry JK, Dean JC, Prevention of intractable partial seizures by intermittent vagal stimulation in humans: preliminary results. Epilepsia; 1990;31 (Suppl 2):S40-43).

COMMENT. Five patients age 20 to 59 with complex partial seizures received vagus nerve stimulation at the Neurology Service and Neurological Surgery Section, Department of Veteran's Affairs Medical Center, Gainesville, Florida (Uthman, BM, Wilder BJ et al. Epilepsia 1990;31 (Suppl 2):S44-S50). Three patients had a greater than 50% reduction in seizure frequency. The battery life of the stimulator is approximately two years and cost of replacement is comparable to that of a five year supply of antiepileptic drugs. Vagal stimulation may offer an option of treatment before temporal lobectomy and in patients with bilateral independent epileptogenic foci. -Editor. *Ped Neur Briefs* March 1991.

CORPUS CALLOSOTOMY FOR INTRACTABLE SEIZURES

The results of corpus callosotomy in 18 patients 16 years old and younger are reported from the Sections of Neurology and Neurosurgery, Dartmouth-Hitchcock Medical Center, Hanover, NH. A significant improvement with a decrease in seizure frequency of greater than 80% occurred in 83% of patients having generalized atonic, tonic, or tonic-clonic seizures. There was no postoperative deterioration in behavior, memory, or language function when the callosotomy was performed as a two stage procedure. Some patients had a very mild and transient hemiparesis that resolved in a few days but none developed persistent mutism, a reported complication in other series. Many generalized seizures were converted to focal seizures postoperatively. Partial seizures are usually not responsive. Patients with evidence of unilateral disease tend to have the best results from callosotomy while those with generalized infantile spasms, Lennox-Gastaut syndrome, or anoxic encephalopathy have less predictable results. Mental retardation is not a contraindication and improvement in control of the seizures may improve behavior and cognitive functioning. (Nordgren RE et al. Corpus callosotmy for intractable seizures in the pediatric age group. Arch Neurol April 1991;48:364-372).

COMMENT. Callosotomy may be considered in

young patients with frequent generalized atonic, tonic, and tonic-clonic seizures. Early surgical intervention may prevent the adverse effects of frequent recurrent seizures and the possibility of kindling. -Editor. *Ped Neur Briefs* April 1991.

PROGNOSIS AFTER CORPUS CALLOSOTOMY

The response to corpus callosal section in 64 patients with intractable epilepsy was evaluated in a multicenter study in Australia. Age at time of operation ranged from 3 years to 47 years (mean age 20 years); 43% underwent callosotomy during childhood, at age <16 years. Mean age of onset of epilepsy was 5 years, and mean duration of epilepsy before surgery was 15 years. The most common seizure patterns were generalized tonic-clonic (GTC) (83%) and drop attacks (73%). Focal seizures occurred in 42%, of whom half had seizures of frontal lobe origin. The rate of favorable outcome was 60% for drop attacks, 47% for tonic seizures, 49% for GTCs, and 55% for complex partial seizures. Outcome for drop attacks was more favorable with unilateral seizure activity or generalized slow spike and wave, characteristic of Lennox-Gastaut syndrome; bilateral independent spikes, and severe mental retardation carried a poor prognosis. Improvement followed complete callosotomy in 6 of 10 patients not benefited by anterior callosotomy. (Reutens DC et al. Corpus callosotomy for intractable epilepsy: Seizure outcome and prognostic factors. Epilepsia Sept/Oct 1993;34:904-909). (Reprints: Dr SF Berkovic, Department of Neurology, Austin Hospital, Heidelberg, Victoria, Australia 3084).

COMMENT. In children with medically intractable epilepsy, especially drop attacks of focal or Lennox Gastaut types and complex partial seizures of frontal lobe origin, corpus callosotomy should be considered when focal resection is not appropriate. Surgical complications are reported to be mild, and include transient hemiparesis and mutism.

Satisfactory seizure control is reported in 25 (74%) of 34 children following corpus callosotomy performed at the Institute of Neurology, Goiania, Brazil. (Cendes F et al. Epilepsia Sept/Oct 1993;34:910). The majority had mental retardation. Atonic seizures responded best, followed by tonic, GTC, and atypical absence seizures. Complex partial and myoclonic seizures were not controlled. Of 26 patients with behavior problems, 81% had a significant decrease in aggressiveness, hyperactivity, and/or attention deficit. Total section was complicated by interhemispheric disconnection symptoms. Mutism, dysarthria, or gait dyspraxia persisted in 5 of 13 patients affected. Section limited to the anterior two thirds was uncomplicated. The neurophysiological basis for corpus callosotomy is the interruption of bilateral ictal synchrony.-Editor. *Ped Neur Briefs* Nov 1993.

OUTCOME OF EPILEPSY SURGERY

The surgical outcome in 34 patients between 2 and 15 years of age who were operated on for medically intractable seizures is reported from the Neurosurgical Clinic, University Clinical Center, Visegradska 26, Belgrade, Yugoslavia. Temporal epileptic foci were present in 9 patients, extratemporal foci in 6, infantile hemiplegia in 16 and epilepsia partialis continua in 3. Detectable brain lesions were present in 30 (88%). At 1-14 years postoperative follow-up (mean, 4 years), 21(62%) are seizure free, 8 (23%) have improved, and 5 (15%) have shown no improvement. Patients with temporal foci had a partial temporal lobectomy or restricted temporofrontal resection; those with extratemporal foci had cortical resection; and patients with infantile hemiplegia had a partial hemispherectomy, extensive cortical resection or functional hemispherectomy of Rasmussen type. (Ribaric II et al. Surgical treatment of epilepsy: our experiences with 34 children. Child's Nerv Syst Nov 1991;7:402-404.) (Reprints Dr Ribaric, University Clinical Center, Visegradska 26, YU-11000 Belgrade, Yugoslavia.).

COMMENT. Of 16 patients with infantile hemiplegia who were subjected to hemispherectomy, 12 (75%) were seizure free. Lindsay J et al. from the Park Hospital for Children, Oxford, England, found a similar incidence of seizure control following hemispherectomy in 17 children with hemiplegic epilepsy (Dev Med Child Neurol 1987;29:592). See "Surgery and Epilepsy" in Progress in Pediatric Neurology, Millichap JG ed, 1991, pp 131-138). Editor. *Ped Neur Briefs* Jan 1992.

POST-OPERATIVE EPILEPSY RECURRENCE

Post-operative seizures occurred in 72 patients after resective procedures for epilepsy at The Epilepsy Surgery Program, Departments of Neurology and Neurological Surgery, The Cleveland Clinic Foundation, Cleveland, OH. The patients ranged in age from 2-47 years (mean 26 years). Temporal lobe resection had been performed in 74 % and extratemporal resections in 26%. The post-operative seizures were similar to preoperative patterns in 74%. 86% of patients had their first seizure occurrence within 1 year of surgery. Of 21 patients with recurrences in the first week after operation, none had subtherapeutic antiepileptic drug levels. Those with first recurrences from 1 week to more than 1 year after operation had subtherapeutic levels in 10 to 50% of patients. One-half of the patients had more than 1 seizure a month. In temporal resection patients half of the recurrences were controllable, whereas patients with extratemporal resections had a greater likelihood (96%) of persistent seizures and seizures became intractable in 74%. The age at operation, the duration of epilepsy, and associated structural lesions did not influence the likelihood of persistent seizures or intractability after recurrence. (Wingkun EC, Awad IA et al. Natural history of recurrent seizures after resective surgery for epilepsy. Epilepsia Nov/Dec 1991;32:851-856.) (Reprints: Dr. Awad, Department of Neurological Surgery, Cleveland Clinic Foundation, 9500 Euclid Ave, Cleveland, OH 44195.)

COMMENT. After the first seizure recurrence there appears to be a predictable trend of persistent seizures over the next 5 years. A decrease in seizure recurrence in the first 3 years after the first episode of relapse may reflect a more careful attention to antiepileptic drug therapy. Seizures recurring within 1 week postoperatively are not benign and have the same likelihood of subsequent intractability as other recurrent seizures in the first postoperative year. The outcome of resective surgery in extratemporal regions was less encouraging than temporal resections. If seizure recurrences are delayed until after the first postoperative year the outlook is better and seizures rarely become intractable. Changes in antiepileptic drugs, dosages, or poor compliance may be important factors in recurrence of seizures. The maturing epileptogenicity at the scar of a previous resection does not appear to contribute to intractability of seizures but may be a factor in later recurrences .

Details of the anticonvulsant drug regimens used before and after operation were not provided and the comparative efficacy of phenytoin and carbamazepine in postoperative epilepsy would be of interest. A comparative study of the cognitive effects of phenytoin and carbamazepine in healthy young adults has shown no significant clinical differences between the two drugs. (Meador KJ et al. Comparative cognitive effects of carbamazepine and phenytoin in healthy adults. Neurology, 1991;41:1537.) -Editor. *Ped Neur Briefs* Jan 1992.

ANTICONVULSANTS FOLLOWING CRANIOTOMY

A randomized prospective clinical trial of carbamazepine or phenytoin for 6 or 24 months including a control no-treatment group is reported in 276 post-craniotomy patients at the Walton Hospital, Liverpool, England. 103 (37%) patients suffered at least 1 seizure. Of those who developed status epilepticus in the first week after operation, 8 % were treated with carbamazepine, 5 % with phenytoin, and 2 % had no treatment. Serum anticonvulsant levels were not monitored in all patients. In those who were monitored the levels were never in the optimal range, particularly in the phenytoin treated group. Early anticonvulsant treatment did not affect the long-term response of epilepsy to anticonvulsant drugs. The occurrence of seizures within the first post-operative week did not increase the likelihood of late epilepsy.

Acute allergic skin rashes occurred in 28 (13%) patients. The authors concluded that prophylactic anticonvulsants should not be recommended routinely following supratentorial craniotomy. (Foy PM et al. Do prophylactic anticonvulsant drugs alter the pattern of seizures after craniotomy? J Neurol Neurosurg Psychiatry Sept 1992;55:753-757.) (Correspondence: Dr. P.M. Foy, Mersey Regional Department of Medical and Surgical Neurology, Walter Hospital, Liverpool, England.)

COMMENT. The authors admit that the small and uncertain effect of antiepileptic drug treatment in this study might be related to noncompliance and failure to achieve optimal blood levels. Of those blood levels available a significant proportion of phenytoin levels were suboptimal, and it could be argued that the more rigorous monitoring might have improved results. In contrast, satisfactory carbamazepine levels were achieved and yet, there was no difference in outcome. These findings suggest that phenytoin has a greater prophylactic action than carbamazepine in postcraniotomy seizure control. According to Drs. Wingkun and Awad at the Cleveland Clinic, changes in antiepileptic drugs, dosages, or poor compliance may be important factors in postoperative recurrence of seizures (see Ped Neurol Briefs Jan 1992;6:8). The unusually high incidence of skin rashes associated with anticonvulsant treatment in this study suggests that postcraniotomy patients are more susceptible than non-surgical epilepsy patients. The respective frequency of skin rash with the two anticonvulsants used in this study was not stated. It would be of interest to know if the antibiotic Cefotaxim was administered to these surgical patients in conjunction with the anticonvulsant, since this combination of drugs is known to increase the risk of serious skin reactions (see Ped Neurol Briefs May 1992;5:37).-Editor. *Ped Neur Briefs* Oct 1992.

SURGICAL TREATMENT OF EPILEPSY: 40 YEARS EXPERIENCE

The results of surgical treatment between 1940 and 1980 of 118 children with frontal or temporal lobe epilepsy were reviewed at the Montreal Neurological Illstitute. The mean age of seizure onset was 5.1 years, the mean age at operation 11.7 years, and the follow-up was 15 years (range 2-31 years). Outcome was excellent in 13 of 45 (29%) frontal surgery patients and 43 of 73 (59%) temporal surgery patients. A history of prolonged febrile seizures in 22 (30%) of the temporal surgery group was associated with a good prognosis. Secondarily generalized seizures occurring in 60 (50%) patients usually predict a poor prognosis. (Fish DR et al. Surgical treatment of children with medically intractable frontal or temporal lobe epilepsy: Results and highlights of 40 years' experience. Epilepsia March/April 1993;34:244-247). (Reprints: Dr Luis F Quesney, 3801 University St, Montreal, Quebec, Canada, H3A 2B4).

COMMENT. Surgical epilepsy candidates with a history of febrile convulsions and without secondarily generalized seizures are most likely to benefit from temporal lobe resection. -Editor. *Ped Neur Briefs* April 1993.

EPILEPSY SURGERY AND TUBEROUS SCLEROSIS

The results of operation for treatment of epilepsy in 5 male and 4 female patients with tuberous sclerosis in a 5-year period from 1986-1990 are reported from the Mayo Clinic. Pathological examination of resected lesions demonstrated 7 cortical tubers and 2 astocytic hamartomas. MRIs correlated with clinical and focal EEG findings. Seven patients are free from seizures and 2 are partially controlled. In selected tuberous sclerosis patients with single or multiple cerebral lesions, both the primary and secondary epileptogenic lesions were modified by removal of the primary ictal focus. (Bebin EM, Kelly PJ, Gomez MR. Surgical treatment for epilepsy in cerebral tuberous sclerosis. Epilepsia July/Aug 1993;34:651-657). (Reprints: Dr MR Gomez, Dept of Neurology, Mayo Clinic, 200 First St, SW, Rochester, MN 55905).

COMMENT. Results of surgery for epilepsy due to cortical dysplasia (CD) are reviewed in 17 patients treated at the Maudsley Hospital, London (Hirabayashi S et al. J Neurol Neurosurg Psychiatry July 1993;56:765). Only 6 became free or almost free from seizures, and 8 had no relief. Outcome related to the extent of the pathology but not to histology. Lesions outside the temporal and frontal lobes and generalized interictal EEG abnormalities, reflecting extensive or multiple lesions, correlated with poor surgical outcome. MRI was abnormal in 5 of 7 patients examined, contrasting with a low detection rate of abnormalities by CT scan. The use of MRI and PET should improve the identification of CD patients amenable to surgery. -Editor. *Ped Neur Briefs* Sept 1993.

MRI ABNORMALITIES IN PARTIAL EPILEPSY

The incidence of cerebral abnormalities on MRI in 30 consecutive children, aged 0.9-15.5 years, presenting with intractable complex partial seizures, is reported from the Institute of Child Health and Hospital for Sick Children, London, UK. A clinical diagnosis of a temporal lobe focus was made in 19 patients, and all showed hippocampal, temporal lobe abnormalities, or both, on the MRI. Surgery performed in 2 confirmed the radiological diagnosis of hippocampal sclerosis in one and astocytoma in the other. Of 7 children without localizing features clinically, 5 had a hippocampal abnormality, one had atrophy of the right temporal lobe, and one had diffuse cortical change. Lateralizing features by EEG were recorded in 12 (41%), and 7 had an MRI abnormality on the same side. (Cross JH et al. Early detection of abnormalities in partial epilepsy using magnetic resonance. Arch Dis Child July 1993;69:104-109). (Respond: Dr Helen Cross, Neurosciences Unit, The Wolfson Centre, Mecklenburgh Square, London WClN 2AP, UK).

COMMENT. An MRI finding of hippocampal sclerosis was documented as early as 4 years of age in one patient in this study, and progressive hippocampal abnormalities over a six month period were apparent in one other. The MRI as employed in this study can separate the causes and effects of seizures and help to clarify the relationship between early hippocampal damage in children and subsequent temporal lobe epilepsy.

Studies of hippocampal neuron loss and memory scores, before and after temporal lobe surgery for epilepsy at the Reed Neurological Research Center, University of California, LA, support a role for the left hippocampus in rote verbal memory. Patients with severe as compared with minimal left hippocampal neuron loss may be at risk for lower memory functioning postoperatively (Rausch R, Babb TL. Arch Neurol Aug 1993;50:812-817). -Editor. *Ped Neur Briefs* Aug 1993.

ICTAL SPECT IN LOCALIZING EPILEPTOGENESIS

Ictal single-photon emission computed tomography (SPECT) was used successfully in the localization of an epileptic focus in two children, ages 9 and 7 years, with intractable epilepsy reported from the University of Alabama at Birmingham Epilepsy Center. CT and initial MRIs were normal, and repeated EEG-video monitoring studies failed to localize the seizures. Resection of the abnormal areas shown by SPECT as hyperperfusion in the frontal lobes revealed a cortical dysplasia. The children had no neurological deficits and remained seizure free 1 year after surgery. (Kuzniecky R et al. Ictal single-photon emission computed tomography demonstrates localized epileptogenesis in cortical dysplasia. Ann Neurol Oct 1993;34:627-631). (Respond: Dr Kuzniecky, Department of Neurology, UAB Station, Birmingham, AL 35294).

COMMENT. Ictal SPECT performed exactly at the onset of a clinical seizure precisely localized the primary epileptogenic area in the cortical dysplasia and permitted a discrete resection of the focus without neurologic deficit. -Editor. *Ped Neur Briefs* Oct 1993.

PROGNOSIS OF BRAIN TUMOURS WITH EPILEPSY

The prognosis of 560 patients with a clinical and CT diagnosis of intrinsic supratentorial brain tumor was examined retrospectively at the Department of Neurosciences, Walton Hospital, Liverpool, England. Epilepsy was the first symptom in 164 patients. Patients presenting with epilepsy had a median survival of 37 months compared to 6 months in those presenting with other symptoms; they were more likely to have a normal clinical examination, a non-enhancing low density lesion on CT scan and a low grade tumor. Significant independent variables which adversely affected prognosis were increasing age, focal neurological signs, an enhancing CT lesion at diagnosis, surgical biopsy, and male sex. Primary intracerebral tumors presenting with epilepsy were relatively benign. They were less likely to receive radiotherapy or biopsy, but more likely to undergo resective surgery. No beneficial effects from either early resective surgery or radiotherapy were demonstrated. The average duration of symptoms before CT diagnosis was 28 months (range 2 days - 232 months in those presenting with epilepsy) and 4 months (range 1 day - 175 months in those with other presentations). Seizures were refractory to anti-epileptic drugs with only 11 of 164 patients ever achieving a 1 year remission (Smith DF et al. The prognosis of primary intracerebral tumours presenting with epilepsy: the outcome of medical and surgical management. J Neurol Neurosurg and Psych Oct 1991;54:915-920).

COMMENT. Backus RE and Millichap JG analyzed the records of 291 consecutive children treated for intracranial tumor at the Mayo Clinic from 1950-1959 with particular attention to patients with seizures (Pediatrics June 1962;29:978-984). Seizures occurred in 17% of the total group - in 25% of patients with supratentorial tumors and in 12% of those with infratentorial tumors. They were the initial symptoms in 15% of patients with supratentorial tumors and in 1% of those with infratentorial tumors. The average age at onset was 4.9 years in the supratentorial group and 4. 8 years in the infratentorial group . The diagnosis of supratentorial tumors was delayed for an average of 2 years, whereas infratentorial tumors were diagnosed within an average time of 3 months of the initial seizure. The electroencephalogram was of localizing value in 92% of tumors that involved the cerebral cortex. The histologic type of tumors was verified in 46 of the 50 patients who had seizures. Seizures were more common in patients with slowly growing astrocytomas grades 1 and 2 (67 % incidence) than in those with rapidly expanding astrocytomas grades 3 and 4 (10% incidence). Symptoms of increased intracranial pressure were present at the time of the first seizure in 20% of patients with supratentorial tumors and in 79 % with infratentorial tumors. A delta pattern in the EEG indicative of an expanding lesion occurred in 50 % of patients, and spike, sharp wave, or spike and wave seizure discharges compatible with a static lesion were recorded in 32% of patients with supratentorial tumors (Millichap JG et al. The electroencephalogram in children with intracranial tumors and seizures. Neurology May 1962;12:329-336).

With the increasing availability of neuroimaging techniques and particularly the MRI, the early diagnosis of tumor in patients with focal epilepsy will be facilitated and may lead to earlier surgical resection. The present study questions the advisability of resective surgery in patients with primary brain tumors presenting with seizures. A prospective, randomized study of aggressive versus conservative management is required. -Editor. *Ped Neur Briefs* Nov 1992.

NONEPILEPTIC PAROXYSMAL DISORDERS

HYPEREXPLEXIA OR HEREDITARY STIFF BABY SYNDROME

The stiff baby syndrome and its diagnostic distinction from epilepsy is reviewed from the Service de Neuronatologie, Pavillon de la Mere et l'Enfant, Nantes, France. The disease hyperexplexia was first described in 1962 by Kok and Bruyn in 29 members of one family and occurred as a dominant autosomal transmission. It was distinguished by a permanent hypertonia that is heightened by the slightest stimulus. The hypertonia was noted at birth and became less pronounced during the first year of life but later could lead to repeated falls. The electromyogram showed persistent activity even at rest and the activity was abolished by diazepam. Lingam S, Wilson J, and Hart E named the condition "hereditary stiff baby syndrome" (Am J Dis Child 1981;135:909). The child has a fixed stare and an expresslon of anxiety. The hypertonia diminishes during sleep and increases with the slightest psychic or tactile stimulus. Attacks of hypertonia may involve respiratory muscles and lead to apneas which can endanger the child's life. Digestive disorders including vomiting are usually associated with a hiatal hernia. The electroencephalogram is normal. (Tohier C et al. Hyperexplexia or stiff baby syndrome. Arch Dis Child April 1991;66:460-461).

COMMENT. In addition to myoclonic epilepsy, the differential diagnosis includes the stiff man syndrome which is not hereditary but which may occur in children, the Isaacs Mertens syndrone with distal hypertonia and fasciculations, the jumping Frenchmen of Maine syndrome with violent starts induced by slight stimuli and associated with echolalia and echopraxia, and Gilles de la Tourette syndrome. The pathology of stiff man syndrome has been localized to the spinal interneurons but the mechanism of hyperexplexia is controversial. Treatment with diazepam is effective in both syndromes. -Editor. *Ped Neur Briefs* May 1991.

HYPEREKPLEXIA; RESPONSE TO CLONAZEPAM

Sixteen patients, including 1 neonate, in a large 5 generation family with hyperekplexia (startle disease or congenital stiff-man syndrome) were treated with clonazepam at the University of Texas Health Science Center, San Antonio, TX. All showed dramatic and sustained improvement. Clonazepam was introduced at a dose of 0.5 mg (0.125 - 0.25 mg for children at bedtime). The total daily dose in children did not exceed 1.5 mg and increases of .125 to .25 mg were made every third day until the symptoms improved. (Ryan SG et al. Startle disease, or hyperekplexia: response to clonazepam and assignment of the gene (STHE) to chromosome 5q by linkage analysis. Ann Neurol June 1992;31:663-668.) (Correspondence: Dr Ryan, Department of Pediatrics, the

University of Texas Health Science Center, 7703 Floyd Curl Drive, San Antonio, TX 78284-7814.)

COMMENT. Hyperekplexia is a distinctive clinical syndrome of hypertonia and exaggerated startle responses that is inherited as an autosomal dominant. This familial form of hyperekplexia responds to clonazepam whereas the less frequent nonfamilial form sometimes fails to respond. A late onset variant with symptoms arising in adolescence responded dramatically to valproate and was not benefited by clonazepam. (Andermann F et al. Brain 1980; 103:985.)

Of 15 patients with hyperekplexia identified in 3 families at the Departments of Neurology and Pediatrics, Wayne State University School of Medicine, Detroit, MI, 3 infants died unexpectedly during the neonatal period. Patients treated with clonazepam (0.1-0.2 mg/kg/day) had no serious apneic episodes and startle reflexes induced by nose tapping were diminished (Nigro MA, Lim HCN. Hyperekplexia and sudden neonatal death. Pediatr Neurol May/June 1992;8:221-225). Hyperekplexia is included in the differential diagnosis of neonates with apnea, aspiration pneumonia, episodic muscular rigidity and near miss SIDS. Nose tapping to elicit the hyperekplexic startle response should be included in the routine examination of newborns. (Ped Neurol Briefs May 1991;5:36). The primary pysiological abnormality in hyperekplexia involves spinal as well as brainstem hyperexcitability (Matsumoto J et al. Ann Neurol July 1992;32:41-50). -Editor. *Ped Neur ОBriefs* Aug 1992.

HYPEREKPLEXIA REVISITED: CSF GABA LEVELS

The August 1992 issue of Ped Neur Briefs included 3 articles on hyperekplexia. An additional report from the Hammersmith Hospital, London illustrates the difficulties of clinical diagnosis of startle disease (hyperekplexia). At 1 hour after birth the infant had generalized jerks diagnosed as convulsions and treated with phenobarbitone. She had pronounced truncal hypotonia, but on day 3 she developed hypertonia in the limbs, exaggerated tendon reflexes, and jitteriness. The hypertonia diminished during sleep but increased when she was touched. Jerks and stiffening were precipitated by handling, tapping, and especially by turning to the prone position. Pyridoxine and phenobarbitone reduced the frequency and severity of the attacks but did not relieve the touch-induced myoclonus. Clonazepam introduced on day 28 controlled the symptoms. Forcible flexion of the infant also stopped the jerks and stiffening. The measurement of CSF GABA concentration may be helpful in the diagnosis. (Dubowitz LMS et al. Low cerebrospinal fluid concentration of free gamma aminobutyric acid in startle disease. Lancet July 11, 1992;340:80-81.) (Correspondence: Dr. L.M.S. Dubowitz, Department of Paediatrics and Neonatal Medicine, Hammersmith Hospital, Du Cane Road, London W12 OHS, UK.)

COMMENT. I am startled by the unexplained rash of recent articles on hyperekplexia! Ryan SG et al. have studied 4 large clonazepam responsive families with a hereditary hyperekplexia, using a panel of chromosome 5q polymorphic DNA markers. Multilocus linkage analysis in each family confirmed the previous chromosomal assignment of hyperekplexia to chromosome 5q. A mutation in a GABA-receptor subunit proposed as a cause of hyperekplexia is supported by the benzodiazepine responsiveness of the disorder.- Editor. *Ped Neur Briefs* Oct 1992.

TONIC UPGAZE OF CHILDHOOD

A child with intermittent upward deviation of the eyes is reported fron the Neuropediatric Unit CHUV, Lausanne, Switzerland. The boy was normal until nine months of age when brief intermittent upward eye deviation was noted and one month later these movements occurred for very long periods. At 14 months, vertical jerking of the eyes was associated with difficulty in downward gaze. He walked late at 16 months and fell often. When first examined at 21 months, the intermittent tonic upgaze lasted hours or days and was associated with a compensatory posture of the head, tilted with chin down. A downbeat nystagmus occurred when attempting to look down. His gait was wide-based and unsteady. The EEG, CT scan, NMR, and CSF exams were normal. The symptoms fluctuated and increased with fatigue and intercurrent illness. They were less marked in the morning on awakening from sleep. Treatment with acetazolamide was without effect. When last seen at 39 months of age the abnormal eye movements and head posture had almost resolved and the ataxia was mild. Since age 18 months he had had episodes of cyanosis, loss of contact, hypotonia, and falling, sometimes triggered by an emotional situation and resembling breathholding spells. (Deonna T et al. Benign paroxysmal tonic upgaze of childhood - a new syndrome. Neuropediatrics Nov 1990;21:213-214).

COMMENT. This syndrome was first described by Ouvrier RA and Billson MD (J Child Neurol 1988;3:177-180). These authors reported four cases. Ahn and Hoyt reported three infants with a similar syndrome (See Ped Neur Briefs Jan 1989). The eye movements are not seizures and improvement following levodopa therapy in one child suggests a closer analogy with dopa-sensitive dystonia. -Editor. *Ped Neur Briefs* May 1991.

PAROXYSMAL OCULAR DOWNWARD DEVIATION

Paroxysmal ocular downward deviation in 13 children with spastic quadriplegia, mental retardation and cortical visual impairment is reported from the Department of Pediatric Neurology, Seirei-Mikatabara General Hospital, Hamamatsu, Shizuoka, Japan. The ocular abnormality was observed in infancy, predominantly in pre-term infants and it resolves spontaneously in many by 2 years of age. The movement differed from the setting sun sign or tonic downward deviation and was not accompanied by retraction of the eyelids. No patient had hydrocephalus or kernicterus (Yokochi K. Paroxysmal ocular downward deviation in neurologically impaired infants. Pediatr Neurol Nov/Dec 1991;7:426-428).

(Correspondence: Dr. Yokochi, Department of Pediatric Neurology, Seirei-Mikatabara General Hospital, Mikatabara 3453, Hamamatsu, Shizuoka 433, Japan.)

COMMENT. The CT and MRI in these patients showed periventricular leukomalacia or multicystic encephalomalacia with involvement of optic radiations. Paroxysmal ocular downward deviation is proposed as a new sign of brain damage with central visual impairment, particularly in preterm infants.

Transient chronic upgaze differs from that of the transient variety of tonic downgaze deviation of the eyes in newborns, being more persistent and exacerbated by fatigue or illness (see Progress in Pediatric Neurology, Millichap JG,ed. 1991, p.139). -Editor. *Ped Neur Briefs* Feb 1992.

SHUDDERING ATTACKS

The successful treatment of shuddering attacks with a beta-adrenergic blocker (propranolol) in a 3 year old girl is reported from the Division of Pediatric Neurology, Children's Hospital of Philadelphia, University of Pennsylvania, Philadelphia PA. The girl was admitted with a 3 week history of shaking episodes described as jerking and shivering 5 to 6 times a day. There was no loss of consciousness. The problem was first diagnosed as a tic since eye blinking had also been present for several months. The family history was negative for tremor or other movement disorders. The neurological exam showed episodes of head flexion with adduction and flexion of the arms and knees without loss of consciousness or postural tone. Within 2 weeks of starting propranolol 0.5 mg/kg/d the movements had ceased. When therapy was discontinued 2 months later, the shuddering resumed within a week and responded once again to propranolol therapy at 1/2 the original dose. A second attempt to discontinue therapy resulted in a prompt return of the shuddering attacks and the necessity for further treatment (Barron TF, Younkin DP. Propranolol therapy for shuddering attacks. Neurology Jan 1992;42:258-259). (Reprints: Dr. Todd F. Barron, Division of Pediatric Neurology, The Milton S. Hershey Medical Center, P.O. Box 850, Hershey, PA 17033.)

COMMENT. It is proposed that the etiology and response to therapy of both essential tremor and shuddering attacks may be mediated by similar mechanisms. This appears to be the first report of successful treatment of shuddering attacks with propranolol. A family history of essential tremor has previously been reported in patients with shuddering spells and some manifested both shuddering and tremor (Vanasse M et al. Neurology 1976;26:1027). Shuddering attacks have also been related to an intolerance to monosodium glutamate in children (Reif-Leahrer L, Stemmermann MG. N Engl J Med 1975;293:1204). -Editor. *Ped Neur Briefs* Feb 1992.

FAMILIAL PAROXYSMAL ATAXIA: ACETAZOLAMIDE THERAPY

A dramatic response to acetazolamide in 3 patients with familial paroxysmal ataxia is reported from the Ipswich Hospital, Neurological Centre, Suffolk, England. Case 1 developed mild squint at 3 years and nystagmus at 6 years. Subsequently she experienced episodes of dysarthria, ataxia and vertigo often accompanied by nausea and vomiting and followed by headache and drowsiness. The attacks lasted from 2 to 24 hours and occurred every 2 weeks. When assessed at 26 years of age the attacks were occurring up to 5 times a week. The EEG was normal and an MRI showed atrophy of the superior cerebellar vermis. Acetazolamide 250 mg bid reduced attacks dramatically over an 8 month observation period. Cases 2 and 3, sons of Case 1, developed identical episodes at 1 year and 6 weeks of age, respectively. Both responded to acetazolamide. The father of the index case was ataxic and then chairbound for 13 years and died at age 67. This family was the first described in the U.K. but many may be mislabeled as epilepsy or migraine (Hawkes CH Familial paroxysmal ataxia: report of a family. J Neur Neurosurg and Psych March 1992;55:212-213.) (Correspondence: Dr. CH Hawkes, Ipswich Hospital, Neurological Centre, Heath Road, Ipswich, Suffolk IP4 5PD, England.)

COMMENT. Provisional diagnoses of basilar migraine and epilepsy had been made initially in two of these cases. The accurate diagnosis in one individual will often reveal similarly affected family members.

Inheritance is autosomal dominant. Acetazolamide is also effective in the treatment of paroxysmal dystonia (tonic seizures) as a presenting manifestation of multiple sclerosis (Sethi KD et al. Neurology April 1992;42:919-921). Koller W et al. have used acetazolamide successfully in the treatment of essential tremor (Neurology April 1992;42(Suppl 3):322). -Editor. *Ped Neur Briefs* May 1992.

FAMILIAL ALTERNATING HEMIPLEGIA

The familial occurrence and autosomal dominant inheritance of alternating hemiplegia of childhood is reported from Children's Hospital, and Massachusetts General Hospital, Harvard Medical School, Boston. Hemiplegic attacks without preceding seizure activity occurred in the proband, a 9-year old, developmentally retarded boy, during the first year of life. Choreoathetosis and dystonic posturing were noted between attacks. Father, brother, paternal uncle, and paternal grandmother had histories of- alternating hemiplegia. Stroke, neurodegenerative disease, and other causes were excluded. The karyotype showed a translocation, 46,XY,t(3;9)(p26;q34) in the patient and affected relatives. Flunarizine decreased attack frequency >70%. (Mikati MA et al. A syndrome of autosomal dominant alternating hemiplegia: Clinical presentation mimicking intractable epilepsy; chromosomal studies; and physiological investigations. Neurology Dec 1992;42: 2251-2257). (Reprints: Dr Mohamad Mikati, Department of Neurology, Division of Neurophysiology, Hunnewell 2, Children's Hospital, Boston, MA 02115).

COMMENT. This is the first description of truly familial alternating hemiplegia, a syndrome of unknown etiology. The authors favor neurovascular or metabolic, rather than epileptic mechanisms.

Sakuragawa N reports 23 cases in an excellent review article from the National Institute of Neuroscience, Ogawa Higashi-cho, Kodaira-shi, Tokyo 187, Japan (Brain Dev Sept 1992;14:283-8). The classification of alternating hemiplegia as a migraine variant is discussed. -Editor. *Ped Neur Briefs* Jan 1993.

NONEPILEPTIC SEIZURES DURING SLEEP

Nonepileptic (psychogenic or pseudo) seizures (NESs) were documented by video-electroencephalographic monitoring during apparent sleep in 12 patients reported from New York University School of Medicine, NY. Onset was in childhood in 6 patients, and age at testing ranged from 11 to 67 years (mean, 33 yr). In addition to NESs unassociated with ictal EEG changes, 3 patients had EEG interictal epileptiform discharges and 1 had a complex partial seizure during monitoring, distinct from NES. Most NESs occurred within 2 hours of falling asleep or awakening. Provocative testing with suggestion reproduced nocturnal attacks in 9 patients. Seizures reported during sleep are not necessarily epileptic in nature. (Thacker K et al. Nonepileptic seizures during apparent sleep. Ann Neurol April 1993;33:414-418). (Respond: Orrin Devinsky MD, Dept of Neurology, Hospital for Joint Diseases, 301 E 17th St, New York, NY 10003).

COMMENT. One-half of these patients had a history of childhood abuse. Four patients had evidence of epilepsy in addition to NESs.

The differential diagnosis in pseudoepileptic seizures is illustrated by case-reports from the Department of Neurology, University of Virginia Health Sciences Center, Charlottesville, VA. (Ozkara C, Dreifuss FE. Epilepsia March/April 1993;34:294-298). Epilepsy and pseudoepileptic seizures frequently coexist; the combination occurs in 20% before age 10 years and 60% after 10 years. Munchausen's syndrome often presents as pseudoepilepsy. Frontal lobe seizures have atypical patterns and may masquerade as pseudoseizures; these consist of thrashing, pedaling, kicking, or thrusting movements, an agitated appearance and utterance of loud expletives during sleep. -Editor. *Ped Neur Briefs* May 1993.

CHAPTER 2

MIGRAINE AND OTHER HEADACHES

INTRODUCTION

Advances in pediatric migraine and other headaches have involved studies of epidemiology, diagnostic criteria, pathophysiology, precipitating factors, including diet, and medical management. The sensitivity of the International Headache Society criteria for diagnosis of headache when applied to children and adolescents is restrictive, and modifications are necessary to accommodate certain symptomatologies and headache syndromes peculiar to children.

The management of headache in children is different from that in adults and requires a knowledge of the child's concepts of illness and pain. The long-term use of medication is undesirable, and relaxation techniques and dietary modification may be more effective and appropriate.-*Editor.*

DIAGNOSIS

INCIDENCE OF MIGRAINE HEADACHE

A population based study at the Mayo Clinic and

Olmsted County, Minnesota identified 629 residents with newly diagnosed migraine headache between 1979 and 1981. The age adjusted incidence was 137/100,000 person-years for males and 294/100,000 person-years for females. The highest incidence in females was at 20-24 years (689/100,000), and in males 10-14 years (246/100,000). The incidence increased 34% in women and 100% in men from 1979 to 1981. The majority of the cohort (81%) had migraine with aura or migraine without aura. The onset was associated with head trauma in 4% of male and 3% of female patients; it was associated with a particular food or drink in 3% of females and 7% of males . In 10 % of females the migraine attacks were related to menstruation, 2% had headaches associated with pregnancy, and 11% of females stated that oral contraceptives increased or initiated their migraine attacks. A childhood onset of migraine was found in 25% of males and in 12% of females affected. Of the 629 newly diagnosed patients in the study, 100 (15%) were less than 15 years of age. (Stang PE et al. Incidence of migraine headache: a population-based study in Olmsted County, Minnesota. Neurology Sept 1992;42:1657-1662.) (Reprints Dr. Paul E. Stang, Applied Healthcare Research, Glaxo Inc. Research Institute, 5 Moore Drive, CS 1130, Research Triangle Park, NC 27709.)

COMMENT. Bille in a 14 year longitudinal study of over 9000 school children found 11% (71 per 100,000 per year) to have developed migraine, an incidence in children far below that reported in the present study (Bille D. Migraine in school-children. Acta Paediat (Uppsala, suppl 136,1962)).

In a cross sectional epidemiological survey of a general population reported from Glostrup Hospital, Denmark, the prevalence of migraine without aura (common migraine) in the previous year was 6% and of migraine with aura (classic migraine) 4%. The prevalence of migraine without aura was significantly higher among women than among men, with a male-female ratio of 1:5. Sixty-three percent had episodic tension-type headache and 3% chronic tension-type headache. Tension-type headache in migraineurs was not significantly more prevalent than in non-migraineurs. The results support the view that migraine and tension-type headache are distinct entities. (Rasmussen BK et al. Interrelations between migraine and tension-type headache in the general population. Arch Neurol Sept 1992;49:914-918.)

An interesting article by a PNB subscriber, Dr. E.B. Russo, Western Montana Clinic, Missoula, MT (J Ethnopharmacol 1992;36:193-206), reviews the botanical treatments used for headache by 5 Indian tribes of the Ecuadorian Amazon. Several tribal peoples have developed a varied pharmacopoeia which includes many agents taken internally for headache treatment, a possible source for new antimigraine drugs. -Editor. *Ped Neur Briefs* Oct 1992.

MIGRAINE DIAGNOSES AND SYMPTOM PATTERNS

The diagnostic rates based on various criteria and symptom complexes of children and adolescents with chronic headache were evaluated in 88 consecutive patients who attended the Pediatric Headache Clinic at the University of Maryland School of Medicine, Baltimore, 1989-1991. Thc male/female ratio was 1 (43:45). The mean age 12.5 years; 44 Caucasian and 40 African-American. Clinical migraine was diagnosed in 63 (74%), of which only 14% were classic in type. Migraine versus non-migraine diagnoses were not related to age, gender, or race. When International, Prensky, Vahlquist, and the author's (Gladstein) criteria for migraine were used, the diagnosis was applied in only 50%. Prevalence of migraine diagnosis by the International criteria differed from the other classifications as a function of race, favoring Caucasians over African-American, 61% to 35%. Minority children were less likely to present with nausea, vomiting, lateralized pain, or food as a precipitant of headache. Children older than 12 years complained more often of radiating pain, scalp tenderness, and abdominal pain. Adolescent males reported higher rates of vomiting and decreased appetite than in females, while adolescent females found stress a more frequent precipitant. Older children and adolescents, especially females, used aspirin more frequently than those under 12 years of age. (Gladstein J et al. Diagnoses and symptom patterns in children presenting to a pediatric headache clinic. Headache Oct 1993;33:497-500). (Respond: Jack Gladstein MD, University of Maryland School of Medicine, Department of Pediatrics, Rm N5W70, 22 South Greene St, Baltimore, MD 21201).

COMMENT. These findings suggest that the International Headache Society criteria (1988) should be modified to increase their sensitivity to children and adolescents. Criteria at present proposed for the pediatric headache population should be reexamined.

In 100 consecutive children with chronic, recurrent headaches as a presenting complaint seen in a private office during a 2 year period, 42 were diagnosed as migraine, of which 27 (64%) were classified as classic migraine. These were hemicranial, associated with visual phenomena and/or nausea and vomiting, and the family history was positive in the majority. The 15 patients with common migraine had generalized headaches complicated by visual phenomena, nausea, or vomiting. Phenytoin controlled the migraine in 77%; the beneficial response was unrelated to EEG abnormalities. In this study, a unilateral location and family history were considered important criteria in the diagnosis of classic migraine. The character of the pain, throbbing or pulsating, emphasized in some classifications, was considered unreliable in children and was not included in diagnosis. (Millichap JG. Recurrent headaches in 100 children. Electroencephalographic abnormalities and response to phenytoin (Dilantin). Child's Brain 1978;4:95-104).

An uncommon EEG pattern, characterized by diffuse continuous beta activity, is described in an 8-year-old boy with recurrent migraine aura without headache from Ferrara University, Italy. (Soriani S et al. Headache Oct 1993;33:509-511). Epileptiform EEG discharges are not unusual in pediatric migraine patients. -Editor. *Ped Neur Briefs* Nov 1993.

EPISODIC MYDRIASIS AS MIGRAINE EQUIVALENT

A 14-year-old girl who presented with yearly attacks of bilateral internal ophthalmoplegia, nausea and headache since the age of 9 is the subject of a case report from the Department of Child Neurology, University Hospital Nijmegen, The Netherlands. She complained of blurred near vision when reading, associated with photophobia, phonophobia, nausea and aspirin-resistant bitemporal headaches. Attacks lasted 1 to 7 days. The pupils were symmetrically dilated during the attack and there was no response to direct or consensual light with complete loss of accommodation. The father and paternal aunt had migraine (van Engelen BGM et al. Bilateral episodic mydriasis as a migraine equivalent in childhood: a case report. Headache June 1991;31:375-377).

COMMENT. The authors note that ophthalmoplegic migraine with bilateral mydriasis has not previously been described in children. A single ischemic lesion localized in the central parasympathetic nucleus of Perlia and the Edinger-Westphal nuclei is proposed as the likely mechanism for the bilaterality of the mydriasis. Other causes including drugs, deodorant-antiperspirants, and perfumes were excluded.

Unusual clinical manifestations of migraine are reviewed by Ehrenberg BL in Seminars in Neurology June 1991;11:118-127. Some patients have headaches without aura, some have confusional spells, memory lapses and episodes of speech arrest resembling complex partial seizures. *Basilar migraine* is manifested by auras of vertigo, dysarthria, tinnitus, decreased hearing, diplopia, disturbances in both visual fields, bilateral sensory loss or weakness, or alterations in consciousness. The syndrome of benign epilepsy of childhood with occipital paroxysms is preceded by hallucinations or visual loss and associated with occipital spike-wave activity on interictal EEG. Episodes with auras or hallucinations lasting 5 to 60 minutes resemble migraine attacks. Numerous studies show a high incidence of EEG abnormalities in large populations of migraine patients (Millichap JG Child 's Brain 1978; 4:95-105). A beneficial response to phenytoin in this and other studies does not contraindicate a diagnosis of migraine. Migraine-epilepsy syndromes are reviewed by Andermann F. Boston: Butterworths 1987. These include epileptic seizures induced by a classic migraine aura and seen more often in children than in adults.-Editor. *Ped Neur Briefs* Oct 1991.

HEADACHE AND CHIARI TYPE I MALFORMATION

Headache was the presenting symptom in 5 of 6 patients with Chiari type malformation, reported from the Departments of Neurology and Neurosurgery, Trondheim University Hospital, Norway. Patient 1 had migraine headaches that started at age 22 during a first pregnancy. Patients 2 and 3, monozygotic twin daughters of patient 1, had headache and diplopia or vertigo, starting either at puberty or after the birth of a first child at the age of 20 years. Patients 4 and 5, daughters of patients 2 and 3, had pain in the neck and head. The diagnosis was made by MRI and confirmed at the time of surgery in 1 twin. The mother of patient 1 had severe headaches of undetermined cause. Whooping cough at the age of 2 weeks may have accentuated the degree of cerebellar herniation in 1 twin (Stovner LJ et al. The Chiari type I malformation in two monozygotic twins and first-degree relatives. Ann Neurol Feb 1992;31:220-222). (Correspondence: Dr. Stovner, Department of Neurology, Trondheim University Hospital, 7006 Trondheim, Norway.)

COMMENT. Chiari type I malformation should be considered in the diagnosis of headache presenting at puberty or during first pregnancies. Hormonal changes may accentuate the tonsillar herniation and precipitate the occurrence of symptoms. A herniation of at least 5 mm is clearly pathological and 3-5 mm represents a borderline zone. The significance of minor degrees of herniation in adolescents with recurrent migraine type headaches is a concern and requires careful follow-up .

Chiari type I malformation was the cause of a velopharyngeal insufficiency in a 5 year old girl reported from the Hopital Robert Debre, Paris, France (Gerard CL. Dev Med Child Neur Feb 1992;34:164-181). This child had denervation of the IX, X and XI cranial nerves, absent gag reflex, speech problem, but no complaint of headaches was recorded -Editor. *Ped Neur Briefs* April 1992.

CHILDHOOD CLUSTER HEADACHES

Cluster headaches similar to the typical adult form occurred in 35 patients at or before 18 years of age in a study from the Montefiore Medical Center and Schneider Children's Hospital, New York. The mean age at onset was 14 years (range 5-18). The delay from onset to diagnosis ranged from 0 to 34 years (mean 8 years). Pain was ocular in 88% and lacrimation occurred in 85%. Ptosis was present in 48% and nasal congestion in 60%. A family history of migraine occurred in 9 patients and a family history of cluster headaches in 3. The frequency and duration of cluster periods increased with age in 14. (Maytal J et al. Childhood onset cluster headaches. Headache June 1992;32:275-279) (Reprints: Dr. Joseph Maytal, Division of Pediatric Neurology, Schneider Children's Hospital, Long Island Jewish Medical Center, New Hyde Park, New York 11042.)

COMMENT. Familial cluster headache occurring in 3 generations is reported from the Brigham and Women's Hospital, Boston (Spierings ELH, Vincent AJPE. Neurology July 1992;42:1399-1400). The child, an 8-year-old boy, had suffered from headaches since age 4; the father age 42, and the paternal grandfather age 73, had cluster headache also. Three pairs of identical twins with cluster headache have been reported, suggesting a genetic factor in predisposition. (Roberge C et al. Headache 1987;27:299; Couturier EGM et al. Neurology 1991;41:761). -Editor. *Ped Neur Briefs* Aug 1992.

PATHOPHYSIOLOGY OF HEADACHE

PATHOPHYSIOLOGY OF VASCULAR HEAD PAIN

The mechanism of head pain, provocative stimuli, and receptors involved in drug treatment are reviewed from the Stroke Research Laboratory, Neurosurgery and Neurology, Massachusetts General Hospital, Boston, MA. A primitive defensive fiber network surrounds the brain and its blood vessels which is derived principally from trigeminal ganglia neurons. Headaches develop from activity within the trigeminal vascular system and are controlled by serotonin agonists that couple with 5-HT receptors on unmyelinated C fibers to block activity in the trigemino-vascular system. Neuropeptide release and neurogenic inflammation within the coverings of the brain are inhibited. Altered physiologic states (stress, fatigue), bright lights and sleep deprivation may precipitate migraine and act by modulating neuronal activity and synaptic events within cortical gray matter. Local increases in cortical blood flow modulated by trigemino-vascular fibers facilitate removal of potentially noxious chemicals. (Moskowitz MA. The visceral organ brain: Implications for the pathophysiology of vascular head pain. Neurology Feb 1991;41:182-186).

COMMENT. That vasospasm contributes to monosodium glutamate-induced headache has been demonstrated by Merritt JE and Williams PB in the Department of Pharmacology, Eastern Virginia Medical School, Norfolk, VA. (Headache Sept 1990;30:575-580). The direct effects of glutamate and its metabolite glutamine on arterial contractility were examined using rings of rabbit aorta. High concentrations of glutamate caused significant concentration dependent contractions. At high concentrations the calcium channel blocker Verapamil inhibited the glutamate response. Monosodium glutamate has a direct effect on peripheral arterial tone and may represent a serious health hazard to certain individuals with vascular disease.

A study of treatments used by patients for migraine prior to attending the City of London Migraine Clinic showed that alternative medical treatments were popular including acupuncture, hypnotherapy, homeopathy, feverfew, osteopathy, yoga, and vitamin supplements. The authors emphasize the importance of an accurate history of all medications used, whether prescribed or over-the-counter. (MacGregor EA et al. Headache Sept 1990;30:571-574). -Editor. *Ped Neur Briefs* April 1991.

BLOOD MAGNESIUM LEVELS IN MIGRAINE

Serum and erythrocyte magnesium levels were screened between attacks in patients with migraine without aura (n=38) and with aura (n=6) and for comparison, in a group of patients suffering from chronic tension-type headache (n=25) as well as a group of control patients (n=19) at the Headache Unit, Citadelle University of Liege, Liege, Belgium. Serum magnesium levels were not significantly different between the four groups of patients, whereas magnesium levels in erythrocytes were significantly reduced in the group of migraineurs without aura (1.87) compared with those with aura (2.1), patients with tension-type headache (2.03) and the controls (2.12). Normal values in the laboratory ranged from 2-2.8 mmol/l in erythrocytes (Schoenen J. et al. Blood magnesium levels in migraine. Cephalagia May 1991;11:97-99).

COMMENT. The correlation between magnesium levels and migraine pathophysiology is speculative. The possible importance of magnesium in migraine is suggested by the finding of reduced magnesium in white blood cells in women with premenstrual syndrome and headaches and the benefits of oral treatment with magnesium in premenstrual headaches. The authors hypothesize that the reduction in erythrocyte magnesium may be due to an abnormal regulation of intracellular magnesium in migraine patients.-Editor. *Ped Neur Briefs* July 1991.

ESTROGENS, PROGESTINS, AND HEADACHE

Approaches to the therapy of hormone-related headaches are reviewed from the Department of Neurology, Temple University School of Medicine and the Comprehensive Headache Center at Germantown Hospital, Philadelphia, PA, and the Reproductive Endocrine Unit, National Institute of Child Health and Human Development, NIH, Bethesda, MD. Migraine can occur before, during, or after menstruation, or at the time of ovulation. During menstruation, it is often associated with dysmenorrhea and before or during menstruation, migraine is frequently refractory to treatment. These are the times of greatest fluctuation in estrogen levels. The primary trigger of menstrual migraine appears to be the withdrawal of estrogen rather than progesterone. Changes in the sustained estrogen levels with pregnancy (increased) and menopause (decreased) can result in changes in headache frequency and intensity. Women who have migraine exclusively with their menses can be treated by the perimenstrual use of prophylactic medication (antidepressants, beta-blockers, calcium channel blockers, or methysergide). The efficacy of pyridoxine and diuretics has not been established in double-blind studies. Ergotamine tartrate at bedtime or twice a day is an effective prophylactic agent. Headache associated with oral contraceptive use or menopausal hormonal replacement therapy may be related in part to periodic discontinuation of estrogens. Oral contraceptives can induce, change, or alleviate headache. They can trigger the first migraine attack, most often in women with a family history of migraine. Stopping the contraceptive may not bring immediate headache relief and there may be a delay of one-half to one year or no improvement (Silverstein S D, Merriam G R Estrogens, progestins, and headache, Neurology June 1991;41:786-793).

COMMENT. The influence of the menstrual cycle on migraine in older children and adolescents requires further evaluation and attention. The first migraine attack may be triggered by oral contraceptives and this possible cause should be considered in adolescent girls with migraine. -Editor. *Ped Neur Briefs* July 1991.

MIGRAINE AND EPILEPSY: INFANTILE ONSET

The coexistence of classical migraine, visual phenomena and seizures and occipital spike-wave complexes in the EEG are reported in 14 children from the Department of Neurological Sciences, University La Sapienza, Rome, Italy. The age of onset was 3 to 9 years (mean age 5.4 years) and the clinical and EEG follow-up ranged from 4 to 16 years (mean 11.2 years). Visual phenomena were described as bright rings, bands, red-colored disks, in both visual fields or in the visual hemifield opposite the spike-wave localization. Amaurosis followed the appearance of the phosphenes. In some patients the migraine with aura and epilepsy were chronologically related phenomena; migraine might occur immediately before or after seizures; migraine may act as a triggering factor for epilepsy. In others, visual phenomena either preceded migraine with aura or occurred as an isolated event or even preceded epileptic seizures (De Romanis F et al. Migraine and epilepsy with infantile onset and electroencephalographic findings of occipital spike-wave complexes. Headache June 1991;31:378-383).

COMMENT. In 50% of the patients in this study, migraine with aura, with phosphenes and amaurosis as prodromal symptoms, replaces epileptic seizures when they disappear or improve following antiepileptic treatment. Ergot alkaloids or pizotifen were of little or no benefit whereas migraine with aura responded to antiepileptic treatment. Occipital epilepsy in childhood in this study was not benign and seizures were controlled by antiepileptic treatment in only 2 subjects

Migraine and pregnancy is reviewed by Uknis A and Silberstein SD in the same issue of Headache 1991;31:372-374. A first attack of migraine with unilateral parasthesias and blurred vision occurred in a 27-year-old woman during the first trimester and led to the diagnosis of her pregnancy. Pre-existing migraine usually improves with pregnancy, whereas relapse frequently occurs in the post-partum period.

Children born to migraineurs have no increased incidence of birth defects. -Editor. *Ped Neur Briefs* Oct 1991.

HEADACHE AND DEPRESSION

A history of maternal depression and migraine was significantly more common and proportionately higher in children with abdominal migraine and recurrent abdominal pain in a study from Birmingham, England. At a structured interview with a printed recording sheet, 27% of mothers gave a lifetime history of migraine. Mothers of children in the headache group gave a history of migraine 1.5 times more often than in controls. A total of 21% of mothers gave a lifetime history of depression. Significantly more mothers had a history of depression in the headache, migraine, recurrent abdominal pain and abdominal migraine groups than in controls. (Mortimer MJ et al. Does a history of maternal migraine or depression predispose children to headache and stomachache? Headache July 1992;32:353-355.)

COMMENT. This study emphasizes the need to assess the mother when treating children with headache or recurrent abdominal pain. In a study of 28 patients aged between 13 - 18 years with chronic daily headache seen at The Germantown Hospital, Philadelphia, PA, 86% were diagnosed with depression. Antidepressant medication, biofeedback and psychotherapy were recommended. (Kaiswer RS. Depression in adolescent headache patients. Headache July 1992;32:340-344) Dr. J.N. Blau of the National Hospitals for Nervous Diseases, Queen Square, London comments that "in migraine the plethora of theories provoke profound intellectual dissatisfaction" and that migraine may be a protective phenomenon (JRSM Oct 1992;85:593-594).-Editor. *Ped Neur Briefs* Oct 1992.

HEADACHE AS FIRST SYMPTOM OF CEREBRAL TUMOR

Five children, ranging in age from 10 months to 4 years, all presenting initially with headache, with or without vomiting, and in whom the final diagnosis was intracranial tumor, are reported from Petah Tiqva, Israel. The initial neurologic examination, including the fundi, was normal in three patients with craniopharyngioma, pinealoma, and cerebellar astrocytoma. Two patients with medulloblastoma and fourth ventricle choroid plexus papilloma had abnormal neurologic findings at presentation. The authors stress the need for neuroimaging studies in children younger than 4 years of age who have headache, especially if accompanied by vomiting, even if the neurologic exam is normal. (Straussberg R, Amir J. Headaches in children younger than 7 years: are they really benign? Arch Neurol Feb 1993;50:130 [Letter to the Editor]).

COMMENT. In response, Shinnar S and Chu ML emphasize that a presenting complaint of headache, even in young children, is generally associated with a benign clinical syndrome, and a neuroimaging study is not always necessary or advisable. The heavy sedation required for the MRI in this age group and risks of an adverse reaction to contrast medium with CT must be weighed against the benefits of the study. They agree with Honig PJ and Charney E (AJDC 1982;136:121) that headache as the sole manifestation of brain tumor is very uncommon in young children.

Headache in young children is not only a problem in evaluation but also in recognition as a significant isolated symptom. Clinical acumen and careful judgement are required in decisions, 1) to advise a neurologic consultation, and 2) to order sophisticated or invasive tests. The pediatric neurologist usually has the benefit of a pediatrician's knowledge of the child and family and his decision to seek a second opinion. Notwithstanding the relatively rare occurrence of cerebral tumor in children who present with headache, uncomplicated by some other manifestation, the pediatric neurologist's first duty is to exclude the more serious diagnoses. The value of the electroencephalogram as an important preliminary test in the diagnosis and localization of intracranial tumors of children should not be forgotten. (Millichap JG,

Backus RE et al. Neurology May 1962;12:329).-Editor. *Ped Neur Briefs* March 1993.

MOYAMOYA AND HEMIPLEGIC MIGRAINE

A 6-year-old girl presenting with a 6-month history of classical familial migraine, complicated by transitory hemiparesis and moyamoya disease diagnosed by MRI, is reported from the Kaiser Permanente Medical Center, Hayward, CA. Headaches occurred each week and were associated with nausea, vomiting, and photophobia. She awoke on 3 occasions with right-sided weakness, numbness, and garbled speech. All symptoms resolved after two hours of sleep. Neurologic exam was normal between attacks. MRI showed bilateral occlusion of the carotid arteries and increased vascularity of collateral vessels in the basal ganglia, consistent with moyamoya. (Bernstein AL Hemiplegic migraine and moyamoya disease. AJDC July 1993;147:718-719). (Respond: Dr Bernstein, Dept of Neurology, Kaiser Permanente Medical Center, 27400 Hesperian Blvd, Hayward, CA 94545).

COMMENT. Children with a diagnosis of hemiplegic migraine may have a vascular malformation or moyamoya disease as the underlying pathology. The clinical course depends on the rapidity and extent of vascular occlusion and the ability to develop a collateral circulation. Early diagnosis and surgical revascularization have been advocated because of the risk of permanent neurologic deficits. (See Ped Neur Briefs July 1987, and Progress in Pediatric Neurology, Chicago, PNB Publ, 1991, pp389-391). -Editor. *Ped Neur Briefs* July 1993.

MIGRAINE PRECIPITANTS

CHOCOLATE IS A MIGRAINE-PROVOKING AGENT

Patients with migraine who believe that chocolate could provoke their attacks were challenged with either chocolate or a closely matching placebo in a double-blind parallel group study at the Princess Margaret Migraine Clinic, Charing Cross Hospital,

London, England. The placebo contained no cocoa butter or cocoa powder and the carob powder used in the placebo was also added to the chocolate and successfully disguised by the use of a peppermint-masking flavor. The two groups of patients, all adults, were matched for age and sex and all were drug-free for at least 48 hours prior to investigation. Chocolate ingestion (40 gram bar) was followed by a typical migraine episode in 5 out of 12 patients, while none of the 8 patients challenged with placebo had an attack (P=.051). The median time interval to onset of symptoms following chocolate consumption was 22 hours (range 3.5-27 hours) (Gibb C.M., Rose F.C. et al. Chocolate is a migraine provoking agent, Cephalalgia May 1991;11:93-95)

COMMENT. In a double-blind challenge study in children referred with severe headache, 82 of 99 patients responded to an oligoantigenic diet (Egger J et al. Lancet 1983;2:865). Relapses occurred in 74 on the introduction of one or more food stuffs, with chocolate provoking attacks in 30%. Methyl-zanthine, theobromine and phenolic compounds including catechin are some pharmacologically active compounds found in relatively large amounts in chocolate. The relevant chemical agent responsible for initiating a migraine attack requires to be elucidated. My own clinical experience in children suggests that chocolate is a common precipitating factor in migraine susceptible patients. The effects of eliminating chocolate and caffeine containing drinks should be investigated before long-term drug treatment is considered. -Editor. *Ped Neur Briefs* July 1991.

ICE CREAM HEADACHE

The characteristics of cold induced headaches in a group of migraine patients were compared with the usual migraine headaches and with cold induced headaches in a control population, in a study using a retrospective questionnaire at the City of London Migraine Clinic, London, England. The control patients were preclinical medical and dental student volunteers. Seventeen percent of the migraine patients and 46% of the students developed headache following palatal application or a swallow of ice cream. "Ice cream headache" was less common in migraine patients than the controls, and the pattern of the headache induced by ice cream was similar in the 2 groups. Only 2 of the 12 migraine patients who developed ice cream headache on testing experienced the headache at a similar site to their usual migraines (Bird N, MacGregor EA, Wilkinson MIP. Ice cream headache - site, duration, and relationship to migraine. Headache Jan 1992;32:35-38). (Reprints: Dr. E. Anne MacGregor, The City of London Migraine Clinic, 22 Charterhouse Square, London ECIM 6DX, England.)

COMMENT. This study suggests that ice cream headache is common but may be less common in migraine patients than the general population. These findings are in contrast to some previous studies showing that 93% of migraine patients reported ice cream headaches compared with 31% of non headache controls (Raskin NH, Knittle SC Headache 1976;16:222-225).

The precipitating factors noted in 6 of 51 Nigerian children with migraine were fatigue in 3, lack of sleep in 2, and milk chocolate drink in 1. Ice cream was not noted as migraine precipitant in this study from Kano, Nigeria (Okogbo ME. Migraine in nigerian children: a study of 51 patients. Headache Nov 1991;31:673-676). Haemoglobin genotype obtained in 41 cases was AA in 66% and AS in 34%. The prevalence of haemoglobin AS was higher than in the general population (25%). -Editor. *Ped Neur Briefs* April 1992.

MANAGEMENT OF HEADACHE

A DEVELOPMENTAL PERSPECTIVE OF TREATMENT

Developmental issues related to the assessment and treatment of childhood headache are discussed from the Department of Psychology, University of South Alabama, Mobile, Alabama. The three major areas of development are cognitive, self-regulation, and psychosocial development. Young children use "what", "where", and "who" before they can use "how", "why", and "when". "What is a headache?" is more likely to produce an intelligible response than "How do people get headaches?" Knowing the child's explanation of headache will help provide better explanations of medical and psychological procedures for children. Children's reports of the quality of headache pain are variable and may be exaggerated in the 9 to 11 age group and minimized in the 6 to 8 year olds. The headache record is the predominant outcome measure for determining treatment success, and the diary format should divide the day according to relevant and easily remembered events of meals and bedtime. An open ended format for measuring intensity such as a vertical thermometer scale is preferred to a fixed response scale of 0-5 that assumes equal increments in intensity. Headache duration might be compared to the length of a favorite television show, recess, or other activity rather than actual time estimates which may be problematic for children. "Before" and "after" are confusing for preschoolers although they understand the concepts of "first" and "last".

A shift from an external health locus of control to the acknowledgement of one's own role in headache control occurs with increasing age. Treatments that incorporate self-regulation such as autogenic thermal feedback training require an understanding of an internal control mechanism. From a medical perspective the foundation for self-management and self-regulation of behavior develops as the child applies autonomy to managing the external world. Awareness of autonomy, initiative and industry issues may facilitate successful treatment of childhood headache. A shift in family attention to headache free days could be a strong treatment reinforcer for children, focusing less attention on the headaches. (Marcon RA, Labbe EE. Assessment and treatment of children's headaches from a developmental perspective. Headache Sept 1990;30:586-592).

COMMENT Adding a developmental perspective to

psychological interventions in the management of childhood headache is likely to increase treatment effectiveness. The management of headache in children is different from that of adults and requires an assessment of cognitive and affective development and a knowledge of children's concepts of illness and pain. Factors in precipitating headaches such as diet and exercise may be more important in children than in adults and will require special attention. The use of long-term investigational medications in children is undesirable and relaxation techniques and dietary modification may be more effective and appropriate. -Editor. *Ped Neur Briefs* April 1991.

SUMATRIPTAN IN ACUTE MIGRAINE

The efficacy of oral sumatriptan 100 mg in 61 patients with acute migraine was assessed in a double blind, randomized, placebo-controlled, crossover study at the Department of Neurology, The Prince Henry and Prince of Wales Hospitals, Sydney, and Austin Hospital and Repatriation General Hospital, Melbourne, Australia. The International Headache Society guidelines were used in diagnosis. The youngest patients were 18 years (mean 39 years) and all had 1 to 6 migraine attacks, with or without aura, per month for at least one year. Current prophylactic treatment was continued during the trial in 30% of the 47 patients analyzed. The response rate was significantly greater with sumatriptan than with placebo, 51% vs 10%. Rescue medication was needed at two hours in 41% and 88%, respectively. Of 28 patients who were headache-free at 2 hours after sumatriptan, 11 (39%) had a recurrence of headache within 24 hours. A tight feeling or tingling sensation in the head was the commonest side effect (Goadsby PJ et al. Oral sumatriptan in acute migraine. Lancet Sept 28 1991;338:782-783).

COMMENT. Sumatriptan is a 5-hydroxytryptamine agonist found superior to ergotamine in a previous multi-national study (Eur Neurol 1991;31:314-22). Trials in children are under consideration and FDA approval is in progress (now approved).

The International Headache Society guidelines for diagnosis of migraine used in the above study are complex and have not been widely adopted in clinical practice. Diagnostic criteria for practicing physicians are proposed by Solomon S and Lipton RB (Headache 1991;31:384-387). The criteria proposed for office diagnosis of migraine without aura (common migraine) are as follows (any two of the four features): (1) headache - unilateral; (2) headache - pulsating quality; (3) associated nausea; (4) associated photophobia or phonophobia. If preceded within one hour by visual, sensory, or motor symptoms lasting 5 to 60 minutes the headaches are diagnosed as migraine with aura (classical migraine). Organic disease must be ruled out and the patient should have had several similar attacks in the past. Tension type headache is usually diagnosed by negative criteria and by ruling out migraine, cluster headache and headaches due to organic disease. Cluster headaches are differentiated from migraine by the frequency of attacks (daily) and the associated autonomic symptoms (ipsilateral conjunctival injection, tearing, nasal congestion, ptosis or miosis).- Editor. *Ped Neur Briefs* Oct 1991.

CHAPTER 3

ATTENTION DEFICIT, BEHAVIOR, AND LEARNING DISORDERS

INTRODUCTION

Martha Bridge Denckla, M.D.
Johns Hopkins University, Baltimore, MD

Most research in learning disabilities (LD) continues to focus on reading disability (RD) which remains the prototype. The validity of defining RD or LD by the discrepancy formula approach continues to be questioned. For RD, there is no demonstrable difference in neuropsychological (i.e., information-processing) deficits associated with discrepancy-based as compared with those of poor readers who have IQs close to their reading level. By extension to LD in general, most clinicians and researchers doubt that calculating a "gap" between IQ and achievement will reveal the biological nature of arithmetic or written language disability. The neuropsychological approach to "nonverbal learning disabilities," exemplified by Rourke, is relevant to totally nonacademic (i.e., social) aspects of learning and the autistic-like Asperger's syndrome.

Reading Disability (RD), also called "dyslexia," is generally and consensually understood to be based upon phonological impairments. Despite the many replications of the phonological-linguistic basis of dyslexia and its anatomic-physiologic correlates (anomalous right-left asymmetry, local functional displacement from left temporal to left parietal cortex) a recrudescent issue about visual processes in dyslexia divides the field. Neither the report of *peripheral* (non-central) visual superiority of adult dyslexic subjects nor the report of magnocellular-related transient visual evoked potential deficit in adult dyslexic subjects has withstood attempts to replicate the results. Hence, at present not even these highly sophisticated attempts to define visual system deficits in dyslexia have succeeded in changing the prevailing view (phonolinguistic) of the biological correlates of poor reading. A related and persistent problem is the overlap between RD (or *any* LD) with ADD(H), exemplified by the finding that spelling disability and hyperactivity demonstrate shared genetic etiology.

Attention Deficit Hyperactivity Disorder (ADDH). As of May 1994, in the DSM IV, the "H" will again become detachable (hence the use of ADDH rather than ADHD as abbreviation). Conceptually, there has been a shift towards empasizing deficits in the executive or "top-down" aspects of attention, the executive control and response preparation systems; even "sustained attention" as a basic deficit has lost support. The scrutiny in cognitive neuroscience of such output-related processes has led to a fronto-striatal emphasis in MRI studies of the possible structural basis for ADDH. Several studies still in press, using volumetric approaches to MRI regions of interest, have demonstrated that some portions of basal ganglia are smaller in ADDH population samples (although left versus right and caudate versus globus pallidus are controversies yet to be resolved). Width measurements of MRI sections have revealed that right frontal area fails to be asymmetrically larger (as in normal) in ADDH subjects. PET scans of ADDH adults (but not adolescents) are concordant, with reduced metabolism most prominent right-frontally (interestingly, a small female adolescent ADDH subgroup did show a brain metabolic deficit with frontal prominence). The heterogeneity within the diagnostic category ADDH, even when "H" is again a separable component, continues to be a problem in design and interpretation of anatomic and physiological studies. The overlap with LD means that anterior-posterior ratios cannot be interpreted unless pure subject groups are studied. Many studies of LD are "contaminated" by ADDH-related findings, but the reverse is also true (albeit less openly acknowledged). That is, if LD (especially RD) is referable to left posterior deficits and ADDH to right frontostriatal deficits, inclusion of mixed LD/ADDH subjects obscures localization effects. - *Martha Bridge Denckla, M.D., Learning Disabilities Research Center, Kennedy-Krieger Institute, Baltimore, MD.*

BIBLIOGRAPHY

Bjaalid I-K, Hoien T, Lundberg I. Letter identification and lateral masking in dyslexic and normal readers. Scand J Educ Res 1993;37:151-161.

Castellanos FX, Giedd JN, Eckburg BS, Marsh WL et al. Quantitative morphology of the caudate nucleus in attention-deficit hyperactivity disorder. Am J Psychiatry 1994; in press.

Corkum PV, Siegel LS. Is the continuous performance task a valuable research tool for use with children with attention-deficit-hyperactivity disorder? J Child Psychol Psychiatry 1993;34:1217-1239.

Harnadek MCS, Rourke BP. Principal identifying features of the syndrome of nonverbal learning disabilities in children. J Learning Disab 1994;27:144-154.

Kushch A, Gross-Glenn K, Jallad B, Lubs H et al. Temporal lobe surface area measurements on MRI in normal and dyslexic readers. Neuropsychologia 1993;31:811-821.

Riccio CA, Hynd GW, Cohen MJ, Gonzalez JJ et al. Neurological basis of attention deficit hyperactivity disorder. Special issue: Issues in the education of children with attention deficit disorder. Except Child 1993;60:118-124.

Siegel LS. Phonological processing deficits as the basis

of a reading disability. Special issue: Phonological processes and learning disability. Developmental Rev 1993;13:246-257.

Stevenson J, Pennington BF, Gilger JW, DeFries JC et al. Hyperactivity and spelling disability: testing for shared genetic etiology. J Child Psychol Psychiat 1993;34:1137-1152.

Swanson HL. Executive processing in learning-disabled readers. Intelligence 1993;17:117-149.

Van der Meere JJ, Vreeling HJ, Sergeant JA. A motor presetting experiment in hyperactive, learning-disabled and control children. J Child Psychol Psychiatry 1992;33:1347-1354.

Victor JD, Conte MM, Burton L, Nass RD. Visual evoked potentials in dyslexics and normals: failure to find a difference in transient or steady state responses. Visual Neurosci 1993;10:939-946.

Zametkin AJ, Liebenauer LL, Fitzgerald GA, King AC et al. Brain metabolism in teenagers with attention deficit hyperactivity disorder. Arch Gen Psychiatry 1993;50:333-340.

Zametkin AJ, Nordahl TE, Gross M, King AC et al. Cerebral glucose metabolism in adults with hyperactivity of childhood onset. N Engl J Med 1990;323:1361-1366.

ETIOLOGY AND PATHOPHYSIOLOGY

ETIOLOGY OF ATTENTION DEFICIT DISORDERS

Familial-genetic factors in the etiology of attention deficit disorder (ADDH) were studied in 145 children who met the DSM-III criteria at the Neuropediatrics Unit, Shaare Zedek Medical Center, Jerusalem, Israel. Boys outnumbered girls by 3:1. 30% of ADDH children had siblings with LD, compared to 6.7% in 30 normal children. 34% of ADDH children were of North African descent which comprised only 12 % of the population in Jerusalem. ADDH was correlated with delayed language development and intrauterine growth retardation. No correlation was found between ADDH and numerous pre- and peri-natal factors, IQ, parental age, years of education, profession, and language spoken at home (Gross-Tsur V et al. Attention deficit disorder: association with familial-genetic factors. Ped Neurol July/Aug 1991;7:258-261).

COMMENT. A familial-genetic factor has been implicated in the etiology of ADHD in previous studies and the present report supports this finding. The familial-genetic factor was expressed by the male preponderance, the increased frequency of learning disabilities in siblings and an ethnic propensity. A delay in language development should alert the pediatrician to the possible development of ADHD and the need for early intervention programs. The benefits of early educational programs for parents concerning methylphenidate in the treatment of ADHD are demonstrated in a report from The Children's Hospital of Michigan, Detroit (Liu C et al. Social acceptability of methylphenidate and behavior modification for treating attention deficit hyperactivity disorder. Pediatrics Sept 1991;88:560-565). Before educational intervention, families rated behavior modification as the most acceptable and methylphenidate as the least acceptable method of management. After 3-1/2 months experience with interventions for their children there was a significant increase in acceptability of methylphenidate related to the parental education about ADHD. -Editor. *Ped Neur Briefs* Oct 1991.

ADHD AND THYROID HORMONE RESISTANCE

The presence and severity of attention deficit-hyperactivity disorder (ADHD) in 104 members of 18 families with a history of generalized resistance to thyroid hormone were evaluated at the National Institutes of Health, Bethesda, MD, using structured interviews. Of 49 affected with a mutant thyroid receptor gene and reduced responsiveness to thyroid hormone and 55 unaffected family members, 52 were adults and 52 were children. Among adults, ADHD was present in 11 of 22 (50%) with thyroid resistance and in 2 of 30 (7%) without. Among children, 19 of 27 (70%) resistant to thyroid hormone and 5 of 25 (20%) nonresistant subjects met the criteria for ADHD. The likelihood of having ADHD was 15 times higher for adults with generalized resistance to thyroid hormone than for unaffected family members, and 10 times higher for affected children. Male subjects, both affected and unaffected, had a risk of ADHD three times higher than females. (Hauser P et al. Attention deficit-hyperactivity disorder in people with generalized resistance to thyroid hormone. N Engl J Med April 8, 1993;328: 997-1001). (Reprints: Dr Hauser, Molecular and Cellular Endocrinology Branch, Nat Inst of Diabetes, NIH, Bldg 10, Rm 8D-14, 9000 Rockville Pike, Bethesda, MD 20892).

COMMENT. The criteria for diagnosis of thyroid hormone resistance were as follows: 1) normal or elevated serum thyrotropin concentrations, 2) elevated serum T3 and T4, and 3) resistance of peripheral tissues to thyroid. Although this genetic thyroid disorder may be uncommon in ADHD, studies of thyroid function should be included more frequently in the clinical evaluation of hyperactive children.-Editor. *Ped Neur Briefs* April 1993.

ANATOMY OF MEMORY

Studies of the anatomy and function of the brain system for memory in humans and animal models are reviewed from the Veterans Affairs Medical Center, San Diego and the Department of Psychiatry, University of California, San Diego, La Jolla, CA. Patients who underwent temporal lobe surgery developed memory impairment only when the removal extended far enough posteriorly to include the hippocampus and the parahippocampal gyrus. Horel proposed that memory functions were disrupted not by hippocampal damage but by damage to temporal stem white matter adjacent to the hippocampus. Damage to both the hippocampus and the amygdala was required to produce severe amnesia in monkeys and humans. A circumscribed bilateral lesion involving the entire rostro-caudal extent of the CAl field of the hippocampus caused memory impairment in the absence of other cognitive dysfunction. By use of the high resolution MRI the hippocampal region was found to be shrunken and atrophic in 4 amnesic patients while the temporal lobe was of normal size.

Memory is classified as declarative (explicit) or non-declarative (implicit). *Declarative memory* refers to recollection of facts and events and depends on the integrity of the medial temporal lobe. *Non-declarative memory* refers to a collection of skills, habits, priming, conditioning and non-associated learning, all of which are non-conscious recollections, and is independent of the medial temporal lobe. The medial temporal lobe memory system is essential for establishing long-term memory for facts and events and is needed to bind together the distributed storage sites in neocortex that represent a whole memory. As time passes after learning, memory stored in the neocortex gradually becomes independent of the medial temporal lobe structures and the role of this system in memory is only temporary. More permanent memory develops presumably as a result of slow synaptic change and in concert with normal forgetting. The process by which the burden of long-term permanent memory storage is gradually assumed by the neocortex assures that the medial temporal lobe system is always available for the acquisition of new information. (Squire LR, Zola-Morgan S. The medial temporal lobe memory system. Science Sept 20, 1991;253:1380-1385).

COMMENT: The article refers to a neuropsychological evaluation of a patient, H.M., with a profound and a selective impairment in human memory after bilateral surgical removal of the medial temporal lobe (Scoville WB, Milner B. J Neurol Neurosurg Psychiatry 1957;20:11). A reference to Marcel Proust's novel of the mind "The Remembrance of Things Past," is made in an editorial by Hilts PJ in The New York Times Sept 24, 1991. Proust's memory of a town and gardens was triggered by the pleasures of a morsel of cake soaked in a spoonful of warm tea, a mechanism involving the amygdala.-Editor. *Ped Neur Briefs* Oct 1991.

PREDICTORS OF COGNITIVE AND MOTOR DEVELOPMENT

The relative effects of 4 major areas of adversity on early cognitive and motor development were examined in approximately 1,000 children at age 5 years in the Department of Paediatrics and Child Health, University of Otago Medical School, Dunedin, New

Zealand. The 4 areas of adversity examined were perinatal complications, family background, child rearing practices, and physical health. The effects on cognitive ability were measured by IQ, receptive language and expressive language. Girls' cognitive ability and motor ability in early childhood were not related to the number of perinatal complications present during pregnancy or birth but were affected by adverse family background conditions and child rearing practices. Girls' language ability was unrelated to the number of health problems at age 3. In boys, IQ scores, receptive language and motor ability were related to the index of perinatal complications; and family background and child rearing affected IQ, receptive language and motor ability scores. Health index affected motor ability in both boys and girls. (Stanton WR et al. Indices of perinatal complications, family background, child rearing and health as predictors of early cognitive and motor development. Pediatrics Nov 1991;8:954-959.)

(Reprints Dr Stanton, Dept Paediatrics, University of Otago Medical School, Box 913, Dunedin, New Zealand)

COMMENT. In summary, the perinatal complications index was not generally predictive of cognitive ability and motor ability outcomes and the health index was predictive mainly of motor ability. Family background and child rearing were predictive of IQ and receptive language scores. Boys are more susceptible to biological and psychological stress than girls. The results support a concept of a continuum of adversity in the areas of perinatal complications, family background, child rearing, and health during early development of learning and motor ability.- Editor. *Ped Neur Briefs* Jan 1992.

LEARNING DISABILITIES AND FRONTAL LOBE DAMAGE

Tho adult patients age 31 and 26 years who suffered bilateral prefrontal damage early in life and who subsequently presented with severe aberrant behavior, are reported from the Division of Behavioral Neurology and Neuroscience of the Harvard Neurology

Department and Beth Israel Hospital, Boston, MA. One patient had a subdural hematoma and a collection over the left frontal lobe in the first week of life and the second patient suffered bilateral skull fractures and a right frontal hematoma in an automobile accident at four years of age. Neurological and neuropsychological examinations indicated the principal site of involvement was located bilaterally in the frontal lobes. Both patients had impulsive behavior triggered by stimulus, they performed with childish abandon and shallow foresight and neither was able to learn from negative experience or punishnent. They were socially isolated, had little sense of remorse, empathy, or fairness toward others but instead felt victimized. Environmental factors did not account for their lifelong behavioral problems and prolonged psychotherapy and medications were without benefit. In comparison with severe deficits of conportment. judgment and insight, neither patient displayed limiting deficits of language, memory, or visuospatial skills. The behavioral features were qualitatively similar but quantitatively more intense than behavioral deficits acquired in adulthood as a consequence of bilateral frontal lobe lesions. (Price BH et al. The comportmental learning disabilities of early frontal lobe damage. Brain Oct 1990;113:1383-1393).

COMMENT. A battery of developmental psychology tests showed that social and moral development of these two patients was arrested at an immature stage. The learning disability associated with bilateral prefrontal lesions acquired early in life is characterized by deficits in maturation of judgment, insight, foresight, abstract reasoning, perspective taking, empathy, and moral development. The predominantly behavioral presentation in the absence of focal neurological signs may lead to the erroneous impression that underlying factors are primarily psychiatric or environmental. The EEGs of both patients were normal whereas the MRIs showed bilateral frontal lobe lesions. The WAIS-R was average in one patient and borderline to low average in the second patient.

Mesulan M-Marsel, an author of the above paper, writes in Neurologic Progress (Ann Neurol Nov 1990;28:597-613) on "Largescale neurocognitive networks and distributed processing for attention, language, and memory." The neurons of the CNS operate to receive sensory signals from outside and fron within (input), they plan and execute motor acts (output), and govern intermediary processing between input and output. Thought, language, selective attention, memory, and advanced cognition and comportment are the products of intermediary processing networks located primarily in limbic and association areas. Complex behavior is mapped at the level of multifocal neural systems rather than specific anatomical sites and give rise to brain behavioral relationships that are both localized and distributed. Anatomical channels transfer information content and chemical pathways modulate behavior.-Editor. *Ped Neur Briefs* Jan 1991.

DELAYED COGNITIVE ABNORMALITIES AND FRONTAL LOBE DAMAGE

The consequences of early frontal lobe damage, restricted to the polar and mesial portion of the left prefrontal cortex and deep white matter, on higher cognitive and psychologic development are reported in a 33-year-old woman who sustained injury at 7 years of age and was evaluated at the Division of Behavioral Neurology and Cognitive Neuroscience, University of Iowa College of Medicine, Iowa City. The birth and milestones of development were normal, and academic achievement was average before she sustained a spontaneous intraparenchymal cerebral hemorrhage at 7 years. Her neurologic exam was normal and generalized tonic clonic seizures were controlled with medication. MRI revealed the lesion in the left prefrontal cortex and deep white matter, and cerebral blood flow studies were abnormal in left and right frontal regions. Defects in higher cognition were noted especially in self regulation of emotion and affect and in social behavior. These were of delayed onset and were followed by a period of progression and finally an arrest of development in adolescence. The progressive impairment resulted from a disrepancy between the demands of adolescent development and the altered maturation of frontal lobe neural and cognitive systems. The patient failed to acquire the executive and self regulatory processes associated with frontal lobe function. (Eslinger PJ et al. Developmental consequences of childhood frontal lobe damage. Arch Neurol July 1992;49:764-769). (Reprints: Dr. Eslinger, Division of Neurology, The Milton S. Hershey Medical Center, 500 University Drive, Hershey, PA 17033.)

COMMENT. A variety of neuropsychological syndromes including Gerstmann's syndrome are described as a consequence of lesions or stimulation to the left posterior perisylvian territory (Benton AL. Gerstmann's syndrome. Arch Neurol May 1992;49:445-447). A cortical stimulation study in a 17-year-old epileptic boy had shown that repeated stimulation of different loci in the posterior perisylvian region had elicited diverse cognitive syndromes (i.e. acalculia, agraphia, alexia, anomia, constructional apraxia, finger agnosia, and right-left disorientation). Stimulation of adjacent loci, between the angular and supra-marginal gyri, had produced a complete Gerstmann syndrome without accompanying deficits.-Editor. *Ped Neur Briefs* Aug 1992.

BRAIN DAMAGE AND VIOLENCE

The neurologist's role in understanding violence and brain damage as a neurological defense of violent crime are reviewed by neurologists at Georgetown University, Washington, DC. Pincus stresses the role of biological factors as contributory to aggressive behavior and notes that cognitive impairment, lapses of attention, and psychotic symptoms are more common among violent compared to nonviolent criminals. He concludes that programs of research targeting brain damage and child abuse as causes of violence might lead to more effective preventive methods of management than prison expansion. Resnak points out that the majority of violent criminals have no history or evidence of brain damage and concludes that neurology will not solve the mystery of violent behavior and murder. Admitting that many murderers have a higher incidence of epilepsy, head injury, child abuse, malnutrition, and learning disabilities, but the majority of epileptics, abused, and mentally retarded do not commit violence. Both experts agree that brain damage can decrease the threshold for violent, impulsive behavior, and serve as a mitigating factor in determining responsibility and defense for some crimes. (Pincus JH. Neurologist's role in understanding violence. Arch Neurol Aug 1993;50:867-869. Restak R. The neurological defense of violent crime. 'Insanity defense' retooled. Arch Neurol Aug 1993;50:869-871). (Reprints: Dr Resnak, Neurology Associates, 1800 R St NW C-3, Washington, DC; Dr Pincus, Georgetown University Hospital, 3800 Reservoir Rd NW, Washington, DC 20007).

COMMENT. Three criteria are required by law for alleged brain damage to serve as a mitigating factor in determining responsibility. 1) Is there evidence of *brain damage* (deviation from normal brain structure) and is it reponsible for a *deficit* (impairment or loss or alteration of intelligence and emotion, and behavioral abnormality)?; 2) Is the deficit a contributing cause of the defendant's crime?; 3) Without the deficit and resulting behavior, would the crime not have happened? Of 14 death row juveniles who had committed capital crimes, 11 had suffered head trauma, 9 had abnormal EEGs or neurologic examinations, and 12 gave a history of physical or sexual abuse (Lewis DO, Pincus JH et al. Am J Psychiatry 1988;145:584). Brain damage may unleash violence, but it does not explain it, according to Hachinski V. (Arch Neurol Aug 1993;50:871).

A study of frontal lobe-subcortical circuits in the mediation of a wide range of human behavioral disorders, reported from the Departments of Neurology, Psychiatry and Biobehavioral Sciences, UCLA School of Medicine, Los Angeles, CA (Cummings JL. Arch Neurol Aug 1993;50:873-880) demonstrates that we should not entirely dismiss a possible role of brain damage in crimes of violence. -Editor. *Ped Neur Briefs* Aug 1993.

LEARNING DISABILITIES IN EPILEPSY

Neurophysiological mechanisms by which epilepsy may interfere with learning ability are reviewed from the Department of Clinical Neurophysiology, Maudsley Hospital, and Department of Psychology, Middlesex Hospital, London, England. Five mechanisms are listed: 1)Disruption of ongoing processing by epileptiform activity that interferes with attention to incoming information, its storage or retrieval;2) disruption of storage and retrieval of information by discharges temporally distant from the learning experience; 3) permanent damage to neural tissue; 4) antiepileptic drug toxicity; 5) disruption of brain function by chronic frequent discharges during sleep. Subclinical generalized spike wave discharges may be accompanied by transitory cognitive impairment demonstrable by psychological testing during EEG recording. Left-sided focal spiking produces errors on verbal tasks whereas right-sided discharges impair handling of non-verbal material. Subclinical discharges may disrupt educational skills in children and impair driving performance in motorists. Suppression of discharges by antiepileptic drugs may improve psychological functioning. Spike wave monitors may find a place in special schools to alert teachers to a child's absence attacks. (Binnie GD et al. Learning disabilities in epilepsv: Neurophysiological aspects. Epilepsia 1990;31 (Suppl 4):S2-8).

COMMENT. The above article is the first in a report of the Symposium on Epilepsy and Education at the XVIIIth International Epilepsy Congress, New Delhi, India, October 1989. Other reports in this Epilepsia supplement include references to epileptic syndromes and cognitive functioning (Dam M); effects of antiepileptic drugs (Trimble MR); the EEG in assessing cognitive function (Stores G); and the effects of discontinuation of antiepileptic drugs on cognition (Blennow G et al). Community based studies in the United Kingdom have shown that up to 30% of children with epilepsy underachieved in school and many are referred for special education. -Editor. *Ped Neur Briefs*

Feb 1991.

ATTENTION DEFICIT AND EEG ANALYSIS

Computerized power spectral analysis (PSA), permitting topographic representation and statistical analysis of EEG, of 25 right-handed males, 9-12 years of age with attention deficit hyperactivity disorder was used in studies from the Departments of Psychology, Pediatrics (Neurology) and Computing Center, University of Tennessee and East Tennessee Children's Hospital, Knoxville, TN. When compared with 27 controls matched for age and grade level, children with ADHD had increased theta (4.75 Hz) and decreased beta 1 (12.75-21 Hz). The differences were less when the patients were at rest during visual fixation and greater when tested for reading and drawing skills. The increased theta activity was found in the frontal and central locations and decreased beta in posterior and temporal locations. These differences were enhanced in patients with ADHD during the drawing task, with a difference of more than 20% between groups (P<.01) in premotor and prefrontal regions. The study provided 80% predictability for ADHD group membership and 74% for membership in the control group (Mann CA. Quantitative analysis of EEG in boys with attention-deficit-hyperactivity disorder: controlled study with clinical implications. Pediatr Neurol Jan/Feb 1992;8:30-36). (Correspondence: Dr. Lubar, Department of Psychology, University of Tennessee, Knoxville, TN 37996-0900.)

COMMENT. In a previous study (Flynn JM, Deering WM. Dev Med Child Neurol 1989;31:215-223) PSA was used successfully to differentiate the Boder subgroups of dyslexic children. An increase of theta in the left temporal region was greater for those with dyseidetic dyslexic disorder as compared with the dysphonetic disorder. The present study shows that quantitative EEG may help to characterize the attentive difficulties in children with ADHD and provide more objective and physiologically based data than are currently available from subjective questionnaires or rating scales. -Editor. *Ped Neur Briefs* April 1992.

BEHAVIOR DISORDERS AND EPILEPSY

A longitudinal study of 127 children with epilepsy aged 8-12 years and their mothers, designed to identify factors contributing to behavior problems, is reported from the Indiana University School of Nursing, Indianapolis; the Minnesota Comprehensive Epilepsy Program, Minneapolis; and the Harvard School of Public Health, Boston. Variables that accounted for 30% of the variation in child behavior problems included female gender, seizure frequency, family stress, and family social support. Family stress and seizure frequency were positively related whereas family social support was negatively associated with behavior problems. Children experiencing behavior problems had poorer seizure control and came from troubled families with mothers receiving inadequate support from relatives. (Austin JK et al. Correlates of behavior problems in children with epilepsy. Epilepsia Nov/Dec 1992;33:1115-1122). (Reprints: Dr JK Austin, Indiana University School of Nursing, 1111 Middle Dr, Indianapolis, IN).

COMMENT. Family variables and seizure frequency are important correlates of behavior problems in children with epilepsy. Neurological dysfunction may predispose children to both epilepsy and psychiatric disturbance, but family stress may have a stronger influence on child adjustment than seizure severity. In addition to treatment with antiepileptic drugs, attention to family relationships is important in clinical management of childhood epilepsy. -Editor. *Ped Neur Briefs* Jan 1993.

COGNITIVE EFFECTS OF CABAMAZEPINE AND PHENYTOIN: A REANALYSIS

A previous report from the University of Washington School of Medicine, Seattle, WA, that carbamazepine had fewer adverse neuropsychological effects than phenytoin has been re-evaluated. When patients with disproportionately high phenytoin levels were excluded, the neuropsychological differences originally reported could not be demonstrated by statistical analysis. (Dodrill CB, Troupin AS.

Neuropsychological effects of carbamazepine and phenytoin: A reanalysis. Neurology Jan 1991;41:141-143).

COMMENT. Two additional studies have found no definite adverse cognitive effects that could be related to phenytoin (Meador KJ et al. Neurology 1990;40:391-394; Dodrill CB, Temkin NR. Epilepsia 1989;30:453-457). The authors comment that many studies reporting adverse cognitive effects of phenytoin use computerized tests heavily loaded with motor speed. When the motor speed element is factored out, the cognitive effects also disappear.

Cognitive function in relation to time-of-day variation in serum carbamazepine concentration in epileptic patients is reported from the Neuropsychology Laboratory, Department of Psychosomatic and Behavioral Medicine, Rikshospitalet, Oslo, Norway (Reinvang I et al. Epilepsia Jan/Feb 1991;32:116-121). Patients had been seizure-free for at least one month and took 2 daily CBZ doses. The test battery showed no differences between performance at times of high versus low serum concentrations. A 33% fluctuation in CBZ concentrations during the day was significant. The subjects were mainly adults and different results might be obtained in children. -Editor. *Ped Neur Briefs* Feb 1991.

COGNITIVE IMPAIRMENT AND CARBAMAZEPINE

The effects on cognition of carbamazepine, phenytoin and sodium valproate were compared in 64 new cases of childhood epilepsy treated at the Leeds General Infirmary, England. The children age 5-14 years had no neurological deficit and were allocated randomly and assessed prospectively over a 12 month period. They were seizure-free throughout the 12 months. Psychological tests included visual recall, auditory recall (memory), visual scanning (vigilance), Stroop test (concentration), speed of information processing, and standard scales of intellectual functioning and reading. Serum levels of carbamazepine (CBZ) showed a significant negative correlation with changes in scores on the sum of five memory tests from before medication to 6 months and a year later. No significant correlations with memory scores were found for children treated with phenytoin (PHT). Only 10 of 126 serum level estimations of CBZ gave a value greater than 8.2 mcg/L. In the sodium valproate group significant positive correlations were found between serum levels and the sum of five memory tests at 1 month and at 6 months after starting treatment. The memory test clearly showed that there was impaired recent recall on CBZ apparent by 6 months of treatment and even more definite after a year. Reading scores were also lower in the CBZ compared with the PHT group after a year on drug treatment. Doses of CBZ were usually in the lower half of the accepted therapeutic range of 5-15 mcg/L (Forsythe I et al. Cognitive impairment in new cases of epilepsy randomly assigned to carbamazepine, phenytoin and sodium valproate. Dev Med Child Neurol June 1991;33:524-534).

COMMENT. In this study involving children with epilepsy previously untreated, carbamazepine in moderate dosage adversely affected memory but sodium valproate and phenytoin did not. The tendency to favor carbamazepine in preference to phenytoin on the basis of reported cognitive deficits seems questionable and unfounded. A phenytoin-induced improvement in auditory memory has been demonstrated in children with EEG dysrhythmias (Millichap J G et al. Auditory perceptual deficit correlated with EEG dysrhythmias. Response to diphenylhydantoin sodium. Neurology 1969;19:870-872). -Editor. *Ped Neur Briefs* July 1991.

ANTIEPILEPTIC DRUGS, REACTION TIME, AND IMPULSIVITY

The effects of antiepileptic drugs (AED) on reaction time, attention, and impulsivity in 111 epileptic children, aged 5 to 13 years, are reported from the Children's Hospital of Los Angeles and University of Southern California School of Medicine. Higher total serum levels of AEDs correlated significantly with more impulsive errors. Carbamazepine (CBZ) monotherapy levels in 54 children were negatively correlated with simple and complex reaction times and omission errors, and positively correlated with commission errors. Higher CBZ serum levels were associated with faster responses and fewer omission errors but impulsive errors on complex reaction time tests were increased. Among 73 children receiving phenobarbital monotherapy, minimal slowing of reaction times and increased omission errors were noted with higher serum levels, but changes were not significant. A number of other AEDs were included in the total drug score analysis, but none was large enough to analyze individually as monotherapy, except for phenobarbital and CBZ. (Mitchell WG et al. Effects of antiepileptic drugs on reaction time, attention, and impulsivity in children. Pediatrics Jan 1993;91:101-105). (Reprints: Wendy G Mitchell MD, Neurology, Mail Stop 82, Children's Hospital of Los Angeles, PO Box 54700, Los Angeles, CA 90054).

COMMENT. Contrary to recent concern regarding possible adverse effects of phenobarbital on cognitive function, this study shows no significant effects on reaction time and attention. The authors do not recommend CBZ in preference to other AEDs. -Editor. *Ped Neur Briefs* Jan 1993.

ORGANIC BRAIN DYSFUNCTION AND AUTISM

A population-based neurobiological study of 35 children with autistic disorder (AD) and 17 with autistic-like conditions (ALC) is reported from the Department of Child and Adolescent Psychiatry, University of Goteborg, Sweden. Major indications of brain damage or dysfunction were found in 90%. Etiological groups included Moebius syndrome (9%), fragile X syndrome (6%), chromosomal anomalies (6%), neurocutaneous disorders (6%), congenital hydrocephalus (3%), Rett syndrome (3%), Laurence-Moon-Biedl syndrome (3%), severe perinatal distress (9%), and epilepsy or severe EEG pathology (20%). Genetic factors were implicated in 9% with fathers and a brother with Asperger's syndrome. The EEG was abnormal in 50% and 18(40%) had epileptiform discharges, maximal in the temporal lobes. CAT scan abnormalities in 25% included dilated ventricles, porencephaly, and general atrophy. BAERs were abnormal in 33%. (Steffenburg S. Neuropsychiatric assessment of children with autism: a population-based study. Dev Med Child Neurol June 1991;33:495-511).

COMMENT. Multiple biological etiologies for autism and autistic-like disorders are suggested by this comprehensive study. Despite the extra effort and patience involved, the pediatric neurologist should not dismiss the child with autistic symptoms to the care of the psychiatrist without first attempting a full neurologic evaluation including EEG and CT or MRI. -Editor. *Ped Neur Briefs* July 1991.

ASPERGER'S SYNDROME

The diagnosis of Asperger's Syndrome was made in six children admitted to the psychiatric in-patient Clinic at the Maudsley and Bethlem Royal Hospitals, Denmark Hill, London SE5 8AZ, England. Previous evaluations by mental health professionals focusing on family dynamics had lead to accusations of parental, emotional or sexual abuse and suggestions of fabrication of the child's behavioral disorder. Detailed in-patient psychiatric appraisal clarified the nature of the behavioral abnormalities and the diagnostic key features of Asperger's Syndrome: 1) A formal concrete way of thinking, and 2) an inability to identify and understand human emotions and relationships. Four of the six children were boys. Communication difficulties ranged from a stilted speech to almost robotic manner. Abnormal preoccupations included toy cars, insects, fungi, poisons, violence to babies, ritualistic drawings and orderliness. Developmental delays and learning disorders involved language, spelling, reading and visual memory. Neurologic examination showed motor incoordination and nonspecific EEG abnormalities in one child and dilated ventricles in one. IQ scores varied from 60 to 138 with a mean of 90. Parents made to feel guilty, hostile and defensive were relieved and cooperative when the diagnosis was established and there anxieties were acknowledged. (Perkins M,

Wolkind S N. Asperger's syndrome: who is being abused? Arch Dis Child June 1991;66:693-695).

COMMENT. The syndrome described as an "autistic psychopathy" by an Austrian psychiatrist, Hans Asperger in 1944, includes abnormalities in language, poor social skills, peculiar interests and motor clumsiness.

The clinical characteristics of Asperger's syndrome were reviewed in 34 patients, age 5-35 years (Wing L. Psychol Med Feb 1981;11:115-129). Several children walked at a normal age but were slow to talk and became increasingly odd and withdrawn in personality. A genetic factor is suspected and no specific organic pathology has been identified. The syndrome listed in the ICD-10 but not in DSM-III-R is sometimes classified as a subgroup of the autistic spectrum with motor clumsiness, higher IQ and higher verbal skills (Tuchman R F. Autism: Delineating the spectrum. Int Pediatr 1991:6:161-169). Studies involving MRI and possible genetic or environmental factors require further investigation. In the absence of a specific etiology and biological marker, diagnosis is dependent on clinical criteria, a careful history, and full psychiatric and pediatric neurology evaluations. -Editor. *Ped Neur Briefs* July 1991. ~

SLEEP DISORDERS AND NEUROPSYCHOLOGICAL ABNORMALITIES

The IQ and neurodevelopmental quotients of 17 of 32 children with congenital central hypoventilation syndrome were determined at the Departments of Pediatrics and Psychology, Rush-Presbyterian-St. Luke's Medical Center, Chicago, IL. Sleep hypoventilation was severe in all cases, with an alveolar carbon dioxide pressure of 62+/-2.5 mm Hg and a hemoglobin saturation of 65%. Seizures were associated in 72 %, pulmonary hypertension in 78% and mild cerebral atrophy in 40%. All patients were hypotonic or had major motor delays. Autopsy performed in 6 cases showed diffuse central nervous system astrocytosis, gliosis, and atrophy but no brainstem abnormality. The IQ and developmental quotients varied from greater than the 85th percentile to less than the 5th percentile, with verbal and performance discrepancies. The data support a diffuse central nervous system process but the possible effects of transient hypoxemia on neurodevelopmental test results could not be definitely determined (Weese-Mayer DE, Silvestri JM et al. J Pediatr March 1992; 120:381-7 and 388-93). (Reprints: Dr. Weese-Mayer, Department of Pediatrics, Rush-Presbyterian-St. Luke's Medical Center, 1653 West Congress Parkway, Chicago, IL 60612.)

COMMENT. Congenital central hypoventilation syndrome, characterized by absent ventilatory and arousal sensitivity to hypercapnia and variable sensitivity to hypoxemia, has been reported with Hirschsprung disease, neural-crest tumors, and mild cerebral atrophy on CT or MRI. Many require ventilatory support particularly while asleep. Seizures and neurodevelopmental delays may bring these patients to the attention of the pediatric neurologist.

The effects of phenobarbital on sleep behavior in children with febrile seizures were evaluated by Hirtz DG, Farwell JR et al. at Bethesda, MD and Seattle, WA (Neurology April 1992;42(Suppl 3):367). Night awakenings were not more common in children on phenobarbital except for those who were poor sleepers initially. Lengthy night awakenings were not more frequent and total sleep time was not altered. At least one behavioral disturbance previously assigned to the use of phenobarbital in the prophylaxis of febrile seizures has been negated by this study.

Horne J, from the Sleep Research Laboratory, Loughborough University, Leicestershire, U.K., discusses epilepsy in sleep in a paper on sleep and its disorders in children (J Child Psychol Psychiat March 1992;33:473-487). In addition to febrile convulsions and benign rolandic childhood epilepsy, other paroxysmal disorders that occur during sleep include the complex partial seizures of frontal origin, usually misdiagnosed as nightmares (Stores G, 1991) and sometimes referred to as "nocturnal paroxysmal dystonia" (Lugaresi et al. 1986).-Editor. *Ped Neur Briefs* May 1992.

HEAD SIZE AND COGNITION IN VERY LOW BIRTH WEIGHT (VLBW) INFANTS

The effect of VLBW (<1.5 kg) and subnormal head size at 8 months of age (corrected for prematurity) on neurocognitive abilities at school age was investigated by a longitudinal follow up of 249 children born between 1977 to 1979 and admitted to the neonatal intensive care unit at Rainbow Babies and Children's Hospital, Cleveland, OH. Head size was subnormal at birth in 12%, at term 23%, and at 8 months 13%. As compared with 216 children with normal head sizes, the 33 children with subnormal head sizes at the age of 8 months had significantly lower mean birth weights and higher neonatal risk scores and at 8 years of age had a higher incidence of neurologic impairment and lower IQ scores. A subnormal head size at 8 months of age was predictive of poor verbal and performance IQ scores at 8 years of age; lower scores for receptive language, speech, reading, mathematics and spelling; and a higher incidence of hyperactivity. (Hack M et al. Effect of very low birth weight and subnormal head size on cognitive abilities at school age. N Engl J Med July 25, 1991;325:231-237)

COMMENT. A relation between subnormal head circumference and cognitive functioning has been reported in many different studies, including children with learning disabilities. Improvements in neonatal growth and development may depend on nutrition of chronically ill neonates and environmental enrichment after discharge from hospital. This study shows that the determination of the head circumference at 8 months of age is a useful means of predicting subsequent cognitive deficits and difficulties in school.

Volpe JJ, in an editorial (N Engl J Med 1991;325:276-277), stresses the need for a better method of detection of brain injury in VLBW infants since 77 % of those with normal head circumference at 8 months had IQs below 85 and an academic skill index below 80 in the study by Hack et al. Those infants with a small head circumference at 8 months of age made up only a minority of infants who subsequently had cognitive deficits. Cranial ultrasonography detects overt brain lesions but not the subtle lesions in the periventricular white matter. MRI may detect periventricular injury missed by ultrasound and CT scanning; it is also used to measure the progress and degree of myelination in the human infant in the first months of life. A decreased rate of brain growth in the first months of life might identify a larger proportion of at risk infants and justify further study with the MRI in selected patients.

Collin MF and associates from the Department of Pediatrics, Loyola University Medical Center, Maywood, IL report that normal infant development is poorly predictive of continued normal development in the extremely low birth weight infant (Pediatrics July 1991;88:115-120). Only 11(31%) of 36 children had normal development upon reassessment in early childhood. With or without major complications, extremely low birth weight places children at risk for emerging development problems with age. Head circumference was not addressed in this study. -Editor. *Ped Neur Briefs* Aug 1991.

HEAD SIZE, IQ AND BIRTH WEIGHT

Head growth and IQ were correlated at ages 2, 5 and 8 years in children grouped according to birth weight in the Departments of Obstetrics and Gynecology and Pediatrics, University of Melbourne, Australia, and the Royal Women's Hospital, Melbourne. All children were white and with no signs of moderate or severe cerebral palsy. Using the National Center for Health Statistics reference values more group 1 children (birth weight 500-999 g) than group 2 children (birth weight 1,000-1,499 g) were below the 10th percentile at ages 2 and 8 years. Using the Nellhaus standards the difference between groups 1 and 2 was not significant and head growth appeared to be satisfactory at age 2 years. Comparing group 3 (birth weight greater than 2,500 g) with groups 1 and 2 combined, fewer of the group 3 children were below the 10th percentile at both ages 2 and 8 years, using the NCHS reference and at age 8 years, using the Nellhaus data. The heads of very low birth weight children were progressively narrower but not longer than those of normal birth weight children. Dolichocephaly was unrelated to IQ and the correction of occipitofrontal circumference for dolichocephaly was rarely of clinical importance. Occipitofrontal circumference best correlated with the full scale IQ on the Wechsler Intelligence Scale for Children-Revised. At age 8 years the Wechsler IQ was significantly related to the OFC ratio in both very low birth weight and normal birth weight children. The AP-BP ratio was unrelated to IQ (Kitchen WH et al. Very low birth weight and growth to age 8 years II: head dimensions and intelligence. AJDC Jan 1992;146:46-50.)

COMMENT. The authors concluded that the National Center for Health Statistics data for occipitofrontal circumference measurements were more appropriate than the Nellhaus data in this study. Head growth achieved by age 8 years was progressively reduced in lower birth weight categories in all measurements except the anteroposterior diameter. Occipitofrontal circumference was closely related to IQ and other head measurements are not recommended in routine clinical practice. In a further report the authors found that maternal height and the birth weight ratio were more important than health after birth in predicting a height or weight below the 10th percentile at age 8 years in children with low birth weights. Occipitofrontal head circumference is related to infant development and later intelligence in childhood and is a useful indication of brain size. -Editor. *Ped Neur Briefs* Jan 1992.

PRENATAL HEAVY METAL EXPOSURE AND COGNITION

The effects of prenatal exposure to heavy metals on childhood cognitive skills and health status are reported from the Robert Wood Johnson Medical School, New Brunswick, NJ. Cadmium, chromium, cobalt, lead, mercury, nickel and silver were determined in amniotic fluid taken from 92 pregnant women at 16 - 18 weeks gestation. A prenatal toxic risk score was based on the presence of a detectable level for the various metals. A correlation analysis indicated a negative relation between the toxic risk score and cognitive performance and a significant positive correlation between the toxic risk score and both the total number of atopic illnesses and infections assessed at 3 years of age. These findings indicate that health status as well as cognitive ability may show deficits as a consequence of prenatal heavy metal exposure. (Lewis M et al. Prenatal exposure to heavy metals: effect on childhood cognitive skills and health status. Pediatrics June 1992;89:1010-1015.) (Reprints: Dr. Michael Lewis, Institute for the Study of Child Development, Dept of Pediatrics, UMDNJ-Robert Wood Johnson Medical School, RWJ Professional Bldg. New Brunswick, NJ 08903-0019.)

COMMENT. Lead intoxication in infants is common and is of different origin from that in toddlers (Shannon MW, Graef JW. Lead intoxication in infancy. Pediatrics Jan 1992;89:87-90). Formula preparation with lead contaminated water accounted for 9 of 50 infantile cases whereas paint chip ingestion was the most common cause among 47 children (86%) aged 18 through 30 months. These data support recent recommendations to initiate lead screening in children at 6 months of age.

A maintained average blood level of 25 mcg/dL or more during the second and third year of life was found to be detrimental to the child's attained stature at 33 months of age in a study from the University of Cincinnati (Shukla R et al. Lead exposure and growth in the early preschool child: A follow-up report from the Cincinnati lead study. Pediatrics 1991;88:886-892). -Editor. *Ped Neur Briefs* Aug 1992.

LOW LEVEL LEAD EXPOSURES AND IQ

The Port Pirie cohort study which began in 1979 at the Department of Community Medicine, University of Adelaide, Australia, has been followed into the primary school age range and examines intelligence at the age of 7 years in relation to lifetime exposure to lead. In 494 children from a lead smelting community, the IQ was inversely related to both antenatal and postnatal blood level concentrations. An increase in blood lead concentration from 10 to 30 mcg/dL was associated with a deficit in verbal IQ that varied according to age from 5.5 to 6.4 points. In full scale IQ, the estimated deficit was 4.4 - 5.3 points. (Baghurst PA et al. Environmental exposure to lead and children's intelligence at the age of seven years. N Engl J Med Oct 29, 1992;327:1279-84.) (Reprints: Dr. Baghllrst, CSIRO Division of Human Nutrition, P.O. Box 10041, Gouger St., Adelaide, SA 5000, Australia.)

COMMENT. Mahaffey KR from the National Institute of Environmental Health Sciences, North Carolina, comments in an editorial that the results of 3 longitudinal studies (Australia, Boston and Cincinnati) demonstrate that the lead associated decrements in intelligence are persistent across cultures, racial and ethnic groups, and social and economic classes. They are not limited to socially and economically disadvantaged children (N Engl J Med 1992;327:1308). Meta-analysis of 7 studies showed an average decrease of 0.25 IQ points for each 1 mcg/dL increase in blood lead levels (BPb). This inverse relationship between IQ and BPb continued well below 10 mcg/dL (Rosen JF AJDC Nov 1992;146:1278).

Lead encephalopathy was diagnosed in 10 Saudi Arabian children, ages 8-48 months, during 1984-1988. The mean BPb was 6.1 umol/L (range, 2.5-13 umol/L). (Yaish HM et al. AJDC Nov 1992;146:1257.) In Washington, D.C. 590 (20.8%) of children aged 9 months to 3 years examined showed blood lead concentrations of 0.5 umol/L or more, which exceeded the acceptable CDC limits. At levels between 0.5 and 1.2 umol/L, the free erythrocyte protoporphyrin (FEP) screening test was a very poor predictor of toxic blood lead values (Rifai N et al. AJDC Nov 1992;146:1259).-Editor. *Ped Neur Briefs* Nov 1992.

BRAIN RADIOTHERAPY AND COGNITION

Cognitive function and school achievement were studied prospectively over 3 to 4 years in 19 children treated for brain tumors with whole-brain radiotherapy at the Children's Hospital, Philadelphia, PA. Fourteen children also received adjuvant chemotherapy. A significant drop in IQ was seen among children with non-cortical tumors who received whole-brain radiotherapy with or without chemotherapy and who were treated before age 7. IQ did not decrease significantly in survivors treated after age 7. The IQ fell from a baseline of 104 to 92 at follow-up (Radcliffe J et al. Three- and four-year cognitive outcome in children with noncortical brain tumors treated with whole-brain radiotherapy. Ann Neurol Oct 1992;32:551-554). (Correspondence: Dr. Radcliffe, Division of Child Development and Rehabilitation, Children's Seashore House, 3405 Civic Center Boulevard, Philadelphia, PA 19104.)

COMMENT. All children younger than 7 years in this group were receiving special education at follow-up, and 50% of the children over 7 years at diagnosis were receiving supplemental educational services. Increased fatiguability could be another reason for the poor school performance in these children. -Editor. *Ped Neur Briefs* Dec 1992.

PRENATAL MARIHUANA, CIGARETTES, ALCOHOL AND ATTENTIONAL BEHAVIOR

A follow-up study of attentional behavior in 6 year old children exposed prenatally to marihuana, cigarettes and alcohol is reported from the Department of Psychology, Carleton University, Ottawa, Ontario, Canada. Discriminant function analysis in 126 children revealed a dose response association between prenatal cigarette exposure and impulsive behavior. Performance on memory tasks requiring verbal recall was negatively associated with maternal cigarette use. Prenatal marihuana was associated with omission errors in vigilance tasks reflecting a deficit in sustained attention. The mother's rating of impulsive hyperactive behavior was also higher. Low levels of maternal alcohol consumption were related to decreased impulsive responding, assessed by mothers' reports. (Fried PA et al. A follow-up study of attentional behavior in 6-year-old children exposed prenatally to marihuana, cigarettes, and alcohol. Neurotoxicol Teratol Sept/Oct 1992;*14*:299-311). (Reprints: Dr. Peter A. Fried, Department of Psychology, Carlton University, Ottawa, Ontario, Canada KIS 5B6.)

COMMENT. A negative relationship between prenatal alcohol exposure and attention related variables was not observed in this study. The only differences related to maternal alcohol consumption were in decreased impulsivity: fewer responses were made in the delay tasks and a decreased degree of impulsivity/hyperactivity in the child was reported by the mother. Others have reported an increased reaction time associated with maternal alcohol consumption in 4 and 7 year old children on vigilance tasks. The timing of the exposure to the alcohol was not determined in this present study, and relatively low levels of alcohol were consumed by the mothers. This could account for the absence of negative association between attentional behavior and maternal alcohol use. -Editor. *Ped Neur Briefs* Dec 1992.

CHLORIDE-DEFICIENT DIET AND COGNITIVE DEFICITS

Distinctive cognitive impairments and a specific neurobehavioral syndrome are reported in 11 of 13 children who had failed to thrive on chloride-deficient formula during infancy. They were examined four to nine years later at the Division of Pediatric Neurology, UCLA School of Medicine, Los Angeles, CA and the Department of Neurology, Boston University School of Medicine, Boston, MA. All patients during infancy had developed symptoms of hypokalemic, hypochloremic metabolic alkalosis and/or growth deceleration, concurrently with their exposure to chloride-deficient Neo-Mull-Soy formula. Head circumference at follow-up was within normal limits, three children had hypotonia, two diffuse hyperreflexia, one had choreiform movements and one bilateral intention tremor. The EEG was abnormal in six, with paroxysmal discharges seen in five children. CT and MRI studies were normal. Intelligence was within the average range for 11 of the 13 children tested. All had a neurobehavioral syndrome consisting of a language disorder primarily involving articulation, word finding and naming; visual-motor and fine motor difficulties; and attention deficit disorder often featuring repetitive behaviors, withdrawal and "over-focus." (Kaleita TA, Kinsbourne M, Menkes JH. A neurobehavioral syndrome after failure to thrive on chloride-deficient formula. Dev Med Child Neurol July 1991;33:626-635).

COMMENT. A syndrome characterized by loss of appetite, failure to gain weight, muscular weakness, lethargy, vomiting and severe hypochloremic, hypokalemic, metabolic alkalosis has been described in infants fed chloride-deficient soy-based infant formulas. Clinical features resemble Bartter Syndrome, but the renal biopsy is normal and infants recover when dietary chloride supplements are provided. Previous follow-up reports have drawn attention to developmental delay (Chutorian et al. Pediatr Neurol 1985;1:334-341) and the present study demonstrates specific cognitive, language and attentional deficits in later childhood. -Editor. *Ped Neur Briefs* Sept 1991.

SUGAR AND AGGRESSIVE AND INATTENTIVE BEHAVIOR

The effect of a sucrose challenge on aggressive behavior and sustained attention in a sample of young hyperactive boys and age-matched control subjects was studied at the Schneider Children's Hospital, Long Island Jewish Medical Center, New York, and Albert Einstein College of Medicine, Bronx, New York. The index group met DSM-III criteria for ADD-H and oppositional disorder as determined by interviews using the diagnostic interview for children and adolescents. They also scored at least 14 or above on the hyperkinesis index of parent and teacher revised questionnaires. Baseline testing was followed by a breakfast containing 8 oz of an orange colored and flavored drink containing either 35 g of sucrose or adjusted to equal sweetness with either saccharine (175 mg) or aspartame (175 mg). The sugar and placebo challenges were given with a breakfast high in carbohydrate. There were no significant effects of sugar or placebo on the aggressive behavior of either group. Inattention measured by a continuous performance task increased in the ADD-H group following sugar, but not with saccharine or aspartame control. (Wender EH, Solanto MV. Effects of sugar on aggressive and inattentive behavior in children with attention deficit disorder with hyperactivity and normal children. Pediatrics Nov 1991;88:960-966.) (Reprints: Dr Wender, Schneider Children's Hospital, New Hyde Park, NY 11042).

COMMENT. A deterioration in attention following sugar ingestion has been reported in one other study by Connors et al. in which sugar was administered with a high carbohydrate breakfast. When a negative effect was observed in 3 other studies the sugar was given either in a fasting state or with a protein breakfast. Further studies are indicated. -Editor. *Ped Neur Briefs* Jan 1992.

FOOD-INDUCED HYPERKINESIS

The results of a controlled trial of hyposensitization with intradermal EPD (beta-glucuronidase and food antigens) in 40 children with the hyperkinetic syndrome are reported from the Universitatskinderklinik, Lindwurmstrasse, Munchen, Germany and The Allergy Unit, London, UK. The study was in 3 phases: the first consisted of the oligoantigenic diet; children who responded to the diet entered the reintroduction of foods, phase II; and those with food-induced hyperkinetic syndrome entered phase III, a double-blind, placebo-controlled trial of EPD, 3 intradermal doses at 2-monthly intervals. Of 20 patients who received the hyposensitization active treatment, 16 became tolerant toward provoking foods, compared with 4 of 20 who received placebo ($p<0.001$). The authors conclude that EPD permits children with food-induced hyperkinetic syndrome to eat foods that had previously been identified as responsible for their symptoms (especially chocolate, colorings, cow milk, egg, citrus, wheat, nuts and cheese). Food allergy is considered a possible mechanism of the hyperkinetic syndrome. (Egger J et al. Controlled trial of hyposensitization in children with food-induced hyperkinetic syndrome. Lancet May 9, 1992;339:1150-1153.) (Correspondence: Dr. J. Egger, Universitatskinderklinik, Lindwurmstrasse 4, 8000 Munchen 2, Germany.)

COMMENT: Dr. Egger also reports a beneficial effect of the hypoallergenic diet in 12 children who suffered from enuresis in association with migraine and the hyperkinetic syndrome (Egger J et al. Clin Pediatr May 1992;31:302-307). In an editorial Fitzwater D and Macknin ML (Clin Pediatr 1992;31:308-310) recommend additional studies before dietary therapy can be introduced as a standard therapy for enuresis. Given the hazards of pharmacological therapy and the practical disadvantages of the alarm system, Dr. Egger's dietary and hyposensitization methods deserve attention. For reviews of previous articles on the hypoallergenic diet, see Progress in Pediatric Neurology, Ed Millichap JG 1991, p. 88-89. -Editor. *Ped Neur Briefs* Aug 1992.

STIMULANT MEDICATION IN ADDH

STIMULANT MEDICATION FOR ADHD: THE CHILD'S PERSPECTIVE

The knowledge and attitudes of children receiving stimulant medication for attention deficit hyperactivity disorder were investigated at the Division of Ambulatory Pediatrics, Children's Hospital, Boston, MA. Of 45 respondents and parents who completed separate questionnaires concerning how they felt about receiving stimulant medication, 89% of the children felt that the medication was helpful and 78% either approved or were indifferent to its use. Improved concentration and improved ability to sit still in the classroom were the most frequently reported benefits. Difficulty getting to sleep and decreased appetite were the most common side effects, and at least one negative aspect of therapy was reported in 82% of children. Only five children (11%) would stop taking stimulant medication if they could; these were more likely to perceive medication as unhelpful if they were receiving standard methylphenidate rather than a long-acting preparation. The authors conclude that children's perspectives on medication should be elicited directly, and a sustained release medication may be more acceptable to children with ADHD. (Bowen J et al. Stimulant medication and attention deficit-hyperactivity disorder. The child's perspective. AJDC March 1991;145:291-295).

COMMENT. The need to take stimulant medication while at school may be an important factor in the child's attitude, and compliance for prescribed therapies can be improved by decreasing the complexity or inconvenience of the therapy. Previous studies have shown that standard methylphenidate is superior to sustained release preparations on measures of disruptive behavior and cognitive performance. In contrast to advertising material, the effects of sustained release and standard methylphenidate were not equivalent. Pemoline or slow release dextroamphetamine were recommended in preference to sustained release methylphenidate, if a single daily dose sustained effect is required. (Pelham WE Jr et al. Pediatrics 1987;80:491; Ped Neur Briefs Oct 1987).-Editor. *Ped Neur Briefs* April 1991.

DOSE EFFECT OF METHYLPHENIDATE IN ADD

The clinical response to three dose levels of methylphenidate (5, 10, and 15 mg BID) in 23 children with ADD+H and 17 children with ADD-H is reported from the Department of Psychiatry, University of Massachusetts Medical Center, Worcester, MA. Both groups of children with ADD showed significant improvements in behavior, inattention, self-control, and academic performance. A low dose was as effective as the moderate or high doses in changing the behavior at school but moderate to high doses were needed to produce improved behavior at home and better task performance on the clinic assessment battery. The greatest effect of medication on the ADD-H group occurred at the low dose. In contrast, the drug effect for the ADD+H group was linear, improving with each dose increase. In subsequent clinical recommendations drug treatment was prescribed more often in the hyperactive group (71% of children) than in those without hyperactivity (24%). Children with ADD+H were rated as having more pervasive behavioral problems than the children with ADD-H. Children with ADD+H were impaired in behavioral inhibition and vigilance whereas children with ADD-H were more impaired in the retrieval of verbally learned material. (Barkley RA et al. Attention deficit disorder with and without hyperactivity: Clinical response to three dose levels of methylphenidate. Pediatrics April 1991;87:519-531).

COMMENT. This study confirms previous reports that the most active children with ADD respond better to methylphenidate than those with minimal hyperactivity. (Millichap JG. Learning Disabilities and Related Disorders. Chicago,Yearbook Publishers, 1977). -Editor. *Ped Neur Briefs* June 1991.

TRIAL OF METHYLPHENIDATE AND THIORIDAZINE

A double-blind, placebo-controlled, cross-over study of methylphenidate (0.4 mg/kg/day) and thioridazine (1.75 mg/kg/day) in 27 intellectually subaverage children is reported from The Nisonger Center for Mental Retardation and Developmental Disabilities, Ohio State Univ., Columbus, OH, and the University of Aukland, New Zealand. IQs ranged from 30-90 with a mean of 54 on the Stanford Binet, Form L-M. Ages ranged from 4 to 16 years; 22 boys and 5 girls. ADDH was diagnosed in 21 and the hyperactivity was severe (a score of 19 on the Conners Parent-Teacher Questionnaire). Epilepsy was treated with anticonvulsants in 4. Methylphenidate improved accuracy on a memory task, reduced omission errors on an attentional task, and reduced seat movements on 2 tasks. Thioridazine had no adverse effect on IQ and cognitive-motor performance tests. (Aman MG et al. Methylphenidate and thioridazine in the treatment of intellectually subaverage children: effects on cognitive-motor performance. J Am Acad Child Adolesc Psychiatry September 1991;30:816-824).

COMMENT. Methylphenidate and thioridazine are two of the most commonly used psychotropic drugs in treating mentally retarded children. In this study involving children with mild developmental delays, methylphenidate improved attention and motivation and thioridazine at relatively low dose levels had no adverse effects on learning performance. A combination of methylphenidate AM and Noon and thioridazine PM is sometimes recommended in children with ADHD of normal intelligence who exhibit behavioral problems both during and after school hours. The present study corroborates the probable benefits of this combination therapy. -Editor. *Ped Neur Briefs* Sept 1991.

METHYLPHENIDATE, ADD, AND CLASSROOM PERFORMANCE

The degree to which methylphenidate (MPH) normalized the classroom behavior and academic functioning of 31 children with attention deficit disorder (ADD) was evaluated at Lehigh University, Bethlehem, PA. Children received each of four doses (5, 10, 15, and 20 mg) of MPH and a placebo following baseline measures. In a 6-week double-blind, controlled trial, children with ADD were compared with 25 normal children using teacher ratings of social conduct, direct observations of on-task behavior, and academic efficiency. When analysed as a group, ADD children during treatment with MPH showed 46 to 65% improvements in attention, academic efficiency, and conduct ratings. Doses of 10 - 20 mg were most effective. Significant reductions in day-to-day variability and improved consistency in attention occurred at the 20 mg dose level. Examined individually, 75% of ADD children were responsive to MPH. (DuPaul GJ, Rapport MD. Does methylphenidate normalize the classroom performance of children with attention deficit disorder? J Am Acad Child Adolesc Psychiatry Jan 1993;32:190-198). (Reprints: Dr DuPaul, School Psychology Program, Lehigh University, 111 Research Drive, Bethlehem, PA

18015).

COMMENT. These results complement some previous studies showing that academic efficiency on a daily basis is consistently and significantly enhanced by MPH in a large proportion of treated ADD children. The 25% of children who did not respond would require ancillary classroom interventions and/or alternative therapies. Short-term gains may not translate to long-term improvements, and a multifaceted approach is often emphasized. However, a multimodal intervention program, using behavioral parent training and child self-control instruction in addition to medication, failed to provide greater maintenance of treatment gains than MPH alone, at 9-month follow-up after termination of all treatments. (Ialongo NS et al. J Am Acad Child Adolesc Psychiatry Jan 1993;32:182-189).

ADDH children and adolescents, with and without comormid factors, were responsive to desipramine (4 to 5 mg/daily) in a 6-week randomized, double-blind, placebo controlled trial in 62 children and adolescents evaluated at the Massachusetts General Hospital, Boston. Significant improvements in ratings were observed in patients with ADDH alone and in those with comorbid conduct disorder, major depression, or an anxiety disorder. Response of ADDH was not accounted for by improvements in the comorbid factors. (Biederman J et al. J Am Acad Child Adolesc Psychiatry Jan 1993;32:199-204). -Editor. *Ped Neur Briefs* Feb 1993.

ADHD, CREATIVITY, AND METHYLPHENIDATE

Creativity, measured by the Torrance nonverbal thinking test, was compared in 19 boys with ADHD and 21 control subjects. Boys with ADHD received methylphenidate (mean dose, 0.4 mg/kg) before the first of two test sessions. Torrance scores were 7% lower in boys with ADHD compared to controls. Methylphenidate did not adversely affect creative thinking scores in ADHD boys. (Funk JB et al. Attention deficit hyperactivity disorder, creativity, and the effects of methylphenidate. Pediatrics April 1993;91:816-819). (Reprints: Jeanne B Funk PhD, Dept of

Pediatrics, Medical College of Ohio, PO Box 10008, Toledo, OH 43699).

COMMENT. The results suggest that impulsivity, a characteristic of ADHD children, is not fundamental to creativity; and creativity, as measured by the nonverbal Torrance test, is not impaired by methylphenidate. -Editor. *Ped Neur Briefs* April 1993.

VISUAL EVENT RELATED POTENTIALS, AND EEG, IN ADHD TREATED WITH MEDICATIONS

The effects of methylphenidate (MPH) and sodium valproate (VPA) on the visual event related potentials (VERP) and EEG of children with ADHD were evaluated at the Department of Psychology, Tel Aviv University, Israel, and North Shore University Hospital, Cornell Univ Med College, New York. Two subgroups of ADHD were identified: one with abnormal and the other with normal EEGs and VERPs. The amplitude of the ERP slow negative wave was reduced by MPH and VPA in the abnormal group but was unaffected in the group with normal VERPs. (Frank Y. Visual event related potentials after methylphenidate and sodium valproate in children with attention deficit hyperactivity disorder. Clin Electroencephalogr Jan 1993;24:19-24). (Reprints: Yitzchak Frank MD, Div of Pediatric Neurology, North Shore University Hospital, 300 Community Drive, Manhasset, NY 11030).

COMMENT. The effect of medications in ADHD children appears to be related to electrophysiological findings. A positive effect is expected in patients with abnormal EEGs and VERPs. -Editor. *Ped Neur Briefs* April 1993.

RITALIN SIDE EFFECTS: PLACEBO CONTROLLED EVALUATION

The frequency of side effects of Ritalin was examined in a randomized double-blind placebo-controlled cross-over trial in 206 children aged 5 through 15 years with ADHD at the Marshfield Clinic and Research Foundation, Marshfield, WI. The Barkley Side Effects Questionnaire (BSEQ) was completed by parents at baseline and at the end of each of 4 treatment weeks; 0.3 mg/kg and 0.5 mg/kg per dose of Ritalin were compared to placebo in separate 2-week trials. Each treatment was given three times a day for 7 consecutive days. Five of the side effects studied, (insomnia, decreased appetite, stomachache, headache, and dizziness), were significantly increased by Ritalin, even at the relatively low dose of 0.3 mg/kg; the frequency of appetite suppression was dose-related and was doubled at the higher dose. Four behaviors, (daydreaming, irritability, anxiety, and nailbiting), were all significantly reduced in frequency during treatment with the higher dose of Ritalin. (Ahmann PA et al. Placebo-controlled evaluation of Ritalin side effects. Pediatrics June 1993;91:1101-1106). (Reprints: Peter A Ahmann MD, Dept of Neurology, Marshfield Clinic, 1000 North Oak Ave, Marshfield, WI 54449).

COMMENT. Patients with Tourette's syndrome were excluded from the study. Tics were reported in baseline questionnaires by 12% of parents, but there was no reported increase in either motor or vocal tics and no tics were seen on subsequent evaluations. Parents felt less anxious about potential side effects during close monitoring. The authors advocate the use of the BSEQ in monitoring patients taking Ritalin for ADHD. Ritalin as opposed to generic methylphenidate was prescribed because a difference and less consistency in effectiveness had been noted with the generic drug.-Editor. *Ped Neur Briefs* June 1993.

UNTREATED ADHD AND DRIVING RISKS

A 3- to 5- year follow-up survey of driving-related risks and outcomes in 35 adolescents and young adults with attention deficit hyperactivity disorder (ADHD) and 36 control subjects is reported from the Departments of Psychiatry, Neurology, and Pediatrics, University of Massachusetts Medical Center, Worcester, MA. ADHD subjects had a significantly greater risk than controls for traffic citations, especially for speeding, motor vehicle crashes, automobile injuries, and unsound driving habits. A subgroup of teenagers with ADHD complicated by oppositional defiant and conduct disorders were at highest risk for deviant driving skills/habits and negative driving-related outcomes. Even before receiving a license, the ADHD group was three times more likely to have driven without a valid license than the control group. During their brief driving careers, the ADHD group was involved in a total of 54 crashes compared with 16 for controls, and they were four times as likely to have been at fault. (Barkley RA et al. Driving-related risks and outcomes of attention deficit hyperactivity disorder in adolescents and young adults: A 3- to 5-year follow-up survey. Pediatrics Aug 1993;92:212-218). (Reprints: RA Barkley PhD, Dept of Psychiatry, University of Massachusetts Medical Center, 55 Lake Avenue North, Worcester, MA 01655).

COMMENT. These results corroborate previous studies showing a correlation between ADHD in adolescents and young adults and an increased rate of motor vehicle crashes, especially in those not treated with stimulant medication. (Weiss G, Hechtman LT. Hyperactive Children Grown Up. New York, NY, Guilford Press, 1986). ADHD patients who continued to take stimulant medication as young adults had no more crashes than a control group. Counselling of ADHD patients and their parents regarding risks of driving and increased potential for crashes and injuries is important. The authors suggest that clinicians may wish to consider continued therapy with methylphenidate in adolescents with severe ADHD for the purpose of reducing the risk of driving injuries.- Editor. *Ped Neur Briefs* Aug 1993.

METHYLPHENIDATE AND DESIPRAMINE TOXICITIES

A double-blind controlled study of medications in 12 children with ADHD at New York University and Stony Brook Schools of Medicine showed that nausea, vomiting, dry mouth, tremor, headache, anorexia, lassitude, and tachycardia occurred more frequently when methylphenidate (20 mg) and desipramine (148 mg/day) were combined in therapy compared to either medication alone. (Pataki CS et al. Side effects of methylphenidate and desipramine alone and in combination in children. J Am Acad Child Adolesc Psychiatry Sept 1993;32:1065-1072). (Reprints: Dr Pataki, Department of Psychiatry, New York University School of Medicine, 550 First Ave, New York, NY 10016).

COMMENT. Behavioral improvements found with tricyclic antidepressants and the positive effects of stimulants on cognitive tasks have prompted combined drug therapy of ADHD. The authors advise larger samples and longer trials before the safety of these drug interactions may be established. -Editor. *Ped Neur Briefs* Sept 1993.

DESMOPRESSIN ACETATE AND NOCTURNAL ENURESIS

A literature review of 18 randomized controlled trials of desmopressin for resistant enuresis involving 689 patients is reported from the University of Manitoba, Canada. Frequency of wetting decreased in all studies, ranging from 10% to 91%, and 25% of subjects became completely dry. In the long-term, only 5.7% of responders remained dry after medication was withdrawn. Children older than 9 years do better than those treated at an earlier age. A dose-response effect was apparent, and side-effects consisting of nasal stuffiness, headache, epistaxis, and abdominal pain were infrequent. No cases of water intoxication were reported. In one comparative study, patients treated by conditioning alarms had 10% fewer wet nights and a better long-term result. (Moffatt MEK et al. Desmopressin acetate and nocturnal enuresis: How much do we know? Pediatrics Sept 1993;92:420-425). (Reprints: Dr Moffatt, Univ Manitoba, Room S100-750 Bannatyne Avenue, Winnipeg, Manitoba R3E 0W3, Canada).

COMMENT. If we need to treat, alarms seem superior to drugs. -Editor. *Ped Neur Briefs* Oct 1993.

PERCEPTUAL MOTOR AND SENSORY INTEGRATIVE THERAPY FOR LEARNING DISABILITIES

The effects of sensory integrative therapy (SI), perceptual motor training (PM) and no treatment (NT) were compared in 103 children with learning disabilities at the Department of Paediatrics, Division of Neurology and Department of Rehabilitation Medicine, Hospital for Sick Children, University of Toronto, Canada. After a total of 72 1-hour sessions for 3 hours per week the PM treated subjects showed significant gains over the other 2 groups, primarily in gross motor performance; functional activities, such as copying ability, printing readiness, attention or organizational skills, were not improved. SI treated subjects showed improvement in motor planning. Neither therapy resulted in improvement in cognitive, language or academic performance, attention or self-concept. (Humphries T et al. A comparison of the effectiveness of sensory integrative therapy and perceptual-motor training in treating children with learning disabilities. J Dev Behav Pediatr Feb 1992;13:31-40.) (Reprints: Tom Humphries, Ph.D., Child Development Clinic, Hospital for Sick Children, Toronto, Ontario, Canada M5G IX8.)

COMMENT. Although the claim that occupational therapy may directly improve higher level academic, language, and cognitive performance has not been supported by these studies, perceptual motor and sensory integrative therapy appears to have positive effects on motor planning and gross motor functioning. The possible value of these refinements of motor performance in effecting improvements in functional ability awaits further evaluation. -Editor. *Ped Neur Briefs* May 1992.

CHAPTER 4

DYSLEXIA AND LANGUAGE DISORDERS

INTRODUCTION

Ruth Nass, M.D.
NYU Medical Center, NYC

Advances over the past several years in the investigation of the *developmental language disorders* (DLD) include improved delineation of nosology. Rapin and colleagues have systematized the varying patterns of phonological, semantic, syntactic and pragmatic deficits found in children with DLD. Aram and colleagues, investigating the validity of various current discrepancy criteria for identifying children with DLD, have found that the Stanford Binet IQ versus the Test of Language Development discrepancy score tended to under diagnose the disorder and that the Wechsler Performance IQ versus specific language task discrepancy score tended to over diagnose it, each as compared with experienced clinician's diagnoses.

The association between language disorders (as

well as autistic spectrum disorders) and epilepsy has received increasing attention. Echenne and colleagues (1993), for example, reported epileptiform EEG abnormalities in 30 of 32 children with DLD, most of whom had never had seizures. A sleep EEG in the child with a DLD (particularly those involving comprehension), as well as those with autistic spectrum disorders, may be as standard a part of the screening evaluation as is hearing testing.

The nosology of *dyslexia* has also received attention. (see also Chap 3, p 174). Shaywitz and colleagues (1993) found that the only significant difference between children with an age versus reading achievement discrepancy diagnosis (low reading achievement) and those with an IQ versus reading achievement discrepancy diagnosis of *dyslexia* was the higher IQ of the latter group. While IQ may play a role in determining which child should be considered dyslexic for research purposes, remediation should be provided to those with low reading scores regardless of IQ. Recent studies still suggest that dyslexia is more common among males. However, the less stringent the criteria the more equal the male female ratio. Studies of the genetics of dyslexia have yielded autosomal dominant families, as well as families showing polygenetic inheritance. The genetic pattern appears to depend in part on the strigency of the definition and the presence or absence of other learning disabilities in the families being evaluated. A number of studies have replicated the finding of atypical planum temporale asymmetries among dyslexic individuals. In addition, greater degree of reading and language deficit appears to correlate with the presence of atypical asymmetries.

Livingston et al (1991) proposed, based on visual evoked response results, that dyslexia represents a defect in fast processing of the magnocellular system, but Victor et al (1993) were unable to confirm this. Technical issues are critical here. Metabolic studies suggest that the language tasks most relevant to determining the underlying dynamic pathology of dyslexia involve phonology. Using ^{15}O PET scanning

Rumsey et al (1993) find that adult dyslexics fail to activate posterior regions (left temporal parietal region) during a rhyming task, suggesting that this is the critical neuroanatomic area of dysfunction. - *Ruth Nass M.D., Department of Neurology, NYU Medical Ctr.*

DYSLEXIA

READING ABILITY AND BEHAVIOR IN ADOLESCENTS WITH EPILEPSY

Thirty-four adolescents with epilepsy, and controls matched for age, sex, and general ability, were studied at the University Hospital, Cardiff, Wales. Adolescents with epilepsy had more difficult behavior in class, competitive sports were less popular and comprehension of reading material was significantly lower than that of control groups. The lowest reading scores were found in adolescents with myoclonic seizures, partial seizures with secondary generalization, or generalized tonic-clonic seizures. The low reading scores were also correlated with the EEG findings, including 2 per second spike and wave, photosensitivity, generalized slow waves, or nonspecific generalized spike and wave. Problems in reading comprehension correlated with right focal slow wave, sharp waves, and spikes.

The effects of anticonvulsants on reading and behavior were also investigated. Higher reading scores were seen with ethosuximide and lower scores with benzodiazepines. The Rutter Behavior Scale was significantly higher in patients taking phenytoin indicating less good behavior in this subgroup. The lowest Rutter score occurred in the ethosuximide patients. (Clement MJ, Wallace SJ. A survey of adolescents with epilepsy. Dev Med Child Neurol Oct 1990;32:849-857).

COMMENT. This study shows that adolescents with epilepsy can attend school and lead full lives but they may have problems with comprehension of reading material and with behavior. The value of the EEG in predicting poor reading ability has been demonstrated, and the recognition of localized cerebral lesions by MRI would be of additional interest. Correlations of the behavior and reading ability with degree of seizure control and efficacy of anticonvulsants might be pertinent.

A follow-up study of intractable seizures in childhood is reported by Huttenlocher PR and Hapke RJ (Ann Neurol Nov 1990;28:699-705) from the University of Chicago. There were no clear outcome differences related to seizure type except for a slightly worse prognosis in children with predominantly myoclonic seizures. A major finding of this study was the association between intractable seizures in childhood and mental retardation. The assumption that either seizures themselves or the anticonvulsant drugs may depress intelligence has prompted an increased interest in the effects of surgical treatment early in life. However, the reports of improvement in cognition after surgery are not well documented.-Editor. *Ped Neur Briefs* Jan 1991.

NEUROPATHOLOGY OF DEVELOPMENTAL DYSLEXIA

The brains of three women with dyslexia were examined at the Dyslexia Research Laboratory, Beth Israel Hospital, Harvard Medical School, Boston, MA. The findings were similar to those reported previously from the same laboratory in four men with developmental dyslexia. The planum temporale was symmetrical, multiple foci of cerebrocortical glial scarring were present in two, and all three cases showed brain warts, molecular layer ectopias, and focal dysplasia. Two women had primary brain neoplasms and two showed small angiomas. The microscopic abnormalities were dated to the periods of late neural migration and cortical maturation. A causal connection between the pathoanatomical findings and the cognitive disorder could not be established. However, it is postulated that the dyslexic individual begins with a familial predisposition to dyslexia which is expressed through a propensity to develop symmetrical temporal plana. The presence of many foci of microdysgenesis in the territory of perforating cortical arterioles suggests the possibility of a microangiopathic etiological process. (Humphreys P et al. Developmental dyslexia in women: Neuropathological findings in three patients. Ann Neurol Dec 1990;28:727-738).

COMMENT. The authors invoke an immunopathogenic mechanism for the cortical scars and neuronal ectopias seen in their neuropathological studies of dyslexics. They cite systemic lupus erythematosus in the mother as a possible cause for the microvascular cerebral pathology in the dyslexic offspring. The multifocal microscopic myelinated scars demonstrated in the three dyslexic women subjects were considered similar to the cortical lesions of systemic lupus erythematosus and supportive of an immunopathogenic mechanism for dyslexia.-Editor. *Ped Neur Briefs* Jan 1991.

DYSLEXIA, HANDEDNESS, AND IMMUNE DISORDERS

An association between dyslexia, left-handedness, and immune disorders was investigated in 734 Norwegian grade 6 children, aged 12 years, at the Center for Reading Research, Stavanger, Norway, and the Department of Psychology, University of Bergen. In the sample studied, 10% of students were dyslexic, 8% were left-handed, 3 5% had allergic symptoms, and 6% were asthmatics. 67% of left-handed dyslexic children had immune disorders (P>.05); 42% of left-handed children with immune disorders had dyslexia (P<.01); and 32% of dyslexic children with immune disorders were left-handed (P<.05). Of the three factors, handedness was the most important association. (Tonnessen FE et al. Dyslexia, left-handedness, and immune disorders. Arch Neurol April 1993;50:411-416). (Reprints: Dr Tonnessen, Center for Reading Research, Box 2504, Ullandhaug, N-4004 Stavanger, Norway).

COMMENT. The Geschwind theory postulates a single factor underlying dyslexia, left-handedness, and immune disorders. The results of this study suggest that left-handedness and dyslexia are more important than immune disorders in a possible three-way association of these conditions.-Editor. *Ped Neur Briefs* April 1993.

DYSLEXIA: A VISUAL DISORDER?

Visual evoked potentials were measured with scalp electrodes in eight reading-disabled children aged 8 to 11 years and compared to a control group of 13 age-matched normal readers at the School of Optometry, University of Missouri, St Louis. Using a steady background and a low-spatial-frequency target (0.5 cycle/degree visual angle), the latencies of the early components (Nl and P1) of the VER were longer and the amplitude of the subsequent (P1-N2) component was smaller in the reading-disabled than in normal readers. A flickering background increased the latency and reduced the amplitude of the early components of the VER in normal readers, whereas in reading-disabled children only the amplitude was affected. These differences were most likely due to a sensory deficit and slowed response in the magnicellular visual pathway of reading-disabled children. (Lehmkuhle S et al. A defective visual pathway in children with reading disability. N Engl J Med April 8 1993;328:989-996). (Reprints: Stephen Lehmkuhle PhD, School of Optometry, University of Missouri-St Louis, 8001 Natural Bridge Rd, St Louis, MO 63121).

COMMENT. These findings are supported by previous anatomical and electrophysiological studies that have demonstrated a defective magnicellular visual pathway in dyslexic subjects. A cause-and-effect relation between these slowed visual responses and the reading disability remains to be determined.-Editor. *Ped Neur Briefs* April 1993.

EEG AND SPELLING DISABILITIES

The EEGs in 23 13-year-old Finnish-speaking boys with spelling disabilities and in 21 matched controls were studied in the Departments of Child Neurology, Paediatrics, Clinical Neurophysiology and Psychology, University of Helsinki, Finland. The visual assessment of the records showed an abnormal EEG in

48% of the index group and in 25% of controls. The abnormalities included a general excessive slow activity, temporal slow wave activity and non-paroxysmal slowing. The frequency of paroxysmal activity did not differ significantly in the two groups; 4% in the index group and 9.5% in controls. A neurotic disposition measured by the Tennessee Self-concept scale and clinical subscale was more frequent in the index group than controls and reading was slightly impaired. Arithmetic skills were comparable in the two groups. In covariance analysis the qEEG parameter differences between the index group and controls were partly explained by the neurotic traits and emotional tension, characteristic of the children with spelling difficulties. (Byring RF et al. EEG in children with spelling disabilities. Electroenceph clin Neurophysiol Oct 1991;79:247-255).

COMMENT. Poor rhythmicity and low voltage of the background rhythm have been found in the EEG of children with learning disabilities, and visual EEG analysis has shown a large variety of EEG abnormalities associated with dyslexia (Hughes JR. In: Benton AL and Pearl D (Eds), Dyslexia - An Appraisal of Current Knowledge, Oxford University Press, New York. 1978:205-249. The present authors stress that psychopathology may be a confounding factor in the interpretation of EEG abnormalities in association with spelling disabilities and dyslexia.-Editor. *Ped Neur Briefs* Oct 1991.

LANGUAGE DISORDERS

CEREBELLAR VERMIS ABNORMALITIES IN FRAGILE X SYNDROME, AUTISM, AND POST-SURGICAL MUTISM

Posterior fossa abnormalities measured by magnetic resonance images of the brain were reported in a group of 14 males with fragile X syndrome from the Division of Child Psychiatry, and the Departments of Psychiatry and Radiology, The Johns Hopkins University School of Medicine, and The Kennedy

Institute, Baltimore, MD. The size of the posterior cerebellar vermis was significantly decreased and the fourth ventricle significantly increased in males with fragile X syndrome compared to a group of 17 males with other causes of developmental disability and 18 males with normal IQs. The lack of a significant correlation between age and size of vermis argues against atrophy as the cause but rather a developmental hypoplasia of the posterior vermis. (Reiss AL et al. Neuroanatomy of fragile X syndrome: the posterior fossa. Ann Neurol Jan 1991;29:26-32).

COMMENT. Hypoplasia of the cerebellar vermal lobules VI and VII has also been described in patients with autism |(Courchesne E et al. N Engl J Med 1988;318:1349). Autistic-like behavior occurs frequently in males with fragile X syndrome and the posterior vermis hypoplasia may have a causative relation. The cerebellar vermis plays an important role in the modulation and execution of motor behavior, and hyperactivity and repetitive stereotypic movements are common behaviorisms in fragile X patients. Language dysfunction also occurs with fragile X syndrome and the posterior vermis of the cerebellum is involved in auditory processing of language.

So-called "*cerebellar mutism*" may develop after removal of posterior fossa tumors, particularly medulloblastoma, and this complication has been correlated with the amount of the posterior vermis resected. (Platenberg C et al. AJNR 1989;10:891). A seven year old girl with a midline posterior fossa tumor developed mutism after surgical removal of an astrocytoma that involved the vermis of the cerebellum. Recovery was slow but speech was regained after a two month period of therapy (Millichap JG, McLone D, unpublished case report).- Editor. *Ped Neur Briefs* Feb 1991.

AUTISM, DYSPHASIA, AND EPILEPSY

The prevalence and clinical manifestations of epilepsy in 302 autistic and 237 dysphasic, non-autistic children were studied at the Departments of Neurology and Pediatrics, Albert Einstein College of Medicine and Montefiore Medical Center, Bronx, New York. Epilepsy occurred in 14% of autistic children and 8% of dysphasic children. Girls were affected more frequently than boys (24% cf 11%). The seizure types included generalized tonic-clonic, atypical absence, atonic, myoclonic, infantile spasms and partial. Infantile spasms occurred in 12% of autistic patients with epilepsy. The major risk factors for epilepsy were severe mental deficiency and the combination of mental deficiency with a motor deficit. When cognitive and motor disabilities were excluded, the risk of epilepsy in autistic children was only 6% and similar to that found in dysphasic non-autistic children (Tuchman RF, Rapin I, Shinnar S. Autistic and dysphasic children. II: epilepsy. Pediatrics Dec 1991;88:1219-1225.) (Reprints: Dr Rapin, Rose F Kennedy Center for Research in Mental Retardation, Room 807, 1410 Pelham Parkway South, Bronx, NY 10461)

COMMENT. The rates of epilepsy reported in autistic children have ranged from 11% to 42%. Associated cognitive and motor deficits, a higher ratio of girls, and the complication of verbal auditory agnosia in some series might explain the higher rates of epilepsy. As a group, autistic children are more likely than dysphasic children to have language subtypes affecting central processing and a history of regression of language and behavior. -Editor. *Ped Neur Briefs* Jan 1992.

EEG IN LANDAU-KLEFFNER (ACQUIRED EPILEPTIC APHASIA) SYNDROME

The EEG was studied in five children with Landau-Kleffner syndrome at the Service de Neurologie I, Hopital Central, Strasbourg, France, and Department de Neurologie C.H.U. Sart Tilmman, Liege, Belgium. Day and nighttime EEG video monitoring was performed before and after each change of therapy. One hundred EEGs of 30 minute to two hour duration were recorded on awake patients. Sleep EEGs were obtained during five spontaneous daytime naps, 15 naps induced by amitriptyline, and 65 complete nights of sleep. Spike-wave duration was measured as a percentage of the total sleep period. The EEG in waking patients showed focal and generalized spike-wave discharges on a normal background rhythm. During sleep, discharges increased and bilateral spike-waves occurred more than 85% of the sleep period. The abnormal EEG and the impairment of higher cognitive function developed and regressed together. It was difficult to differentiate the Landau-Kleffner syndrome and "Epilepsy with continuous spike-waves during slow wave sleep". Only the neuropsychological features differed. They are probably variations of a single syndrome. (Hirsch E et al. Landau-Kleffner syndrome: A clinical and EEG study of five cases. Epilepsia Nov/Dec 1990;31:756-767).

COMMENT. In the classical Landau-Kleffner syndrome aphasia is acquired and other higher cortical functions do not usually deteriorate. In the "continuous spike-wave activity during sleep syndrome" speech is disturbed in 50% of cases but intellectual deterioration occurs and psychiatric disorders develop. In three of the five patients studied by the authors, only treatment by corticosteroids had lasting effects in correcting the regression of higher functions and EEG abnormalities. Phenobarbital, carbamazepine, and phenytoin were either ineffective or exacerbated the EEG and neuropsychological abnormalities. (Marescaux C et al. Landau-Kleffner syndrome: A pharmacological study of five cases. Epilepsia Nov/Dec 1990;31:768-777). These authors recommend that high doses of corticosteroids should be administered early at the first appearance of symptoms and preferably before total aphasia or intellectual regression occur; treatment should be maintained at lower doses for a period of months.

An abnormal pattern of cerebral glucose utilization demonstrated in three children with Landau-Kleffner syndrome by PET study is reported by the same group of authors from Liege, Belgium and Strasbourg, France (Maquet P et al. Cerebral glucose utilization during sleep in Landau-Kleffner syndrome: A PET study. Epilepsia Nov/Dec 1990;31:778-783). The specificity of the metabolic abnormalities and their relationship to the aphasia and EEG remain to be determined.-Editor. *Ped Neur Briefs* Jan 1991.

ACQUIRED APHASIA WITH COMPLEX PARTIAL EPILEPSY

The syndrome of acquired aphasia, dementia and behavior disorder in a child with partial complex epilepsy and continuous spike and waves during sleep is reported from the Service de Pediatrie, et Service de Neurologie, CHUV, Lausanne, Switzerland. The child was observed from age three to 18 years and deterioration in behavior and language occurred between the ages of 3-1/2 and 5 years, coinciding with the period of maximal EEG activity and the presence of almost continuous spike waves during sleep (CSWS). Improvement coincided with the disappearance of CSWS, between the ages of 5-1/2 and 6-1/2 years, and the onset of a unilateral focus that persisted throughout the following years. A definite correlation between the paroxysmal EEG abnormalities and the neuropsychological deterioration and improvement was established retrospectively. (Roulet E, Deonna T et al. Acquired aphasia, dementia, and behavior disorder with epilepsy and continuous spike and waves during sleep in a child. Epilepsia July/August 1991;32:495-503).

COMMENT. Complex partial seizures with recurrence in adolescence and the persistence of an epileptic focus on the EEG are atypical features of the Landau-Kleffner syndrome but this diagnosis could not be definitely excluded.-Editor. *Ped Neur Briefs* Sept 1991.

CORTICOSTEROIDS FOR LANDAU-KLEFFNER SYNDROME

Four children between five and nine years of age with Landau-Kleffner syndrome were treated with ACTH or corticosteroids at the Department of Pediatrics, Beilinson Medical Centre, and Sackler Faculty of Medicine, Tel Aviv University, Israel. ACTH in one patient was given for three months starting with 80 units/day followed by a gradual reduction of the dose. An EEG three weeks after the start of the treatment showed complete disappearance of epileptic activity, but the aphasia was initially unchanged. Complete remission of the aphasia occurred eight months after the completion of the ACTH course. Two years later the aphasia recurred with the concomitant appearance of multiple spike discharges on the EEG. Prompt prescription of ACTH therapy led to a recovery of speech and a normal EEG within a few weeks. Prednisone 60 mg/day for two to three months in two patients caused a prompt improvement in the EEG followed by normal speech. Dexamethasone 4 mg/day resulted in full recovery of speech and a completely normal EEG within two weeks of starting treatment in a nine year old child. Three to six years after discontinuing therapy the children are off anticonvulsant medication and free from seizures and language disability. (Lerman P et al. Effect of early corticosteroid therapy for Landau-Kleffner syndrome. Dev Med Child Neurol March 1991;33:257-266).

COMMENT. These results are encouraging and warrant further trials of hormone therapy in children with the aphasic epilepsy syndrome. As in the treatment of West syndrome, corticosteroids administered early are more effective than delayed treatments.

Hypsarrhythmia is not a sine qua non for ACTH therapy. Two children, aged 3 years and 2 years 8 months with status absence and generalized tonic-clonic seizures refractory to anticonvulsant medication were benefited by ACTH 10 units intramuscular daily. Control of seizures, improvement in the EEG, and a dramatic recovery of mental and motor abilities occurred within two hours of the first injection in one patient and seizure control and EEG improvement occurred in the second after a three week course of therapy. Further trials of ACTH in children with seizures other than infantile spasms are recommended. (Millichap JG. Neurology March 1991;41 (Suppl 1):201).-Editor. *Ped Neur Briefs* April 1991.

PROGNOSIS OF LANDAU-KLEFFNER SYNDROME

The long-term follow up of 6 patients and a

review of the recent literature on the Landau-Kleffner syndrome ("acquired aphasia with convulsive disorder") are reported from the Department of Neurology, University Hospital Dijkzigt-Rotterdam, The Netherlands. The age at onset was 3 to 5 years, with epilepsy as the first sign in 3 and comprehension deficit in 3. Seizures were absence, generalized tonic-clonic, partial and complex partial in pattern. Seizures had disappeared at follow-up in 3 and epileptic activity in the EEG was absent in 4. The course of the aphasia was linked to the appearance and disappearance of electrical status epilepticus during slow sleep (ESES) which was found in 3 patients. Lasting EEG abnormalities and persisting clinical seizures, combined with the presence and duration of ESES, may impede language recovery. The disappearance of ESES may be associated with an improvement of language functions. The course of the aphasia was variable: slow and continuous improvement in 3, rapid recovery in 1, fluctuating in 1, and deterioration followed by slow improvement in 1. The follow-up period varied from 3 to 19 years. The response of the seizures and aphasia to anticonvulsants was variable; some benefit was obtained with phenytoin and phenobarbital in 1 patient, and ethosuximide and valproate were helpful in 2. Prednisone in 1 patient had a variable and inconclusive effect. (Paquier PF, Van Dongen HR, Loonen MCB. The Landau-Kleffner Syndrome or "acquired aphasia with convulsive disorder" Arch Neurol April 1992;49:354-359). (Reprints: Dr. Van Dongen, Department of Neurology, Room EE 2287, University Hospital Dijkzigt-Rotterdam, P.O. Box 1738, 3000 DR Rotterdam, The Netherlands.)

COMMENT. The correlation between ESES and acquired epileptic aphasia has been emphasized previously (Jayakar PB, Seshia SS. J Clin Neurophysiol 1991;7:299-311; Deonna TW. J Clin Neurophysiol 1991;7:288-298). See also Ped Neur Briefs Sept 1991;5:71; Jan 1991;5:45). The beneficial effects of ACTH and corticosteroids have been reported from Tel Aviv University (Lerman P et al. See Ped Neur Briefs April

1991;5:28-29). Corticosteroids administered early were more effective than delayed treatments.-Editor. Ped Neur Briefs May 1992.

OUTCOME OF ACQUIRED APHASIA

The effects of age at onset, etiology, severity, and type of aphasia on the course and outcome were investigated in a group of 28 aphasic children at the Department of Neurology, University Hospital Rotterdam-Dijkzigt, The Netherlands. Head injury was the cause in eight patients with onset between 4 and 11 years, vascular diseases accounted for seven cases with age of onset between 3 and 13 vears, infectious diseases were present in 5 patients with onset between 4 and 12 years, Landau-Kleffner syndrome occurred in six cases with onset at 4-6 years, and cerebral tumor was present in four patients 9-13 years of age. There was no difference in recovery for those children aged above or below 11 years. The very young children with Landau-Kleffner syndrome had a bad prognosis. Six of the eight children with head injury had a favorable outcome, in contrast to those with vascular or infectious disease. Only one of six children with Landau-Kleffner syndrome recovered completely despite normal CT scans. The severity and bilaterality of the lesions showed no significant relation to prognosis of the aphasia. The severity of the cerebral lesion was assessed using a rating scale for CT scans. Most of the children had not recovered completely one year after onset of the aphasia. Recovery was significantly different according to etiological categories. (Loonen MCB, van Dongen HR. Acquired childhood aphasia. Outcome 1 year after onset. Arch Neurol Dec 1990;47:1324-1328).

COMMENT. In general the outcome of acquired aphasia in childhood is good after mild head injury and a poor outcome may be expected in aphasia due to infectious disorders or Landau-Kleffner syndrome. Bilateral lesions on CT scan are frequently found in patients with infectious and vascular diseases in which aphasia is associated with a poor outcome.-Editor. *Ped Neur Briefs* Jan 1991.

CHAPTER 5

TOURETTE SYNDROME AND OTHER MOVEMENT DISORDERS

INTRODUCTION

Harvey S. Singer, M.D.
The Johns Hopkins Hospital, Baltimore, MD

Tourette syndrome (TS) is a relatively common neuropsychological disorder that provides a unique model for studying the interactions among clinical behaviors, genetics, and brain function. New and interesting neurobiological information has been acquired about TS, but the much anticipated identification of the gene(s) that influence inherited vulnerability has remained elusive [1].

Although the existing range of tic symptoms in affected individuals is already extensive, reports now include a young woman with "signing" tics (swore, echoed what others said and repeated her own phrases in sign language) [2]. Several authors have emphasized the presence of premonitory (sensory) experiences occurring prior to and perhaps initiating tics [3], although in my experience these are relatively uncommon. A new classification for tics has been published in order to improve the accuracy of diagnoses: categories now include "definite", "probable", and "by history" [4], [Ped Neur Briefs Nov 1993]. New clinical rating instruments have been developed for following the severity of tics [5]. Investigators have pursued the natural history of TS [6] [Ped Neur Briefs Oct 1993] and have sought to identify prognostic characteristics [7] [Ped Neur Briefs May 1992].

Studies continue to suggest an autosomal dominant mode of genetic transmission for tic disorders [8]. However, since some genetic studies in monozygotic twins have shown a concordance rate for these disorders of less than 100% as well as a variability in tic severity despite the inheritance of similar genetic material [9], non-genetic (environmental) factors may be operating. Recent environmental hypotheses proposed to influence the appearance of tics include prenatal factors, anabolic steroids, and antineuronal antibodies induced by streptococcal infection [9-12]. [Ped Neur Briefs July 1993].

For the child with a tic disorder, problems often extend beyond the presence of motor and vocal tics with co-morbid features including attention deficit hyperactivity disorder (ADHD), obsessive compulsive behaviors, learning disorders, and other psychopathologies. A genetic relationship between TS and ADHD remains controversial [13, 14], but there are emerging suggestions of two types of individuals with TS+ADHD: ADHD that is genetically related and ADHD that is independent of TS. Although psychostimulant medications are generally regarded as the treatment of choice for ADHD, their use in children with TS generates debate [15, 16] and has lead to ongoing studies of alternative medications. Tics are more prevalent in children attending special education classes [17] and formal psychometric evaluations suggest that many learning problems are associated with comorbid features rather than tics per se [18].

Neurobiological data continue to support proposals that TS is a disorder of fronto-subcortical circuits. Volumetric MRI studies in both children and adults have shown significant differences in the putamen and lenticular regions [19, 20]. [Ped Neur Briefs June 1993]. These findings are consistent with reported functional imaging studies. Furthermore, neuroimaging has identified putative anatomical abnormalities of the basal ganglia in individuals with ADHD and OCD [19, 21]. [Ped Neur Briefs June 1993]. Several of the numerous neurotransmitter systems present in the brain have been proposed as the underlying pathophysiological mechanism in TS. Despite ongoing speculations [22], which transmitter(s) is most essential remains under investigation. - *Harvey S. Singer, M.D., Department of Pediatric Neurology, The Johns Hopkins Hospital, Baltimore, MD.*

REFERENCES

1. van de Wetering BJ, Heutink P. The genetics of the Gilles de la Tourette syndrome; a review. J Lab Clin Med 1993;121:638-645.

2. Lang AE, Consky E, Sandor P. "Signing-tics"...insights into the pathophysiology of symptoms in Tourette syndrome. Ann Neurol 1993;33:212-215.

3. Leckman JF, Walker DE, Cohen DJ. Premonitory urges in Tourette's syndrome. Am J Psychiatry 1993;150:98-102.

4. The Tourette Syndrome Classification Group. Definition and classification of tic disorders. Arch Neurol 1993;50:1013-1016.

5. Walkup JT, Rosenberg LA, Brown J, Singer HS. The validity of instruments measuring tic severity in Tourette syndrome. J Am Acad Child Adolesc Psychiatry 1992;30:472-477.

6. Parks S, Como PG, Cui L, Kurlan R. The early course of Tourette's syndrome clinical spectrum. Neurology 1993;43:1712-1715.

7. Goetz CG, Tanner CB, Stebbins GT, Leipzig G, Carr WC. Adult tics in Gilles de la Tourette's syndrome: description and risk factors. Neurology 1992;42:784-788.

8. Carter AS, Pauls DL, Leckman JF, Cohen DJ. A prospective longitudinal study of Gilles de la Tourette's

syndrome. J Am Acad Child Adolesc Psychiatry 1994;33:377-385.

9. Hyde TM, Aaronson BA, Randolph C, Rickler KC, Weinberger DR. Relationship of birth weight to the phenotypic expression of Gilles de la Tourette's syndrome. Neurology 1992;42:652-658.

10. Leckman JF, Peterson BS. The pathogenesis of Tourette's syndrome: Epigenetic factors active in early CNS development. Biol Psychiatry 1993;34:425-427.

11. Peterson BS. Leckman JF, Scahill L et al. Hypothesis: steroid hormones and CNS sexual dimorphisms modulate symptom expression in Tourette's syndrome. Psychoneuroendocrinology 1992;17:553-563.

12. Kiessling LS, Marcotte AC, Culpepper L. Antineuronal antibodies in movement disorders. Pediatrics 1993;92:39-43.

13. Knell ER, Comings DE. Tourette's syndrome and attention deficit hyperactivity disorder: Evidence for a genetic relationship. J Clin Psychiatry 1993;54:331-337.

14. Pauls DL, Leckman JF, Cohen DJ. The familial relationship between Gilles de la Tourette's syndrome, attention deficit disorder, learning disabilities, speech disorders and stuttering. J Am Acad Child Adolesc Psychiatry 1993;32:1044-1050.

15. Gadow KD, Nolan EE, Sverd J. Methylphenidate in hyperactive boys with co-morbid tic disorder: II. Short-term behavioral effects in school settings. J Am Acad Child Adolesc Psychiatry 1992;31:462-471.

16. Robertson MM, Eapen V. Pharmacologic controversy of CNS stimulants in Gilles de la Tourette's syndrome. Clin Neuropharm 1992;15:462-471.

17. Kurlan R, Whitmore D, Irvine C, McDermott MP, Como PG. Tourette's syndrome in a special education population: A pilot study involving a single school district. Neurology 1994;44:699-702.

18. Yeats KO, Bornstein RA. Attention deficit disorder and neuropsychological functioning in children with Tourette's syndrome. Neuropsychology 1994;8:65-74.

19. Singer HS, Reiss AL, Brown JE, Aylward EH, Shih B, Chee E, Harris EL, Reader MJ, Chase GA, Bryan RN, Denckla MB. Volumetric MRI changes in basal ganglia of children with Tourette's syndrome. Neurology 1993;43:950-956.

20. Peterson B, Riddle MA, Cohen DJ, et al. Reduced

basal ganglia volumes in Tourette's syndrome using three-dimensional reconstruction techniques from magnetic resonance images. Neurology 1993;43:941-949.

21. Insel TR. Toward a neuroanatomy of obsessive-compulsive disorder. Arch Gen Psychiatry 1992;49:739-744.

22. Singer HS. Pathobiology. In Kurlan R, ed. Handbook of Tourette's Syndrome and Related Tic and Behavioral Disorders. New York, Marcel Dekker, 1993:267-288.

TOURETTE SYNDROME CLASSIFICATION

A task force (The Tourette Syndrome Classification Study Group), organized by the Tourette Syndrome Association, has expanded the DSM-IIIR definitions of Tourette syndrome and is developing a quantitative rating scale for tics to be used by clinicians in practice and in genetic and other research activities. Each of the four basic DSM definitions (*Tourette syndrome, chronic tic disorder, transient tic disorder, and non-specified tic disorder) is* divided into two categories; "definite," tics witnessed by a reliable observer, and "historical," putative tics not reliably witnessed. Additional tic categories have been included: *chronic single tic disorder; definite tic disorder-diagnosis deferred* (symptoms less than 1 year); and *probable Tourette syndrome* (some criteria for diagnosis absent). (Fahn S et al. Definitions and classification of tic disorders. Arch Neurol Oct 1993;50:1013-1016). (Reprints: Dr Fahn, Neurological Institute, 710 W 168th St, New York, NY 10032).

COMMENT. A similar classification was proposed by a TSA workshop in a previous report (Kurlan R. Neurology Dec 1989;39:1625; see Progress in Pediatric Neurology, Chicago, PNB Publishers, 1991;230-232).

Most tics are idiopathic but some are symptomatic of head trauma, encephalitis, or other etiologies. Three children with *carbamazepine-induced tics* are reported from the Departments of Pediatrics and Neurology, University of Michigan Medical Center, Ann Arbor, MI (Robertson PL et al. Epilepsia Sept/Oct 1993;34:965-968). The temporal association of repetitive blinking, jaw opening or clenching, and tongue movements with the initiation of CBZ treatment for complex partial seizures, and the absence of other etiologies, suggests that CBZ was the likely cause. Additional cases of carbamazepine-related tics and other movement disorders have been reported.

The contingent negative variation (CNV), a slow brain potential which may reflect the level of central dopamine and is a measure of arousal and attention, has been studied in patients with Tourette syndrome (Weate SJ, Drake ME Jr et al. Clin Electroencephalogr Oct 1993;24:188-191). Patients had higher CNV amplitude and more frequent postimperative negative variation than controls, possibly explained by dopaminergic excess. Medication was not a factor.-Editor. *Ped Neur Briefs* Nov 1993.

EARLY SIGNS OF TOURETTE'S SYNDROME

The early course of tics and behavioral disturbances in 101 children with Tourette's syndrome, aged 12 years (range, 8 to 21 years), are reported from the University of Rochester School of Medicine, Rochester, NY. The age at onset was 6.4 +/- 3.1 years. At initial evaluation, 45% already had ADHD and 50% had obsessive-compulsive disorder (OCD). During the observation period of 1.6 years (range, 0.5 to 7 years), tics became controlled with medication in 81%, 13% developed ADHD, 8% OCD, 28% disruptive behavior, and 25% school problems. Of those with behavioral disorders initially, about 50% were controlled over time with treatment. Tic suppressants were withdrawn from 12% of patients. (Park S, Kurlan R et al. The early course of the Tourette's syndrome clinical spectrum. Neurology Sept 1993;43:1712-1715). (Reprints: Dr Kurlan, Department of Neurology, University of Rochester School of Medicine, 601 Elmwood Avenue, Rochester, NY 14642).

COMMENT. If ADHD and OCD are absent at the onset of tics, it is unusual for these behaviors to develop later. Disruptive behavior and school problems are more likely to develop over time.-Editor. *Ped Neur Briefs* Oct 1993.

POSTENCEPHALITIC TOURETTE SYNDROME

A six year old girl who developed a Tourette-like syndrome following herpes encephalitis is reported from the Division of Child Neurology, Walter Reed Army Medical Center, Washington, DC and Departments of Neurology and Pediatrics, Johns Hopkins University School of Medicine, Baltimore, MD. A three day prodrome of headaches, malaise, nausea and vomiting was followed by fever and focal motor seizures involving the left side of the face and the left arm. Lumbar puncture showed 122 WBCs (80% lymphocytes) and a protein of 31 mg/dl. A repeat lumbar puncture within 24 hours showed 750 WBCs, 43 RBCs, and protein 85 mg/dl. CT on hospital day three and subsequent MRIs showed a small hemorrhagic lesion in the right mesial temporal region and progressive edematous changes in the right temporal lobe, basal ganglia and thalamus. EEG showed focal slowing over the right temporal and frontal lobes. A presumptive diagnosis of herpes encephalitis was made and Acyclovir was given for ten days. At two weeks after discharge she developed eye blinking and sudden rapid recurrent purposeless nonrhythmic stereotyped motor movements and vocalizations. The tics were characterized by facial grimacing, head twitching, and shoulder shrugging plus eye rolling, facial contorsions, jumping, touching objects and body parts and making obscene gestures. Vocal tics included grunting, sniffing, and snorting sounds . The tics were suppressed after several weeks on Pimozide (Orap 1 mg b.i.d.). (Northam RS, Singer HS. Postencephalitic acquired Tourette-like syndrome in a child. Neurology April 1991;41:592-593).

COMMENT. The authors refer to reports of acquired Tourette syndrome in adults. Tics followed withdrawal from neuroleptic medications or in association with herpes and other encephalitides, toxic and metabolic encephalopathies, strokes, cerebral tumors, trauma, multiple sclerosis, syphilis, Huntington's, Alzheimer's, and Creutzfeldt-Jakob diseases.-Editor. *Ped Neur Briefs* June 1991.

BASAL GANGLIA AND MRI IN TOURETTE'S SYNDROME

Volumetric MRI changes in the basal ganglia of 37 children with Tourette's syndrome (TS), with and without ADHD, compared to 18 controls are reported from Johns Hopkins University School of Medicine, Baltimore, MD. Major findings were 1) right-handed control children had asymmetry of the putamen with left-sided predominence; 2) 13 TS patients had a reversal of putamen asymmetry compared to controls; and 3) ADHD in TS patients is associated with reduction in volume of the left globus pallidus and lenticular asymmetry. (Singer HS, Denckla MB et al. Volumetric MRI changes in basal ganglia of children with Tourette's syndrome. Neurology May 1993;43:950-956). (Reprints: Dr Harvey S Singer, Department of Neurology-Harvey 811, Johns Hopkins Hospital, 600 N Wolfe Street, Baltimore, MD 21287).

COMMENT. The basal ganglia appear to be involved in the pathogenesis of TS. ADHD in TS patients is associated with additional anatomic changes in the globus pallidus and lenticular region that differ from those primarily associated with tics.

Reduced basal ganglia volumes on MRI of TS patients are also reported from the Yale Child Study Center, New Haven, CT (Peterson B et al. Neurology May 1993;43:941-949). The left lenticular nuclei in TS patients were significantly reduced in volume, and the left globus pallidus and putamen mean volumes showed a 10% reduction. TS basal ganglia lacked the volumetric asymmetry (left greater than right) seen in normal controls.

Five of 7 patients with concurrent Tourette's (TS) and Asperger's (AS) syndromes showed developmental cortical anomalies on MRI, whereas normal MRI scans were found in 8 of 9 TS patients without AS, in a report from the Neurology Service, Hospital Clinic and Provincial, Barcelona, Spain (Berthier ML et al. J Am Acad Child Adolesc Psychiatry May 1993;32:633-639). The group with concurrent TS and AS had more clinical signs of CNS dysfunction and were more impaired on complex problem-solving and spatial tests than did TS patients without AS.-Editor. *Ped Neur Briefs* June 1993.

PATIENT PERCEPTION OF TICS

The subjective perception of abnormal movements was determined in 170 patients with various hyperkinesias at the Movement Disorders Clinic, Toronto Western Hospital, Toronto, Ontario. 102 of 110 patients with non-tic disorders thought that the abnormal movements were entirely involuntary whereas 41 of 60 tic disorder patients stated that all of their motor and phonic tics were intentional or voluntary. A "voluntary response" could be used to predict the correct diagnostic category (tic versus non-tic) in 8 of 9 patients for whom the initial diagnosis was incorrect. A large proportion of the motor and phonic symptoms experienced by tic patients are irresistably, but purposefully executed and resemble compulsions rather than involuntary hyperkinesias. (Lang A. Patient perception of tics and other movement disorders. Neurology Feb 1991;41:223-228)

COMMENT. This recategorization of tics as intentional and purposeful actions is similar to that of compulsions which may be linked genetically.-Editor. *Ped Neur Briefs* April 1991.

TIC SEVERITY AND PSYCHOLOGICAL FUNCTION

The relationship between tic severity and neuropsychological function was examined in 12 monozygotic twin pairs with Tourette's syndrome at the National Institute of Mental Health, Bethesda, MD. Children with more severe tic symptoms had poorer overall performance on psychological tests, and differences were significant on individual tests of attention, visuospatial perception, and motor function. In each twin pair, the twin with more severe tics had poorer global neuropsychological function. (Randolph C et al. Tourette's syndrome in monozygotic twins. Relationship of tic severity to neuropsychological function. Arch Neurol July 1993;50:725-728). (Reprints: Dr Randolph, Experimental Therapeutics Branch, National

Institute of Neurological Disorders and Stroke, Bldg 10, Room 5C104, 9000 Rockville Pike, Bethesda, MD 20892).

COMMENT. Tic severity and psychological function in children with Tourette's syndrome appear to be influenced by nongenetic factors with a common pathophysiology. The authors found that disturbances of attention were a cardinal psychological feature of TS, but most neuropsychological measures were close to normal means.-Editor. *Ped Neur Briefs* July 1993.

STREPTOCOCCAL INFECTION AND TOURETTE SYNDROME

Serum antibodies against human caudate nucleus sections and antistreptococcal titers were determined in 83 ADHD children, 45 with and 38 without an associated movement disorder, at Brown University School of Medicine, Rhode Island. Those with movement disorders [Tourette syndrome (7), tics (23), choreiform movements (15)]. were significantly more likely to have antineuronal antibodies (44%), determined by immunofluorescent staining, and elevated antistreptococcal titers (43%) than those without movement disorders (21% and 27%, respectively). The percentage of children with a movement disorder whose sera were strongly positive for antineuronal antibodies (44%) was similar to that found in children with Sydenham's chorea (46%). (Kiessling LS et al. Antineuronal antibodies in movement disorders. Pediatrics July 1993;92:39-43). (Reprints: LS Kiessling MD, Dept of Pediatrics, Memorial Hospital of Rhode Island, 111 Brewster St, Pawtucket, RI 02860).

COMMENT. The authors are to be congratulated on following up their observation of a temporal relationship between streptococcal infection and the abrupt onset of tics in children seen in their clinic for ADHD. Tics as a sequel to Sydenham's chorea was a recognized complication or continuum more than 60 years ago (Guttmann E (1927) et al; In Wilson SAK, Neurology. Baltimore, Williams and Wilkins, 1955, p 1924), and the association between antecendent group A B-hemolytic streptococcal infection and tics demonstrated in this study might be expected. The resolution of the tics following treatment with amoxicillin requires further investigation.-Editor. *Ped Neur Briefs* July 1993.

HORMONAL INFLUENCES ON TOURETTE SYNDROME

A survey of 47 women with Tourette syndrome reported from the Section of Pediatric Neurology, Children's Hospital of Wisconsin, Milwaukee, WI had an increase in tics beginning at menarche and recurring premenstrually. A comparable number of patients had a decreased tic frequency during the postmenstrual period. The average age of symptom onset was 8 years and the average age of diagnosis was 13.8 years. No significant relationship was found between a change in tic frequency and other non-menstrual cycle-related female hormonal states such as premenstrual syndrome, oral contraceptive use, pregnancy and menopause (Schwabe MJ, Konkol RJ. Menstrual cycle-related fluctuations of tics in Tourette syndrome. Pediatr Neurol Jan/Feb 1992;8:43-46). (Respond: Dr. Konkol, Department of Neurology, MACC Fund Research Building, Watertown Plank Road, Milwaukee, WI 53226.)

COMMENT. Thermal stress is another factor that might exacerbate Tourette syndrome and cause an increase in the frequency of tics (Lombroso PJ et al. Exacerbation of Gilles de la Tourette's syndrome associated with thermal stress: a family study. Neurology Dec 1991;41:1984-1987). When challenged with heat or exercise in climate controlled conditions a 17 year old boy showed a marked increase in frequency of tics. The patient reported that his tics became more severe whenever the weather became warmer, when he had a fever, or after vigorous exercise. He would have difficulty standing and often had to lie down because of the severity of head jerks and other tics.-Editor. *Ped Neur Briefs* April 1992.

PROGNOSIS OF TOURETTE'S SYNDROME

A retrospective study of 58 adults with a diagnosis of Gilles de la Tourette's syndrome (TS) during childhood is reported from the Department of Neurological Sciences,

Rush-Presbyterian-St. Luke's Medical Center, Chicago, IL. The 41 men and 17 women had a mean current age of 27.1 years and a mean age of tic onset of 6.9 years. Forty six percent had a first degree relative with tics. All patients had tics as adults and most had both motor and phonic tics. Coprolalia occurred in 4% of adults. No patient experienced extreme adult disability and tics caused minimal to mild intrusion into private and professional life. All had received specialized medical care for TS in childhood, but only 26% were currently seeing a physician for tic disorders. Maximal disability had occurred during adolescence in most subjects, but 98% graduated high school, and 90% were full time students or fully employed. Childhood tic severity and coprolalia during development had no predictive value for risk of adult moderate/severe tics. Mild tic severity in adulthood correlated with mild tics during adolescence. (Goetz CG et al. Adult tics in Gilles de la Tourette's syndrome: description and rlsk factors. Neurology April 1992;42:784-788). (Reprints: Dr. CG. Goetz, Department of Neurological Sciences, Rush-Presbyterian-St. Luke's Medical Center, 1725 West Harrison St., Chicago, IL 60612.)

COMMENT. In a study of TS in monozygotic twins, Hyde et al. at the National Institute of Mental Health, Washington, D.C. observed a significant effect of birth weight on the phenotypic expression of TS. Tic scores were greater in the lower birth weight twin as compared with the heavier group. Postnatal factors were not identified and did not play a major role in the subsequent expression of TS (Neurology March 1992;42:652-658). Global neuropsychological performance was more impaired in the more severely affected twin particularly in tests of attention and visuospatial perception (Hyde TM et al. Neurology April 1992;42(Suppl 3):396).

Hypnosis was of benefit in reducing involuntary tics in 6 of 7 unmedicated children age 6 to 15 years with TS (Hollander H et al. Neurology April 1992;42(Suppl 3):239).

Deprenyl, an MAO-B inhibitor, was a safe and effective treatment of attention deficit disorder with hyperactivity in 80% of 20 children with TS. None of the patients noted exacerbation of their tics or other adverse side effects at doses up to 15 mg/day(Jankovic J. Neurology April 1992;42(Suppl 3):238).-Editor. *Ped Neur Briefs* May 1992.

FLUOXETINE IN TOURETTE SYNDROME

An open label trial of fluoxetine (20-40 mg/d) was conducted in 32 Tourette syndrome patients with obsessive-compulsive disorder at the Department of Neurology, University of Rochester School of Medicine, NY. A subjective improvement in obsessions and compulsions occurred in 81% of 26 patients (13 children and 13 adults) who were treated for 3-8 months, and a significant reduction in scores on the Leyton Obsessional Inventory occurred for both the adult and child groups. No serious adverse reactions were reported in either group. Side-effects included dyspepsia and nausea (4), skin rash (2), drowsiness (1) and mild hypomanic behavior (1) (Como P G, Kurlan R An open-label trial of fluoxetine for obsessive-compulsive disorder in Gilles de la Tourette's syndrome. Neurology June 1991;41:872-874).

COMMENT. Fluoxetine is a new antidepressant that inhibits serotonin reuptake and is effective for psychiatric patients with obsessive-compulsive disorder. It appears to produce fewer and less toxic side-effects than clomipramine. The improvement in obsessive-compulsive disorder was most dramatic for the child sample of patients and may be a useful addition to the treatment of obsessive-compulsive disorder in Tourette syndrome.-Editor. *Ped Neur Briefs* July 1991.

DYSTONIA AND CHOREOATHETOSIS

DYSTONIA DUE TO PERINATAL ASPHYXIA

Delayed onset dystonia associated with perinatal asphyxia in two patients and asphyxia in early childhood in two patients is reported from the Neurological Institute of New York. In the perinatal group the mean age of onset was 12.9 years; dystonia progressed for a mean of 7 years and as long as 28 years. The patients had moderate motor disability and none was wheelchair bound. The prognosis was better than that of childhood onset idiopathic torsion dystonias. In the absence of any identifiable cause of dystonia the authors considered the asphyxia as related either directly or indirectly to the development of dystonia. (Saint Hilaire MH et al. Delayed onset dystonia due to perinatal or early childhood asphyxia. Neurology Feb 1991;41:260-222).

COMMENT. Despite the known difficulties in relating adverse perinatal events to static encephalopathies of childhood, the authors claim a relationship between perinatal asphyxia and late onset dystonia based on exclusion of other causes of dystonia and documentation by birth records or a verbal history that asphyxia occurred.-Editor. *Ped Neur Briefs* March 1991.

DYSTONIA AND CYTOCHROME B DEFICIENCY

An 18 year old female with idiopathic torsion dystonia associated with mitochondrial encephalomyopathy is reported from the Departments of Neurology, Pediatrics and Biochemistry, Wayne State University School of Medicine, Detroit, Michigan. At the age of 2 1/2 she developed weakness and disuse of the right leg with a febrile illness. Within one week the weakness extended to the right upper limb. During the next six months she developed progressive dysarthria and dystonia of the right leg and trunk. The dystonia progressively involved all extremities over the next four years. At the age of 7 years CT revealed bilateral putaminal hypodensities. Mitochondrial encephalomyopathy was suspected because of persistent lactic acidemia and myopathy. Studies of oxidative metabolism on skeletal muscle mitochondria revealed partial cytochrome b deficiency indicating a defect in cytochrome b-Cl complex (Nigro MA et al. Partial cytochrome b deficiency in generalized dystonia.

Pediatr Neurol Nov/Dec 1990;6:407-410).

COMMENT Children with Leigh encephalopathy may develop dystonia and putaminal degeneration. H magnetic resonance spectroscopy was used to demonstrate regional variation in brain lactate in an 11 month old infant with Leigh syndrome at the University of Pennsylvania, Philadelphia. (Detre JA et al. Regional variation in brain lactate in Leigh syndrome by localized H magnetic resonance spectroscopy. Ann Neurol Feb 1991;29:218-221). Elevations in brain lactate were observed through out the brain, but were most pronounced in the basal ganglia and brain stem regions with an abnormal MRI appearance. The increase in lactate was consistent with a deficiency in oxidative substrate utilization. The measurement of brain lactate is significant in patients where blood lactate levels may not always be elevated.

Symptomatic dystonias secondary to birth asphyxia, birth trauma, Wilson's disease, other degenerative disorders, encephalitis, neuroleptic drugs and mitochondrial disorders are distinguished from idiopathic or primary torsion dystonias. A genetic study of *idiopathic* focal dystonias has shown that 25% of index patients had relatives with dystonia. The results of segregation analysis suggested an autosomal dominant gene or genes with reduced penetrance as a common cause for focal dystonia and a single autosomal dominant gene mutation responsible for inherited dystonia in the majority of patients, irrespective of distribution or severity. Severity is largely determined by age of onset, with generalized idiopathic dystonia developing before the age of 20 and focal dystonias developing in adult life. (Waddy HM et al. Ann Neurol March 1991;29:320-324).-Editor. *Ped Neur Briefs* April 1991.

STRIATAL SYNDROMES AND DYSTONIA

The clinical manifestations and outcome in 13 patients with bilateral basal ganglia lesions and neurological dysfunction are reported from the Child Neurology Unit, Vall D'Hebron University Hospital,

Barcelona, Spain. Lesions were demonstrated by CT, MRI, or ultrasound, and in 4 patients who died the pathology was subacute necrotizing encephalomyelopathy (SNE) (2), hypoxic-ischemic encephalopathy (HIE) (1) , and intracranial hemorrhage (1). Extrapyramidal signs included dystonia in 9 patients, athetosis 1, and rigidity 1. Consciousness was altered in 5, and seizures occurred in 3. The outcome was poor in the majority, with motor sequelae and/or cognitive impairment. (Roig M et al. Bilateral striatal lesions in childhood. Pediatr Neurol Sept/Oct 1993;9:349-358). (Respond: Dr Roig, Child Neurology Unit, Hospital Materno-Infantil Vall D'Hebron, Paseo del Vall D'Hebron s/n, Barcelona, Spain).

COMMENT. Based on a review of the literature, the authors tabulate the causes of infantile bilateral striatal syndrome (IBSS) under acute and subacute/chronic categories. *Acute* causes include SNE, HIE, trauma, hemolytic-uremic syndrome, infections, and MELAS. *Chronic* causes include SNE, Huntington disease, Wilson disease, acanthrocytosis, SSPE, glutaric aciduria, and familial metabolic disorders. The pathological findings were necrosis and neuronal loss. CT demonstrated hypodensities and the MRI showed hyperintense T2 weighted images in the basal ganglia. The physiology of basal ganglia disorders is reviewed and an hypothesis for basal ganglia function is proposed by Hallett M, Clinical Director, NINDS, NIH, Bethesda (Can J Neurol Sci Aug 1993;20:177-183). A direct path linking the putamen and globus pallidus is a positive feedback circuit that selects specific motor synergies to carry out a desired action whereas an indirect path inhibits these synergies, eg. dystonia results from overactivity of the putamen and the direct pathway; chorea is explained by underactivity of the indirect pathway.-Editor. *Ped Neur Briefs* Nov 1993.

MRI IN ATHETOTIC CEREBRAL PALSY

The MRI in 22 children with athetotic cerebral palsy was studied in the Department of Pediatric Neurology, Seirei-Mikatabara General Hospital, Hamamatsu, the Department of Pediatrics, National

Rehabilitation Center for Disabled Children, Tokyo, and the Department of Pediatrics, Nagoya City University Medical School, Japan. Perinatal asphyxia had been diagnosed in 16, neonatal jaundice in 2, and no predisposing condition in 4. MRI lesions possibly caused by asphyxia were found in the basal ganglia, thalamus, and/or cerebral white matter in 14 of 16 children. No abnormalities were seen in the cerebral cortex of the subjects. Six children with lesions in both the thalamus and putamen had moderate or severe motor abnormality. Children with lesions in the cerebral white matter only had mild motor abnormality. (Yokochi K et al. Magnetic resonance imaging in athetotic cerebral palsied children. Acta Paediatr Scand Sept 1991;80:818-823.) (Respond: Dr. Yokochi, Soiroi-Mikatabara Gen. Hosp, Mikatabara 3453, Hamamatsu, Shizuoka 433, Japan.)

COMMENT. Brain lesions causing athetosis in CP children may not be revealed by CT scan but high intensity areas in the thalamus, putamen and/or cerebral white matter may be demonstrated in T2-weighted images of the MRI. The evidence of perinatal asphyxia in 16 of the 22 children reported was judged by Apgar scores of 3 and below, generalized hypotonia, and convulsions in the neonatal period. The MR imaging was performed at 2-12 years of age and studies obtained soon after birth might have documented a prenatal timing for the lesions.-Editor. *Ped Neur Briefs* Jan 1992.

DYSKINETIC AND DYSTONIC CEREBRAL PALSY

The records of 794 cases of congenital cerebral palsy (CP) seen between 1955 and 1986 in the Cheyne Centre for Children with Cerebral Palsy, Chelsea, London were analyzed. Of 219 cases with dyskinetic or dystonic CP, 57 had kernicterus and these were excluded from the analysis. Of the remaining 162 patients, birth weight was below the expected mean in two-thirds. The frequency of abnormal births was similar in those born before 37 weeks (32%) and those born at term (30%). Abnormal birth was more common in dyskinetic CP (38%) than in dystonic CP (19%). In kernicterus cases the birth was abnormal in 3.6%. There was a clear positive relationship between abnormal birth and reported asphyxia. A severe outcome was as common in those with an abnormal birth, abnormal neonatal history, or respiratory problems as in those without these complications. The authors concluded that 1) there was no relationship between birth weight or abnormal birth or asphyxia and the ultimate clinical severity of the cerebral palsy, and 2) abnormal birth and asphyxia are not direct causes of cerebral damage, but expressions of a preexisting condition resulting in susceptibility to the stress of birth (Foley J. Dyskinetic and dystonic cerebral palsy and birth. Acta Paediatr Jan 1992;81:57-60). (Correspondence: Dr. John Foley, The Old House, 54 Ashacre Lane, Worthing, W. Sussex BN13 2DE, UK.)

COMMENT. In contrast to the conclusions drawn by Dr. Foley, Hagberg B and Hagberg G, in their invited commentary of this paper, suggest that in the majority of cases of dyskinetic and dystonic CP negative birth events and birth asphyxia in particular are the direct cause with several predisposing factors. They allude to the value of MRI studies in the timing of basal ganglia pathology in these cases (see also Ped Neur Briefs Jan 1992;6:3-4).-Editor. *Ped Neur Briefs* April 1992.

PSYCHOLOGICAL SYMPTOMS OF SYDENHAM'S CHOREA

The psychological symptoms of 11 children with Sydenham's chorea (8 girls and 3 boys, mean age 8.4 years) were evaluated at the National Institute of Mental Health, Bethesda, MD. Subjects had a recent onset of chorea and rheumatic fever. Seven had rheumatic carditis and 3 had arthritis. All were receiving penicillin, and 8 had been treated with haloperidol, without lasting benefit. All had an elevated antistreptolysin O (ASO) titer, greater than 480 Todd units, and 10 had positive antineuronal antibody titers. Psychological symptoms included nightmares, decreased attention, hyperactivity, distractibility, emotional lability, and an acute onset of obsessive-compulsive disorder. The OCD started shortly before the onset of involuntary movements, peaked with the chorea, and disappeared before movements ceased. The mean total duration of chorea symtoms was 7 months. (Swedo SE et al. Sydenham's chorea: Physical and psychological symptoms of St Vitus dance. Pediatrics April 1993;91:706-713). (Reprints: Susan E Swedo MD, Child Psychiatry Branch, National Institute of Mental Health, Bldg 10, Room 6N240, 9000 Rockville Pike, Bethesda, MD 20892).

COMMENT. Of 9 children exhibiting obsessive-compulsive symtoms, 4 met DSM-III-R diagnostic criteria for OCD. The authors hypothesize that certain acute-onset cases of OCD acquired during childhood may represent an autoimmune cerebral disorder similar to Sydenham's chorea, and affecting the basal ganglia. A trial of intravenous immunoglobulin in children with Sydenham's chorea is in progress at the NIH.-Editor. *Ped Neur Briefs* April 1993.

BENIGN HEREDITARY CHOREA

The clinical manifestations, differential diagnosis, and treatment of benign hereditary chorea (BHC) are reviewed from the Indiana University and University of Minnesota Medical Schools. The diagnosis of BHC is by exclusion. The most common age of onset is about 1 year and walking is often delayed because of clumsiness and falling. After a short period of progression in severity, movements reach a plateau and may sometimes appear to improve. IQ is normal or low-average. In most reported families, the inheritance is autosomal dominant. Treatment with various drugs, eg. haloperidol, chlorpromazine, and prednisone, is only partially effective, and the chorea is usually refractory. (Wheeler PG, Weaver DD, Dobyns WB. Benign hereditary chorea. Pediatr Neurol Sept/Oct 1993;9:337-340). (Respond: Dr Wheeler, Dept of Medical and Molecular Genetics, IB 130, Indiana University Medical Center, 975 West Walnut St, Indianapolis, IN 46202).

COMMENT. BHC is an uncommon form of childhood chorea that has been mistaken for Huntington disease. The recognition of this benign, nonprogressive form of chorea of early onset and without dementia will avoid unnecessary prolonged hospitalization and the risk of invasive diagnostic procedures.-Editor. *Ped Neur Briefs* Nov 1993.

CHAPTER 6

NEUROMUSCULAR DISORDERS

INTRODUCTION

John B. Bodensteiner, M.D.
West Virginia University, Morgantown, WV

The last few years have been tremendously exciting for those interested in neuromuscular disease in children. The multitude of advances have been largely due to the application of molecular genetic techniques: 1) Identification of gene locus; 2) Recognition and delineation of new genetic mechanisms; and 3) Identification of the mechanism of diseases resulting in the recognition of new diseases and better understanding of familiar conditions.

The identification of the gene locus and gene product is followed by the mapping of the gene and delineation of the molecular structure of the protein coded. For example, the delineation of the gene locus in potassium sensitive periodic paralysis on 17q 23.1-25.3. Mapping the gene led to the recognition that substitution of a single base pair in the DNA sequence causes an alteration of the structure and therefore the function of the sodium channel. Other diseases for which the gene loci have been discovered in recent years include facioscapulohumeral muscular dystrophy, spinal muscular atrophy, several types of Charcot-Marie-Tooth disease, nemaline myopathy, central core disease and malignant hyperthermia and myotonia congenita. In several of these diseases the gene mapping has been completed and in some cases the gene product has been determined.

The role of newly recognized genetic mechanisms in the production of neuromuscular diseases is just beginning to be appreciated. The expansion of repetitive nucleotide sequences in unstable regions of DNA as the fundamental genetic mechanism in some diseases has solved a number of conundrums for Mendelian geneticists. An example is the recognition of expanding trinucleotide repeats in the gene coding for protein kinase (located at 19q 13.3) causing myotonic muscular dystrophy. The expansion of the repetitive trinucleotide sequence correlates with the severity of the disease. Thus this mechanism helps to explain the phenomenon of genetic anticipation long recognized in myotonic dystrophy. Another disease which may be related to expansion or duplication of nucleotide sequences is type 1a Charcot-Marie-Tooth disease wherein a duplication of a DNA sequence in the gene for peripheral myelin protein appears to be the underlying defect.

The identification of the mechanism of disease occurs on several different levels. For example, the identification of dystrophin deficiency as the fundamental defect in Duchenne type muscular dystrophy represents the mechanism of disease on one level. However, deficiency of the dystrophin in the myofiber occurs in nonhuman species where the deficiency does not cause the progressive degenerative changes seen in the muscle of young boys. Clearly we do not yet understand the mechanism of this disease on all levels.

Several variations of the molecular structure of the acetylcholine receptor and the associated ion pore have recently been delineated. These conditions present with myasthenia gravis like symptoms and are collectively referred to as the congenital myasthenic syndromes. Although unimportant in terms of disease incidence, the congenital myasthenic syndromes have already provided considerable information about the structure and function of the neuromuscular junction. This information may eventually lead to effective therapeutic approaches for these and other disorders.

The new developments in the field of neuromuscular disease are numerous and selected developments are addressed in this chapter. The papers included should give the reader a sense of the range of the many new advances in the field.-*John B. Bodensteiner, MD, Professor of Neurology and Pediatrics, West Virginia University School of Medicine, Morgantown, WV.*

MUSCULAR DYSTROPHIES

FACIOSCAPULOHUMERAL DYSTROPHY: GENETICS

More than 500 subjects from 41 families with dominantly inherited facioscapulohumeral muscular dystrophy (FSHD) were studied at the Royal Hospital for Sick Children, St. Michael's Hill, Bristol and the University of Wales College of Medicine, Heath Park, Cardiff, Wales. 168 subjects were affected and 330 were unaffected. Dominant inheritance was proven in 28 families and no evidence for recessive inheritance was found in the remainder. New mutation accounted for six isolated cases. The prevalence of FSHD in Wales was estimated at 2/100,000. Estimates of penetrance values were less than 5% at 0-4 years, 21% at 5-9 years, 58% at 10-14 years, 86% at 15-19 years and 95 % at 20 years and over. Early onset is associated with the greatest chance of disability in later life. Proximal lower limb weakness was present in 39% aged less than 20 years, 46% aged 20-40 years, and 68% aged more than 40 years.

Asymmetry of scapular and upper limb involvement was evident in 65% of 113 affected subjects. Creatine kinase is elevated in 80% of affected males under 40 year and 48% of affected women, but use of CK as a presymptomatic test for FSHD is limited. There was no clinical evidence of significant genetic heterogeneity between the 11 largest families studied. (Lunt PW, Harper PS. Genetic counselling in facioscapulohumeral muscular dystrophy. J Med Genet Oct 1991;28:655-664).

COMMENT. The genetic homogeneity for FSHD demonstrated in this study facilitates genetic counseling and answers to questions raised by family members. Different modes of presentation, particularly with respect to pelvic and peroneal involvement may be observed in various members of large kindreds. The recent assignment of the gene for FSHD to chromosome 4 will help to clarify some of the counseling issues, including families diagnosed as FSH type spinal muscular atrophy where the same genetic locus is involved. The risk of disability and wheelchair requirement in later life can be assessed by the reported age of onset and the occurrence of proximal lower limb weakness by age 20 years. The authors estimate that 19% of FSHD heteroxygotes will require a wheelchair by 40 years or over and 30% remain only mildly affected throughout life. Since asymmetry of weakness correlates with handedness, the overuse of limbs and particularly body building exercises should be discouraged.-Editor. *Ped Neur Briefs* Nov 1991.

HEAD CIRCUMFERENCE AND IQ IN DUCHENNE MD

The head circumferences of 64 patients with Duchenne muscular dystrophy were greater than normal and the intellectual performance tested by the Wechsler was significantly impaired in a study performed at The Royal Liverpool Children's Hospital, Alder Hey, Liverpool and The University of Newcastle upon Tyne, UK. There was no correlation between head circumference and intellectual performance. Subsequent studies in 19 patients monitored with CT suggested that the large head was related to increased brain size.(Appleton RE et al. Head circumference and intellectual performance of patients with Duchenne muscular dystrophy. Dev Med Child Neurol Oct 1991;33:884-890).

COMMENT. These patients with DMD had relative and, less frequently, absolute macrocephaly which was unrelated to height and showed some familial tendency, the fathers having larger heads. The cause of the macrocephaly and increased brain size was not determined. Macrocephaly was defined as relative if the head circumference was disproportionately large for height or absolute, if greater than the 97th centile. There was no correlation between the head circumference and intellectual performance of either the entire group of 47 patients or of the 12 patients with absolute macrocephaly.

The predictive value of a reduction in the size of the brain in the first year for mental retardation at 7 years has been investigated in 41 term infants with microcephaly. Half the microcephalic children were mentally retarded at the age of 7. Head size 2 standard deviations below the mean had a very low predictive value for mental retardation (11%). Disproportionate head-to-height ratio did not significantly affect outcome (Dolk H. Dev Med Child Neurol Nov 1991;33:974983). The study was based on the US National Collaborative Perinatal Project Data of over 50,000 pregnancies and was performed at the Department of Epidemiology, Catholic University of Louvain, Brussels, Belgium.-Editor. *Ped Neur Briefs* Nov 1991.

DYSTROPHIN IN LIMB-GIRDLE DYSTROPHY

Dystrophin content in muscle was analyzed by both immunofluorescence and immunoblot in 41 patients with a clinical diagnosis of limb-girdle muscular dystrophy seen at the National Institute of Neuroscience, Tokyo, Japan over a 12-year period. 17% showed a dystrophinopathy consistent with Becker (5 male patients) or carrier of Duchenne (2 female patients) muscular dystrophy. The misclassification of isolated male patients was 31% while that of isolated female patients was 13%. DNA analysis confirmed a dystrophin gene deletion in all five male Becker dystrophy patients identified. By analysis of this study together with two additional reports in the literature, the authors calculate that approximately 40 % of isolated limb-girdle/Becker patients cannot be differentially diagnosed on the basis of clinical and histopathologic criteria. Dystrophin protein and gene studies are required for the accurate diagnosis of these patients and before appropriate genetic counseling can be provided (Arikawa E et al. The frequency of patients with dystrophin abnormalities in a limb-girdle patient population. Neurology Sept 1991;41:1491-1496).

COMMENT. The study demonstrates the clinical overlap between limb-girdle muscular dystrophy and dystrophinopathies and emphasizes the necessity of dystrophin protein and gene studies for accurate diagnosis of isolated cases of muscular dystrophy.

Hoffman, EP et al, from the University of Pittsburgh School of Medicine, describe a novel, severe case of Duchenne muscular dystrophy with biochemical findings that were consistent with a Becker muscular dystrophy. The muscle contained substantial amounts of abnormal dystrophin and a unique intragenic gene deletion resulting in a dystrophin protein missing the carboxyl-terminal domain. This abnormal protein was more damaging to the myofibers than the absence of dystrophin would have been and supports the hypothesis that an intact carboxyl-terminus is crucial for correct dystrophin function. Previous studies have suggested that the carboxyl-terminus of dystrophin is important for normal dystrophin function. The patient described here had dystrophin that lacked the carboxyl-terminus domain yet it was clearly associated with the plasma membrane (Ann Neurol Oct 1991;30:605-610).

Matsumura K et al, from the Department of Neurology, Shimoshizu National Hospital, Chiba, Tokyo, Japan, describe a Japanese family with both Fukuyama type congenital muscular dystrophy and Duchenne muscular dystrophy (J Child Neurol July 1991;6:251-

256). DNA analysis and the dystrophin test showed that dystrophin was expressed normally at the sarcoplasmic membrane of the Fukuyama phenotype patient but was completely absent in the Duchenne phenotype patient. Two different childhood muscular dystrophies coexisted in this family. The dystrophin test assisted in the differential diagnosis of the two diseases when DNA analysis by Southern blotting was not informative.- Editor. *Ped Neur Briefs* Nov 1991.

DYSTROPHIN IN FETAL MUSCLE

Dystrophin, the product of the Duchenne muscular dystrophy gene, was studied in human fetal skeletal muscle from 9 to 26 weeks of gestation at the Jerry Lewis Muscle Research Centre, Hammersmith Hospital, London. Dystrophin was localized to the sarcolemma of myotubes in fetal muscle from at least 9 weeks of gestation. Dystrophin immunostaining increased and became more uniform with age and sarcolemmal staining of myotubes was intense by 26 weeks of gestation. Western blot analysis showed a lower relative molecular mass protein in fetal tissue compared to adult tissue. This persisted until 26 weeks of gestation but switched to the adult form by 9 months of age. The data demonstrated several specific isoforms of dystrophin present in developing skeletal muscle (Clerk A et al. Characterisation of dystrophin during development of human skeletal muscle. Development Feb 1992;114:395-402).

COMMENT. Tome FMS et al. in Paris, France and Boston, MA report on the distribution and localization of dystrophin and dystrophin-related protein during skeletal muscle development and changes in Duchenne muscular dystrophy fetuses. Dystrophin of the same size as in adults was present in normal fetuses as soon as 8 weeks gestation in this study. It was absent in Duchenne muscular dystrophy fetuses. The dystrophin-related protein was quantitatively and qualitatively comparable in normal and Duchenne fetuses. The authors concluded that the prenatal diagnosis of Duchenne muscular dystrophy can be confirmed by immunocytochemical or biochemical analysis of muscular dystrophin in aborted fetuses. Dystrophin-related protein has a particular role in synaptic function which is not disturbed in Duchenne muscular dystrophy (Neurology April 1992;42(Suppl 3):227-228).-Editor. *Ped Neur Briefs* May 1992.

DYSTROPHINOPATHY IN FEMALES

Dystrophin immunocytochemistry was used to study muscle biopsies from 505 girls and women with neuromuscular disease seen at the National Institute of Neuroscience, Tokyo, the University of Pittsburgh School of Medicine, and the Columbia Presbyterian Medical Center, New York. The laboratory findings of 25 (54%) of 46 isolated cases with muscle biopsies were consistent with the familial cases and all showed myopathic histopathology and abnormal elevations of serum CK. The clinical presentations of the isolated cases were consistent with familial cases and included proximal limb weakness before age 10 (40%), myalgias or cramps (24%) and grossly elevated CK levels (24%). About 10% of the isolated cases of hyperCKemic myopathy were proven by dystrophin analysis to have a dystrophinopathy as the cause of their disease (manifesting carriers of Duchenne dystrophy). (Hoffman EP et al. Dystrophinopathy in isolated cases of myopathy in females. Neurology May 1992;42:967-975.) (Reprints: Dr. EP Hoffman, University of Pittsburgh School of Medicine, Biomedical Science Tower, Pittsburgh, PA 15261; Dr. K Arahata, National Institute of Neuroscience, 4-1-1 Ogawahigahi-cho, Kodaira, Tokyo 187, Japan; or Dr. E Bonilla, Department of Neurology, Columbia-Presbyterian Medical Center, New York, NY 10032.)

COMMENT. All isolated female dystrophinopathy patients had had other diagnoses prior to dystrophin testing, the most common being the limb girdle muscular dystrophy. The clinical criteria that implicate a dystrophinopathy in isolated nonfamilial cases in girls and women include a serum CK level in excess of 1,000 IU/l and a myopathic histopathology. The exclusion of dystrophinopathy by dystrophin analysis is necessary in confirming a diagnosis of isolated limb girdle muscular dystrophy. A dystrophin test is also recommended in patients with idiopathic cardiomyopathies since cardiomyopathy was found as the only clinical manifestation in two Duchenne muscular dystrophy carriers reported from Rome, Italy (Mirabella M et al. Neurology April 1992;42 Suppl 3:281). There was no muscle weakness and serum CK was only mildly increased.-Editor. *Ped Neur Briefs* June 1992.

PREDNISONE IN DUCHENNE DYSTROPHY

The results of a randomized controlled trial of daily Prednisone conducted in 99 boys aged five to 15 years with Duchenne dystrophy are reported from the Department of Neurology, University of Rochester, NY and five collaborating institutions. Prednisone at 0.3 mg/kg or 0.75 mg/kg and placebo were administered for six months. Patients were evaluated at ten days, one month, two months, three months, and six months of treatment. At the three month visit those receiving 0.75 mg/kg were significantly strongly than those given 0.3 mg/kg Prednisone and both Prednisone groups were stronger than those treated with placebo. At six months side-effects occurred in the group treated with 0.75 mg/kg and these included weight gain, Cushingoid appearance, and excessive hair growth. This study confirmed previous reports from these Centers showing that Prednisone produces a significant increase in muscle strength, pulmonary function, and functional ability in patients with Duchenne dystrophy. The present study also defines the minimum Prednisone dose required to produce the maximal increase in strength at 0.3 to 0.75 mg/kg. Improvement is rapid occurring within ten days and is maximal by two months of treatment. The authors recommend that a Prednisone dosage of 0.75 mg/kg/day be considered for patients with Duchenne dystrophy who experience functional decline. (Griggs RC et al. Prednisone in Duchenne dystrophy. A randomized, controlled trial defining the time course and dose response. Arch Neurol April 1991;48:383-388).

COMMENT. Clinical trials of myoblast transfer are investigational and limited in application. Studies of the benefits and mechanism of Prednisone in muscle protein synthesis are important particularly in young children showing a rapid functional decline. Alternative schedules of Prednisone administration such as pulse dosage are under investigation and may have fewer side effects. The beneficial effects of prednisone, 0.65 mg/kg/day, extending over a two year observation period has been demonstrated in 89 boys with DMD. (Fenichel GM et al. Neurology March 1991;41 (Suppl 1):166).-Editor. *Ped Neur Briefs* April 1991.

PREDNISONE-TREATED DUCHENNE MUSCULAR DYSTROPHY

The immunosuppressant/antiinflammatory effects of prednisone were studied in 33 patients with Duchenne muscular dystrophy (ages 5 to 15 years) at the conclusion of a six month treatment trial at the Department of Neurology, Division of Neuromuscular Disease, Ohio State University College of Medicine, Columbus, OH. Immunohistochemical analyses were carried out on muscle biopsies: 12 from the placebo group, 9 from the low-dose prednisone group (0.75 mg/kg/d), and 12 from the high-dose group (1.5 mg/kg/d). The number of T cells and the number of muscle fibers focally invaded by T cells were significantly decreased in the prednisone treated groups compared with controls. Prednisone may improve strength in Duchenne muscular dystrophy through primarily immunologic mechanisms involving T lymphocytes. (Kissel JT et al. Mononuclear cell analysis of muscle biopsies in prednisone-treated and untreated Duchenne muscular dystrophy. Neurology May 1991;41:667-672).

COMMENT. The possibility that clinical improvement was related to prednisone-induced alterations in skeletal muscle dystrophin was disproved by a further study from Ohio State University (Burrow KL et al. Dystrophin expression and somatic reversion in prednisone-treated and untreated Duchenne dystrophy. Neurology May 1991;41:661-666). Dystrophin content was analyzed at the conclusion of a six month trial of prednisone, using Western blots and antibody staining of tissue sections. There was no significant difference in dystrophin content between treatment and placebo groups.-Editor. *Ped Neur Briefs* June 1991.

MYOTONIC DYSTROPHY: SEVERITY AND MATERNAL AGE

The severity of myotonic dystrophy in 17 affected sibling pairs from 15 families in which 2 or more affected children were born to mothers with myotonic dystrophy is reported from the Hospital for Sick Children, London, and the Prince of Wales Children's Hospital, Sydney, Australia. In 13 of 17 sibling pairs the younger child was more severely affected than the older child. Increasing age difference between the affected siblings paralleled increasing age for each mother and showed a positive correlation with the difference in disease severity between siblings. Infants born to older mothers suffered more severe myotonic dystrophy. Maternal age at delivery correlated with the age at which the infant sat alone and walked alone. In addition, the incidence of neonatal feeding difficulties, neonatal respiratory difficulties, surgery for talipes, and scoliosis were directly related to maternal age at delivery. (Andrews, PI, Wilson, J. Relative disease severity in siblings with myotonic dystrophy. J Child Neurol April 1992;7:161-167.) (Correspondence: Dr. P. Ian Andrews, Box 3533, Duke University Medical Center, Durham, NC 27710.)

COMMENT. These findings have relevance in genetic counseling and suggest that maternal age and birth order are important in the relative severity of childhood onset myotonic dystrophy. The authors note that a normal infant born after a neonatally affected child is unlikely to develop myotonic dystrophy.

An increased risk of spontaneous abortion, cesarian section and neonatal death for women with myotonic dystrophy is reported from the Chicoutimi Hospital, Quebec, Canada (Prevost C, Mathieu J. Pregnancy outcome of women with myotonic dystrophy. Neurology April 1992;42 Suppl 3:226). The risk estimate that women with myotonic dystrophy will have a congenitally affected child is 3-9%. Among children surviving the neonatal period, 7.3% had congenital myotonic dystrophy and 7.3% had childhood onset myotonic dystrophy.-Editor. *Ped Neur Briefs* June 1992.

MRI IN CONGENITAL MYOTONIC DYSTROPHY

The results of CT and MRI of the brain were analyzed and neurological development was assessed from the neonatal period in 7 children with congenital myotonic dystrophy aged 2-8 years at the Division of Neurology, Chiba Children's Hospital and Department of Pediatrics, Chiba University School of Medicine, Chiba, Japan. Ventricular dilatation seen on the first day of life in 2 of 3 infants had not progressed on follow-up CTs at intervals of 1-6 years. Areas of periventricular hyperintensity on T2 weighted MRIs were seen in all children, and an asphyxial episode at birth was responsible for the MRI abnormalities. Low developmental quotients ranging from 12 to 72 were not correlated with the extent of the periventricular hyperintensity or the ventriculomegaly (Tanabe Y et al. Neuroradiological findings in children with congenital myotonic dystrophy. Acta Paediatr Aug 1992;81:613-617). (Correspondence: Dr. Y. Tanabe, Division of Neurology, Chiba Children's Hospital, 579-1 Heta-cho, Chiba, Japan 280-02.)

COMMENT. The mental retardation commonly found in children with congenital myotonic dystrophy was not attributable to brain damage due to perinatal asphyxia. There was no significant correlation between the severity of mental impairment and the degree of structural change in the brain assessed by periventricular hyperintensity on the MRI.

The frequency of cerebral atrophy, large ventricles, and dysmyelination in patients with *Fukuyama's congenital muscular dystrophy* and *occidental congenital muscular dystrophy* are compared in a study from Riyadh, Saudi Arabia (Cook J, Gascon G et al. Ann Neurol Sept 1992;32:439 (abstr)). In 37 children with Fukuyama's congenital muscular dystrophy, 75% were mentally retarded, 62% had cerebral atrophy, 81% large ventricles and 53% dysmyelination. The mental retardation in this disorder is attributed to a brain dysgenesis.-Editor. *Ped Neur Briefs* Oct 1992.

CEREBRAL HYPOPERFUSION IN MYOTONIC DYSTROPHY

Cerebral blood flow and perfusion measured by SPECT (Xenon and Tc-HMPAO), MRI findings, and neuropsychological function in 22 patients with myotonic dystrophy (MD) were studied at the Departments of Neurology, Radiology, Psychiatry, and Pediatrics, Harbor-UCLA Medical Center, Torrance, CA. Results in 8 patients with maternal (mMD) inheritance were compared with those in 11 with paternal (pMD) inheritance, and in 10 normal controls. Patients with mMD had significantly lower scores on IQ tests and more extensive cerebral hypoperfusion when compared to those with pMD. Decreases in cerebral blood flow, most severe in frontal and temporoparietal association cortex, correlated strongly with lower scores on IQ tests. Patients with mMD had earlier onset of illness than the pMD group (means, 6.3 vs 32 yrs). Cerebral hypoperfusion patterns in the mMD patients were consistent with diffuse brain injury, whereas pMD patients showed only minor changes. (Chang L et al. Cerebral abnormalities in myotonic dystrophy. Cerebral blood flow, magnetic resonance imaging, and neuropsychological tests. Arch Neurol Sept 1993;50:917-923). (Reprints: Dr Chang, Dept Neurology, Harbor-UCLA Medical Center, 1000 W Carson St, F-9, Torrance, CA 90509).

COMMENT. Mothers with myotonic dystrophy should be warned that their children would have a high probability of mental retardation. Hypoxic injury in utero is suggested as the likely explanation for the brain injury. Milder abnormalities in cerebral blood flow seen in the pMD group were attributed to possible sleep apnea, since many had hypersomnolence.-Editor. *Ped Neur Briefs* Oct 1993.

MYASTHENIA GRAVIS

ELECTRODIAGNOSTIC TESTS FOR MYASTHENIA GRAVIS

The value of electrodiagnostic tests in 21 children with myasthenia gravis (MG) is reported from the EMG Department, Hospital Neurologique et Neurochirurgical Pierre Wertheimer, Lyon, France. Repetitive stimulation (RS) of the ulnar nerve induced a significant decrement in 3 of 4 patients with neonatal MG tested between 3 and 30 days of age. The overall percentage of positive RS tests was 88% in 12 patients with juvenile MG. Standard ulnar nerve RS and ischemic test (IT) procedures were positive in 41% and 66% of childhood patients, respectively. The proximal RS (spinal or axillary nerves) or facial RS was performed in 10 patients and was positive in 7. (Vial C et al. Myasthenia gravis in childhood and infancy. Usefulness of electrophysiologic studies. Arch Neurol August 1991;48:847-849).

COMMENT: This study demonstrates the usefulness of electrodiagnostic methods in both infants and children with myasthenia gravis. The RS test is particularly valuable in infants suspected of MG who have negative edrophonium chloride tests.

The aggravation of myasthenia gravis by erythromycin is described in a 15 year old girl at the Departments of Neurology and Pediatrics, University of Iowa College of Medicine, Iowa City (Absher JR, Bale JF Jr. J Pediatr July 1991;119:155-156). Acute respiratory failure occurred during intravenous infusion of erythromycin given for a bacterial respiratory infection. A neurologic consultation revealed a gradually increasing weakness during the preceding 6-12 months, with diplopia on several occasions and a nasal voice. Endrophonium chloride 1 mg IV caused dramatic improvement in ptosis, arm strength and speech, and pyridostigmine provided a substantial benefit initially. She relapsed six months later and underwent thymectomy. A close temporal relationship between erythromycin and worsening of myasthenia gravis was reported in one previous patient (May EF, Calvert PC. Ann Neurol 1990;28:577-9).-Editor. *Ped Neur Briefs* Aug 1991.

PROGNOSIS OF MYASTHENIA GRAVIS

The prognosis of myasthenia gravis (MG) was assessed retrospectively using life table analysis in 844 patients followed up for a mean period of 5 years in 3 neurological centers in Milan, Rome and Pavia, Italy. The patients were aged from 2 to 90 years with a mean of 45 years. The onset of symptoms peaked in the young and middle age groups, and the commonest age at onset was between 20 and 39 years. The proportion of females progressively decreased with age. Sixty-two percent of patients received steroids, 30% anticholinesterase, 21% immunosuppressant drugs (azathioprine), and 66% had thymectomy. There was an inverse correlation between age at onset of symptoms and disease duration at diagnosis and complete remission of MG. Patients with symptoms for less than 1 year at diagnosis had the best outlook with 15-25% remissions by 5-10 years. Thymectomized patients had a significantly higher chance of complete remission than non-thymectomized (15% vs. 8% at 5 years). The earlier the operation, the better the chance of remission. The cumulative probability of complete remission was 1% by 1 year, 8% by 3 years, 13% by 5 years, and 21% by 10 years (Beghi E et al. Prognosis of myasthenia gravis: a multicenter follow-up study of 844 patients. J Neur Sci Dec 1991;106:213-220). (Correspondence: Dr. Ettore Beghi, MD, Instituto di Ricerche Farmcologiche "Mario Negri", Via Eritrea 62, I-20157 Milan, Italy.)

COMMENT. Seventeen percent of the patients in this study were less than 20 years of age at the onset of symptoms. The chance of complete remission is greater in younger patients with mild symptoms at onset and with shorter disease duration at diagnosis. The efficacy of thymectomy might be partly related to the younger age of the patients and the shorter disease duration at the time of operation.

In a series of 35 patients with juvenile myasthenia gravis reported from the Massachusetts General Hospital, Boston, MA (Millichap, JG, Dodge PR. Diagnosis and treatment of myasthenia gravis in infancy, childhood and adolescence a study of 51 patients. Neurology 1960;10:1007-1014), 21 underwent thymectomy and of these 18 (86%) showed complete or partial, type A (drug therapy discontinued) and type B (drug therapy continued) remissions. A similar response to medical therapy alone was obtained in 13 (93%) of 14 patients of this series, and the results were comparable with those observed in patients treated surgically. Drug therapy was discontinued and the remission was complete in 6 (29%) of thymectomized patients compared to 2 (14%) of the patients treated only with cholinergic drugs. Until patients may be allocated for thymectomy at random and a large control series is followed, the merits of surgical therapy cannot be assessed with certainty. Spontaneous remission is another factor that complicates the selection of MG patients for surgery.

An unusual association of early onset juvenile myasthenia gravis and premature birth is reported by Evans OB et al. (Pediatr Neurol Jan/Feb 1992;8:51-53). In a series of patients reported by Fukuyama Y et al. (Paediatr Univ Tokyo 1970;18:57-68), 34 of 76 children had an early onset of juvenile myasthenia gravis.

In contrast to juvenile myasthenia gravis which generally responds to anticholinesterase medication, congenital or hereditary myasthenia is often refractory. A trial of 3,4 diaminopyridine, a drug that enhances acetylcholine release from motor nerve terminals, showed benefit and a highly significant increase in muscle strength in 16 patients treated. The drug was useful when given alone or in combination with anticholinesterase medication (Palace J et al. 3,4-diaminopryidine in the treatment of congenital (hereditary) myasthenia. J Neurol Neursurg Psychiatry Dec 1991;54:1069-1072).-Editor. *Ped Neur Briefs* April 1992.

JUVENILE MYASTHENIA GRAVIS: DIAGNOSIS AND OUTCOME

The usefulness of various diagnostic tests, treatment, and outcome in 27 juvenile myasthenics seen over a 25 year period are reported from the Departments of Pediatrics, Neurology, and Anatomy, University of Iowa. The age of onset in 56% was after 10 years of age. One fourth had ocular myasthenia, one fourth presented with ocular signs and progressed to generalized myasthenia, and half had generalized myasthenia from onset. Ptosis, the most common presenting sign (81 %), was unilateral in 3 3%. In order of descending frequency, the other presenting signs were generalized weakness, dysphagia, diplopia, facial weakness, dysarthria, ophthalmoplegia, and na.sal speech. One patient's mother had MG. The comparative yield of tests showed positive neostigmine and edrophonium tests in 92%, serology was positive for acetylcholine receptor-binding antibodies in 63%, and repetitive distal nerve stimulation showed decrement in 33%. The yield of serology and nerve stimulation tests increased with generalization of myasthenia and when proximal nerves were also tested. Ocular myasthenics responded to pyridostigmine bromide monotherapy, while generalized myasthenia required additional medical and/or surgical therapy. Patients receiving corticosteroids had thymectomy at a later date. Those with normal thymus had a greater chance of remission without medication than patients with thymic hyperplasia. (Afifi AK, Bell WE. Tests for juvenile myasthenia gravis: comparative diagnostic yield and prediction of outcome. J Child Neurol Oct 1993;8:403-411). (Respond: Dr Afifi, Division of Child Neurology, Department of Pediatrics, University of Iowa Hospitals and Clinics, Iowa City, IA 52242).

COMMENT. Thirty-eight percent of these patients were in complete remission and without drugs when followed for more than 4 years (range, days to 20 years). The outcome was better for ocular than generalized myasthenia, 57% cf 30% in remission without drugs. A lower rate of remission in thymectomized (35%) compared to non-thymectomized

(43%) patients was a reflection of disease severity and poor response to medication.

In the study of 35 juvenile myasthenics at the Massachusetts General Hospital, the overall frequency of complete or partial remission in patients treated by thymectomy or with medication alone was not significantly different but a higher rate of complete remission and drug withdrawal was obtained in the thymectomized group (29% v 14%). (Millichap JG, Dodge PR. Neurology 1960;10:1007). The earlier the surgery, the better the chance of remission (see Ped Neur Briefs April 1992;6:30).-Editor. *Ped Neur Briefs* Nov 1993.

CONGENITAL MYOPATHIES

MYOPATHY WITH COMPLEX I DEFICIENCY: RIBOFLAVIN AND CARNITINE THERAPY

A six year old boy with progressive myopathy and motor neuropathy associated with complex I deficiency is reported from the Institutes of Neurology, Pediatrics and Cell Biology, St. Radboud University Hospital, Nijmegen, Netherlands. There was a three month history of weakness in the legs, sudden falling, inability to run and difficulty in climbing stairs. Within two months he developed weakness in his hands, a wobbling gait and a positive Gowers' sign. Muscle tone was impaired and proximal muscles were wasted. Biochemical studies on muscle tissues showed a defect of NADH dehydrogenase (complex I). Dramatic improvement followed oral treatment with L-carnitine 2 g daily and riboflavin 9 mg daily. Seven months later the complex I activity was normal, Gowers' sign was negative, deep tendon reflexes had returned and muscle weakness was limited mainly to the peroneal muscles. Nine further cases of a pure myopathy associated with complex I deficiency are reviewed (Bernsen PLJA et al. Successful treatment of pure myopathy, associated with complex I deficiency, with riboflavin and carnitine. Arch Neurol March 1991;48:334-338).

COMMENT. The present case report of a

mitochondrial myopathy differed fron nine other reports. There was no history of excessive fatiguability or exercise intolerance, the serum lactate concentration was normal, and the muscle biopsy did not show ragged red fibers. The dramatic improvement with riboflavin and carnitine and the return to normal of complex I activity were unusual findings. The authors stress the clinical, biochemical and morphological heterogeneity in complex I deficiency. Biochemical studies of mitochondrial metabolism in the muscle are advisable in children with progressive weakness and exercise intolerance when a precise diagnosis is unclear.-Editor. *Ped Neur Briefs* March 1991.

MITOCHONDRIAL MYOPATHY AND HYPOTONIA

Three children with hypotonia, cardiac impairment, and defects of the mitochondrial respiratory chain complexes, but no ragged red fibers, are reported from the Hopital de la Timone, Chemin de l'Armee, d'Afrique, Marseille, France. Case 1 shared clinical and metabolic features with fatal infantile myopathy associated with cytochrome c oxidase deficiency as described by DiMauro: neonatal hypotonia and weakness, respiratory failure, and severe lactic acidosis. Post-mortem studies at age 7 weeks showed complex IV reduced in the liver but not in the heart and quantitative analysis of mtDNA showed depletion in muscle. Case 2 showed intractable cardiomyopathy, cyclic neutropenia, and 3-methylglutaconic aciduria. The boy died suddenly at age 27 months. Case 3 presented at age 16 months as an acute hypokinetic hypertrophic cardiomyopathy with transient hypotonia and mild lactic acidosis. After the acute episode the boy gradually improved and the neurological and cardiac examinations were normal at the age of 3 years. All cases showed lipid storage myopathy and decreased cytochrome c oxidase. Biochemical studies confirmed the cytochrome c oxidase deficiency in muscle in all cases (Figarella-Branger D et al. Defects of the mitochondrial respiratory chain complexes in three pediatric cases with hypotonia and cardiac involvement. (J Neurol Sci

March 1992;108:105-113.) (Correspondence: Dr. D. Figarella-Branger, Laboratoire d'Anatomie Pathologique, Hopital de la Timone, Chemin de l'Armee d'Afrique, F-13005 Marseille, France.)

COMMENT. Histochemical staining of cytochrome c oxidase may be used for the diagnosis of mitochondrial myopathy when ragged red fibers are lacking. Schon EA et al. and Munnich A et al. review the mitochondrial myopathies and the clinical aspects of mitrochondrial disorders in the current issue of International Pediatrics 1992;7:23-33. The diagnosis of mitochondrial disorder should be considered with (1) an unexplained association of symptoms; (2) an early onset and a rapidly progressive course; and (3) involvement of unrelated organs which share no common embryologic origin and no common biological functions. Determination of lactate/pyruvate and ketone body molar ratios in plasma may help to select patients at risk for further investigation.

In a family with infantile mitrochondrial myopathy and cardiomyopathy reported from Rome, Italy, no correlation was found in the muscle between biochemistry and severity of the clinical intrafamilial phenotype (Bertini E et al. Neurology April 1992;42(Suppl 3):267).-Editor. *Ped Neur Briefs* May 1992.

FATAL AND BENIGN CONGENITAL MYOPATHIES: DIFFERENTIAL DIAGNOSIS

Muscle biopsies from four infants with fatal myopathy and four with benign myopathy were examined using biochemical, histochemical and immunohistochemical techniques in the Departments of Neurology, Pathology and Genetics, Columbia University, New York; Universita Cattolica del Sacro Cuore, Rome, Italy; and Fachbereich Chemie, Philipps-Universitat, Marburg, Germany. At early stages the clinical picture failed to provide clues for differential diagnosis; both fatal and benign myopathies presented with hypotonia, generalized weakness, lactic acidosis, failure to thrive and severe respiratory insufficiency, often requiring assisted ventilation. Patients with benign myopathy gain strength and show an increase in the number of fibers with COX (cytochrome c oxidase) deficient activity. In contrast, patients with fatal myopathy die before one year of age and muscle histochemistry shows no increase in the number of fibers with COX activity. The subunit composition of COX was studied directly on frozen muscle sections using immunologic probes. The fatal type was characterized by absence of the nuclear DNA-encoded subunit VIIa,b of COX while in the benign myopathy both VIIa,b and the mitochondrial DNA-encoded subunit II were absent. From a practical standpoint, immunohistochemistry of COX-II should suffice for differential diagnosis because this subunit was present in the fatal myopathy but absent in the early stages of the benign myopathy (Tritscler HJ, DiMauro S et al Differential diagnosis of fatal and benign cytochrome c oxidase deficient myopathies of infancy: an imnunohistochemical approach. Neurology Feb 1991;41:300-305).

COMMENT. The diagnosis of COX-deficient myopathies of infancy relies on histochemical and biochemical evaluation of COX activities in muscle biopsies. These tests fail to distinguish the fatal and benign phenotypes at early stages because both show lack of COX activity. COX is a complex enzyme composed of 13 subunits with three larger subunits (I, II and III) which are synthesized in the mitochondria, and the ten smaller subunits manufactured in the cytoplasm. COX VIIa,b is absent in the fatal myopathy and both COX-II and COX VIIa,b are absent in the early stages of benign myopathy. Thus, the immunohistochemistry of COX-II is sufficient for the differential diagnosis.-Editor. *Ped Neur Briefs* March 1991.

NEMALINE MYOPATHY: RESPIRATORY FAILURE

A Japanese boy with nemaline myopathy diagnosed at three years of age and complicated by severe respiratory failure at 8 years is reported from the Division of Child Neurology, National Center Hospital for Mental, Nervous, and Muscular Disorders, Kodaira, Tokyo, Japan. The histologic findings of the respiratory muscles obtained during thoracic surgery for pneumothorax showed marked variation in fiber size with increase in fibrous tissue, type II fiber deficiency, elevated acid phosphatase activity, and disorganized intermyofibrillar network. Truncal and biceps muscles showed little variation in fiber size, numerous nemaline bodies and type I fiber predominance. The sudden onset of severe respiratory failure was related to the preferential and progressive involvement of the respiratory muscles. (Saski M et al. Respiratory muscle involvement in nemaline myopathy. Pediatr Neurol Nov/Dec 1990;6:425-427).

COMMENT. Severe respiratory insufficiency is an uncommon development in nemaline myopathy, but a frequent complication of Duchenne's muscular dystrophy. Miller RG et al from the Children's Hospital of San Francisco have made serial measures of respiratory function in 17 patients with Duchenne's muscular dystrophy who underwent segmental spinal fusion and in 22 patients without operations. Declining rcspiratory function was observed in both groups, but operated patients showed improved sitting comfort (Neurology Jan 1991;41:38-40).-Editor. *Ped Neur Briefs* March 1991.

MUSCLE HYPOTONIA IN LOWE'S SYNDROME

As part of a comprehensive evaluation of 23 patients with the oculocerebrorenal syndrome of Lowe at the Section on Human Biochemical Genetics, National Institutes of Health, Bethesda, MD, concentrations of muscle enzymes and carnitine metabolism were studied in addition to special reference to growth and renal function. The diagnostic findings included congenital cataracts, neurologic involvement (cognitive impairment, areflexia, and a history of infantile hypotonia), and renal tubular dysfunction in male patients with typical facies (deep set eyes and frontal bossing). Patients ranged in age from four months to 31 years. Muscle involvement was indicated by an elevation of serum creatine kinase concentration in conjunction with substantial concentrations of MB isoenzymes, elevated aspartate aminotransferase and lactate dehydrogenase in the setting of normal liver function. One-third of the patients had plasma free carnitine concentration below 20 mcmol/L, a concentration associated with depletion of carnitine in tissues. Linear growth decreased after one year of age and head circumferences, normal in the first three to four years of life, then fell to the third percentile in mid-childhood. Longevity was reduced because of renal disease and the oldest patient examined was 33 years. (Charnas LR, Gahl WA et al. Clinical and laboratory findings in the oculocerebrorenal syndrome of Lowe, with special reference to growth and renal function. N Engl J Med May 9, 1991;324:1318-25).

COMMENT. The oculocerebrorenal syndrome of Lowe, an X-linked recessive disorder, is a rare cause of neonatal hypotonia or the limp infant syndrome. Both muscle and central abnormalities may contribute to the hypotonia and areflexia.-Editor. *Ped Neur Briefs* June 1991.

WERDNIG-HOFFMANN: DOMINANT INHERITANCE

A family in which both Werdnig-Hoffmann disease and chronic distal spinal muscular atrophy occurred, with apparent autosomal dominant inheritance, is reported from the Department of Neurology, Mayo Clinic Jacksonville, FL and Johns Hopkins University School of Medicine, Baltimore, MD. The female proband developed symptoms of Werdnig-Hoffmann disease at 2 months of age and died at 10 months. The proband's father and his 2 brothers developed bilateral progressive atrophy and weakness of the hands and legs in their second decade of life. The mother had no symptoms or signs of motor neuron disease, but EMG revealed distal denervation of the limbs. Family studies suggested autosomal dominant inheritance, although the Werdnig-Hoffmann disease may have been influenced by a maternally derived trait. (Boylan KB, Cornblath DR. Werdnig-Hoffmann disease and chronic distal spinal muscular atrophy with apparent autosomal dominant inheritance. Ann Neurol Sept 1992;32:404-407.) (Correspond: Dr. Boylan, Mayo Clinic, 4500 San Pablo Road, Jacksonville, FL 32224.)

COMMENT. Werdnig-Hoffmann disease is generally regarded as an autosomal recessive disorder with linkage to chromosome 5ql1.2-13.3. Other studies have suggested genetic heterogeneity.

The prognosis of patients with Werdnig-Hoffmann disease and a clinical scoring system are evaluated by Russman BS et al. (Ann Neurol Sept 1992;32:439 (abstr)). The 7 criteria for a poor prognosis were poor movement in utero, presence of tongue fasciculation, a poor cry, inability to hold the head at 3 months, inability to roll over by 6 months, loss of function, and diaphragmatic breathing. Five patients with scores of 4-7 died prior to 15 months of age, while 1 patient with a score of 1 died at 31 years. Patients whose scores during the first 6 months of life were 0 or 1 are living and range in age from 3-27 years. Death prior to age 2-4 years is not invariable.

A unique presentation of neonatal adrenoleukodystrophy as a progressive spinal muscular atrophy is reported in 2 siblings who later developed the symptoms and signs of encephalopathy (Miles DK et al. Ann Neurol Sept 1992;32:466 (abstr)). Peroxisomal diseases must be considered in the differential diagnosis of Werdnig-Hoffmann disease.-Editor. *Ped Neur Briefs* Oct 1992.

CONGENITAL BRACHIAL ARTHROGRYPOSIS

Two patients with congenital cervical spinal muscular atrophy and arthrogryposis limited to the upper limbs are reported from the Hospital Enschede, The Netherlands, and University Hospital RWTH Aachen, Germany. A girl, aged 1 year, born with congenital arthrogryposis multiplex, had severe bilateral hypotonia, weakness and wasting of shoulder girdles, arms and hands. Tendon reflexes were absent in the upper limbs. EMG of the triceps was silent, and a biopsy showed severe neurogenic muscle atrophy. A 31 year old man, born with severe muscle weakness and congenital contractures of the upper limbs, had herniations of the intervertebral discs C2-C4 and C5-C7 but normal signal intensity of the cord on T2-weighted images of the MRI. Both patients had normal sensory modalities, and lower limbs were not involved. (Hageman G et al. Congenital cervical spinal muscular atrophy: a non-familial, non progressive condition of the upper limbs. J Neurol Neurosurg Psychiatry April 1993;56: 365-368). (Respond: Dr G Hageman, Department of Neurology, Medical Spectrum Twente, Hospital Enschede, PO Box 50000, 7500 KA Enschede, The Netherlands).

COMMENT. The absence of sensory deficits and normal motor nerve conduction velocities point to involvement of the anterior horn cells. The etiology of the prenatal pathology with loss of anterior horn cells in cases of neurogenic arthrogryposis is unknown, except for one case cited of rubella exposure. The limitation to the upper limbs is unusual.-Editor. *Ped Neur Briefs* May 1993.

NEUROPATHIES

GUILLAIN-BARRE SYNDROME: AGE VARIATIONS

The medical records of 83 children with Guillain-Barre Syndrome were reviewed with reference to the age associated changes at the Department of Pediatrics, University of Tokyo, Japan. Children between 3 and 9 years were most susceptible and summer was the most common time of onset. Limb pain was the initial symptom for 53% of all patients and for 24% in the younger age group (P<0.05). Muscle weakness was the most frequent initial symptom in the younger age group. Upper respiratory infections were the most common preceding illnesses; the interval between the previous illness and the onset of disease was significantly shorter for the older age group. The total duration of the illness was shorter in older children. Cranial nerve involvement occurred in 1/3 of children under 5 years of age and in the same proportion of children over 5 years. In the younger age group bulbar nerves were most commonly affected whereas the facial nerve was involved most frequently in the older age group. Patients with cranial nerve involvement suffered more frequently from respiratory insufficiency; the ages of those affected were distributed evenly between the two groups. The differences in initial symptoms and in interval between preceding illnesses and onset of the disease seemed to be related to the maturational processes of peripheral nerve and spinal root ganglia. It is speculated that the stage of the myelinogenic process might be important in the explanation of age associated alterations in symptomatology (Sakakihara Y, Kamoshita S. Age associated changes in the symptomatology of Guillain-Barre syndrome in children. Dev Med Child Neurol July 1991;33:611-616).

COMMENT. The incidence of Guillain-Barre syndrome increases with age but 25% of cases occur in childhood and adolescence. Since nerve conduction velocity and the thickness of the myelin sheath in peripheral nerves reaches adult levels at around five years of age, some variation in symptomatology between young and older children might be expected. Electrodiagnostic tests have been shown to corroborate the neuropathologic sequence in the Guillain-Barre syndrome and these findings may be modified by age and maturation (Ropper AH et al. Arch Neurol 1990;47:367; McFarland HR Arch Neurol July 1991;48: 678).-Editor. *Ped Neur Briefs* Aug 1991.

HEREDITARY MOTOR AND SENSORY NEUROPATHY MUTATION

A duplication in chromosome 17 responsible for most cases of autosomal dominant HMSN 1 was present as a de-novo mutation in 9 out of 10 sporadic patients examined at the Department of Neurology, Academic Medical Center, Amsterdam, The Netherlands. (Hoogendijk JE et al. De-novo mutation in hereditary motor and sensory neuropathy type 1. Lancet May 2, 1992;339:1081-82.) (Correspondence: Dr. JE Hoogendijk, Department of Neurology, Academic Medical Center, Meibergdreef 9, 1105 AZ Amsterdam, The Netherlands.)

COMMENT. The previous assumption that isolated cases of HMSN I are most frequently autosomal recessive appears to be incorrect and testing for the duplication in chromosome 17 is essential to establish the mode of inheritance for genetic counseling of isolated patients. This duplication of part of chromosome 17 was found in affected individuals from 7 of 8 families with HMSN I. Patients with HMSN type II do not show the duplication (Hallam PJ et al. Ann Neurol May 1992;31:570-572). (Correspondence: Dr. Malcolm, Molecular Genetics Unit, Institute of Child Health, 30 Guilford St., London WCIN IEH UK.)

HMSN type I also known as Charcot-Marie-Tooth disease type I is known to be genetically heterogeneous. At least 5 genetic loci have been identified including 3 dominant genes and 2 X-linked recessive genes. Ionasescu VV et al. from the Department of Pediatrics, University of Iowa Hospitals, Iowa City and the Massachusetts General Hospital present a clinical and genetic linkage study of 8 families with X-linked dominant Charcot-Marie-Tooth neuropathy which supports a localization of the diseased gene between DXS14 and DXYS1 (Neurology April 1992;42:903-908).-Editor. *Ped Neur Briefs* June 1992.

HMSN I: EARLY DIAGNOSIS

The value of nerve conduction velocities in the detection of hereditary motor sensory neuropathy type I (HMSN I) in children at risk was determined in 36 children under 10 years of age at the University of Western Ontario, London, Ontario, Canada. Clinical signs and slowed motor nerve conduction velocities were found in 17 of the 36 children who had 1 parent with HMSN I. Four children had slowed conduction velocities at 1 year of age or less. Clinical signs were subtle and included pes planus, distal foot wasting, weakness of ankle eversion and dorsiflexion, and areflexia. In all but 1 of the 17 affected patients the motor nerve conduction velocities were less than 40 m/s. Sensory potentials were abnormal in 7 children with HMSN I at ages 6-7 years. (Feasby TE et al. Hereditary motor sensory neuropathy type I in childhood. J Neurol Neurosurg Psychiatry Oct 1992;55:895-897). (Reprints: Dr. T.E. Feasby, Department of Clinical Neurosciences, University of Calgary, Foothills Hospital, 1403-29th Street NW, Calgary, Alberta T2N 2T9, Canada.)

COMMENT. These data show that HMSN I can be detected in early childhood. Even at 1 year of age or less the motor conduction velocity is significantly slowed. Abnormal physical findings are found in all children who have slow conduction velocities. The signs may be subtle and not accompanied by disability. Pes planus was the most common foot abnormality in this series. Nerve hypertrophy was uncommon.

Dr. Sghirlanzoni et al., Milan, Italy, report two siblings with HMSN III (Dejerine-Sottas disease) whose parents were both affected with autosomal dominant axonal HMSN II. This family and others cited show the existence of an HMSN III phenotype resulting from the homozygous expressions of HMSN I and II genes. (Neurology Nov 1992;42:2201).

A 4-year-old child with severe hypertrophic peripheral neuropathy had antibodies to myelin glycoprotein of peripheral nerve (Jelloun-Dellagi SB et al. Ann Neurol Nov 1992;32:700). This anti-Po glycoprotein activity may have a role in pathogenesis of the neuropathy.-Editor. *Ped Neur Briefs* Nov 1992.

PROGRESSIVE MONONEUROPATHY

Six patients, aged 10 to 27 years, with insidiously progressive, painless weakness in the distribution of a single major lower extremity nerve are reported from the University of California, San Francisco. The duration at diagnosis varied from 3 months to 8 years. The sciatic nerve was involved in three patients, the common peroneal in two, and the femoral nerve in one. The appearance of the nerve at surgery was normal in two, atrophied in two, and fibrosed in one. EMG revealed a chronic axonal mononeuropathy without conduction block or focal conduction slowing. MRI, CT, and US imaging failed to reveal a nerve mass or compression. (Engstrom JW et al. Idiopathic, progressive mononeuropathy in young people. Arch Neurol Jan 1993;50: 20-23). (Reprints: Dr Engstrom, Box 0114, M794,

Department of Neurology, University of California, San Francisco, CA 94143).

COMMENT. The authors ask the question: Could the patients have had a nerve tumor not uncovered by standard MRI or surgery and too proximal for localization by nerve conduction studies? The diagnosis of neurofibromatosis type 2 was confirmed by a gadolinium MRI in a 14 year-old girl who presented with flaccid weakness and wasting of the left upper limb and EMG evidence of brachial plexopathy (Millichap JG, Gomez MR. Ped Neur Briefs July 1990;4:50-51). The standard MRI was inconclusive whereas the gadolinium imaging revealed enlargement of neural formina C 5-6 on the left side and evidence of a plexiform neurofibroma. Examination of the skin showed depigmented and cafe-au-lait patches, helpful in the diagnosis in this case.-Editor. *Ped Neur Briefs* Feb 1993.

CRITICAL-ILLNESS POLYNEUROPATHY

A review of the neurological complications of sepsis from the University of Western Ontario, London, and Queen's University, Kingston, Ontario, Canada, draws attention to "critical-illness polyneuropathy" as a cause of difficulty in weaning from the ventilator. Patients with major medical, surgical, or traumatic illnesses who are in the recovery phase of septic encephalopathy may develop respiratory difficulties as an early sign of polyneuropathy. Electrophysiological studies, showing reduction of diaphragmatic action potential and denervation of chest wall muscles, may be diagnostic of the neuropathy before weakness of limbs and areflexia develop. In contrast to the central nervous system, damage to the peripheral nervous system is more severe and sometimes persistent in the septic syndrome. (Bolton CF et al. The neurological complications of sepsis. Ann Neurol Jan 1993;33:94-100). (Correspondence: Dr Bolton, Victoria Hospital, 375 South Street, London, Ontario N6A 4G5, Canada).

COMMENT. In addition to encephalopathy and polyneuropathy, patients with sepsis may develop myositis or myopathy and an elevated CPK. The EEG and EMG are sensitive indicators of these complications of the septic syndrome.-Editor. *Ped Neur Briefs* Feb 1993.

HEMOPHILUS INFLUENZAE VACCINE AND GUILLAIN-BARRE

A four-year-old girl with Guillain-Barre syndrome that developed 10 days following H *influenzae* type b conjugate vaccine immunization is reported from Geneva, Switzerland. CSF contained 1 mononuclear cell/cmm and 0.89 g/l protein. Nerve conduction velocities were decreased in upper and lower extremities. Measurements of immunoglobulins against the polysaccharide (PRP) component of the vaccine showed a marked elevation (100 mcg/ml) of the anti-PRP IgM antibody level. Following treatment with two 5-day courses of intravenous immunoglobulins (0.4 g/kg/day) 2 weeks apart, cranial nerve function and muscle strength improved. Apart from absent deep tendon reflexes, the neurological exam was normal at one month follow-up. (Gervaix A et al. Guillain-Barre syndrome following immunization with *Hemophilus influenzae* type b conjugate vaccine. Eur J Pediatr July 1993;152: 613-614). (Respond: Dr A Gervaix, Children's Hospital, University Hospital of Geneva, 30 bvld de la cluse, CH-1211 Geneve 4, Switzerland).

COMMENT. A total of five cases of Guillain-Barre syndrome (GBS) following vaccination with the H *influenzae* type b diphtheria toxoid-conjugate vaccine have been reported. The authors speculate that an excessive anti-PRP IgM antibody response to the vaccine might explain this rare complication.

Treatment of acute GBS is controversial and not without risk, especially in patients with vascular disease. Two adults died from vascular thrombotic complications following gamma globulin therapy for GBS. (McFarland HR. Arch Neurol July 1993;50:687).-Editor. *Ped Neur Briefs* July 1993.

CHAPTER 7

CONGENITAL MALFORMATIONS AND MENTAL RETARDATION SYNDROMES

INTRODUCTION

Harvey B. Sarnat, M.D., F.R.C.P. (C)
University of Washington School of Medicine, Seattle.

The years 1990 through 1993 were enriched with a wealth of exciting new information contributing to an improved understanding of both the pathogenesis and clinical manifestations of dysgeneses of the nervous system. The integration of molecular genetic data with classical embryological observations of morphogenesis was a conceptual advance of major importance; initiated in the previous decade, the relevance of basic developmental neurobiology to clinical pediatric neurology was brought into sharper focus than ever before. This four-year period saw the publication of two major monographs:

Holoprosencephaly: An Overview and Atlas of Cases by JR Siebert and colleagues and Cerebral Dysgenesis: Embryology and Clinical Expression by HB Sarnat.

Hydrocephalus continues to be a major complication of many forms of cerebral malformation ranging from major disturbances of induction such as holoprosencephaly to focal atresia of the cerebral aqueduct; in most cases congenital hydrocephalus was not explained by any demonstrable anatomical aberration. As an alternative to the traditional surgical treatment of hydrocephalus, the medical treatment did not experience the elusive "breakthrough" that had been sought for decades. The carbonic anhydrase inhibitor, acetazolamide, has been used for forty years, and additional reports of its use in the control of hydrocephalus continue to appear, though the drug is successful in only a minority of cases. Nevertheless, it has an established place particularly in early infancy when complications of shunts are more frequent; it is also a viable alternative to ventricular taps or drains in preterm infants whose cranium is still too thin and fragile to support the anchoring of a shunt apparatus. Acetazolamide is not the final or best medical response to this challenge, however, nor were ouabain and other cardiac glycosides that inhibit the Na^{+}/K^{+} ATPase pump essential to CSF secretion. The search for a better drug continues.

The ependyma was a prominent focus of neuroembryological study during the 1990-1993 period, not only because of its importance in the transport of fluids and ions between the cerebral parenchyma and CSF and its still uncertain role in the pathogenesis of hydrocephalus, but because of its increasingly recognized primordial importance in several neurodevelopmental processes, including the arrest of mitotic activity of the neuroepithelium, the guidance of axonal growth cones and the transformation of radial glial cells. The development and maturation of the human fetal ependyma was shown to follow a predictable temporal and spatial sequence including its secretory functions. The roof plate was demonstrated to secrete the glycosaminoglycan *keratan sulfate,* which prevents aberrant decussations of the developing dorsal columns of the spinal cord by strongly repelling axonal growth cones. The floor plate ependyma, which also repels long ascending and descending axons, was demonstrated to actually facilitate the passage of commisural fibers. The pivotal role of the floor plate in neural induction and its mediation of retinoic acid were further clarified, and the floor plate also was shown to influence the differentiation of structures derived from the mesodermal somites, previously thought only to occur as mesodermal induction of ectoderm. A cyclopian zebrafish model of human holoprosencephaly that lacks a floor plate ependyma was discovered and the effects of the lack of a floor plate on axonal guidance was studied in this animal. The early development of the chick spinal cord in the absence of a notochord and floor plate ependyma was described, providing additional clues to the nature of the defects in human midline CNS malformations. The relation of neural induction to neurulation and its relation to spina bifida also was studies experimentally.

New insights into the early ontogenesis of the CNS resulted from intensive studies published during 1990-1993. The arrangement of neuroepithelial cells was found to begin even earlier than suspected, preceding inductive influences of the notochord. The segmentation of the rhombencephalon, directed by homeobox genes, was further documented and explained.

Neuroblast migratory sisorders, including lissencephaly and pachygyria, were better understood at the end than at the beginning of the 1990-1993 period. The Miller-Dieker syndrome was genetically localized to 300 kb microdefect at the 17p13.3 locus and the clinical, electroencephalographic and imaging aspects were further refined. Other radiological and pathological patterns of migratory disorders also were studied. Morphological and metabolic abnormalities of the ependyma were described in infants and children with various types of neuroblast migratory disorders. Lissencephaly secondary to congenital cytomegalovirus infections was documented. Important new experimental data on neuroblast migration mediated by radial glial cells continued to enhance our understanding of the human diseases.

Hemimegalencephaly was studied by EEG, SPECT, MR imaging and histopathologically. Basic studies of reorganization of the corticospinal tract in the fetal rat after ablation of a cerebral hemisphere provided a basis for understanding the lack of asymmetry of muscle tone, movement and stretch reflexes in most human infants with hemimegalencephaly. The importance of the transient subplate neurons in projecting pioneer axons of the corticospinal and thalamocortical connections was demonstrated.

The examples of studies cited and references provided are an arbitrary sampling. The supplements to the body of scientific knowledge of basic and clinical embryology and disorders of ontogenesis during the past three years promise even more expectations in 1994 and beyond. The clinical problem of hydrocephalus remains one of major magnitude in patient care, and the search for a pharmacological means of control of CSF secretion continues. - *Harvey B. Sarnat, M.D., F.R.C.P. (C), Children's Hospital and Medical Center, Seattle, WA.*

BIBLIOGRAPHY

Aicardi J. The agyria-pachygyria complex: a spectrum of cortical malformations. Brain Dev 1991;13:1-8.

Alvarez IS, Schoenwolf GC. Patterns of neuroepithelial cell rearrangement during avian neurulation are dtermined prior to notochordal inductive interactions. Dev Biol 1991;143:78-92.

Artinger KB, Bronner-Fraser M. Delayed formation of the floor plate after ablation of the avian notochord. Neuron 1993;11:1147-1161.

Barkovich AJ, Koch TK, Carrol CL. The spectrum of lissencephaly: report of ten patients analysed by resonance imaging. Ann Neurol 1991;30:139-146.

Barkovich AJ, Kjos BO. Non-lissencephalic cortical dysplasias: correlation of imaging findings with clinical deficits. Am J Neuroradiol 1992;13:95-103.

Bovolenta P, Dodd J. Guidance of commissural growth cones at the floor plate in embryonic rat spinal cord. Development 1990;109:435-447.

Brand-Sabori B, Ebensperger C, Wilting J et al. The ventralizing effect of the notochord on somite differentiation in chick embryos. Anat Embryol 1993;188:239-245.

Bronner-Fraser M, Stern C. Effects of mesodermal tissues on avian neural crest cell migration. Dev Biol 1991;143:213-217.

De Rijk-van Andel JF, Arts WFM, Barth PG et al. Diagnostic features and clinical signs of 21 patients with lissencephaly type 1. Dev Med Child Neurol 1990;32:707-717.

Dobyns WB, Elias ER, Newlin AC et al. Causal heterogeneity in isolated lissencephaly. Neurology 1992;42:1375-1388.

Gadisseux J-F, Kadhim HJ, van den Bosch de Aquilar P et al. Neuron migration within the radial glial fiber system of the developing murine cerebrum: an electron microscopic autoradiographic analysis. Dev Brain Res 1990;52:39-56.

Hatta K, Kimmel CB, Ho RR et al. The cyclops mutation blocks the specification of the floor plate of the zebrafish central nervous system. Nature 1991;350:339-341.

Hayward JC, Titelbaum DS, Clancy RR et al. Lissencephaly-pachygyria associated with congenital cytomegalovirus infection. J Child Neurol 1991;6:109-114.

Ledbetter Sa, Kuwano A, Dobyns WD et al. Microdeletions of chromosome 17p13 as a cause of isolated lissencephaly. Am J Hum Genet 1992;50:182-189.

Keynes RJ, Lumsden A. Segmentation and the origin of regional diversity in the vertebrate central nervous system. Neuron 1990;2:1-9.

Konkol RJ, Maister BH, Wells RG et al. Hemimegalencephaly: clinical, EEG, neuroimaging, and IMP-SPECT correlations. Pediatr Neurol 1990;6:414-418.

Marshall H, Nonchev S, Sham MH et al. Retinoic acid alters hindbrain Hox code and induces transformation of rhombomeres 2/3 into a 4/5 identity. Nature 1992;360:737-741.

McConnell SK, Ghosh A, Shatz CJ. Subplate neurons pioneer the first axon pathway from the cerebral cortex. Science 1990;245:978-982.

Ono K, Shimada M, Yamano T. Reorganization of the corticospinal tract following neonatal unilateral cortical ablation in rats. Brain Dev 1990;12:226-236.

Palmini A, Andermann F, Dulac O et al. Diffuse cortical dysplasia or the "double cortex" syndrome: the clinical and epileptic spectrum in 10 patients. Neurology 1991;41:1656-1662.

Perlman JM, Lynch B, Volpe JJ. Late hydrocephalus after arrest and resolution of neonatal post-hemorrhagic hydrocephalus. Dev Med Child Neurol 1990;32:725-729.

Pouplard F, Pineau P. Use of acetazolamide in external hydrocephalus in infants. Ann Pediatr (Paris) 1990;37:310-12.

Pourquie O, Coltey M, Teillet M-A et al. Control of dorsoventral patterning of somitic derivatives by notochord and floor plate, Proc Natl Acad Sci USA 1993;90:5242-5246.

Sarnat HB. Cerebral Dysgenesis. Embryology and Clinical Expression. New York, Oxford University Press, 1992.

Idem. Role of human fetal ependyma. Pediatr Neurol 1992;8:163-178.

Idem. Regional differentiation of the human fetal ependyma: immunocytochemical markers. J Neuropathol Exp Neurol 1992;51:58-75.

Idem, Trevenen CL, Darwish HZ. Ependymal abnormalities in cerbro-hepato-renal disease of Zellweger. Brain Dev 1993;15:270-277.

Siebert JR, Cohen MM Jr, Sulik KK, Shaw C-M, Lemire RJ. Holoprosencephaly. An Overview and Atlas of Cases. New York, Wiley-Liss, 1990.

Snow DM, Steindler DA, Silver J. Molecular and cellular characterization of the glial roof plate of the spinal cord and optic tectum: a possible role for a proteoglycan in the development of an axon barrier. Dev Biol 1990;138:359-376.

van Straaten HWM, Hekking JWM. Development of floor plate, neurons, and axonal outgrowth pattern in the early spinal cord of the notochord-deficient chick embryo. Anat Embryol 1991;184:55-63.

Wagner M, Thaller C, Jessell T et al. Polarizing activity and retinoid synthesis in the floor plate of the neural tube. Nature 1990;345:819-822.

CONGENITAL HYDROCEPHALUS

CONGENITAL HYDROCEPHALUS AND SEIZURES

The frequency of seizures and long-term outcome in 68 children with congenital hydrocephalus not associated with myelomeningocele were examined at the Washington University School of Medicine, St. Louis, MO. Mental retardation was a risk factor for the development of seizures and was diagnosed 4 times more frequently in children with seizures (76% compared to 17%). Cerebral malformation diagnosed on CT, such as agenesis of the corpus callosum, was another seizure predictive factor (48% v. 17%). The absence of mental retardation, older age and non-paroxysmal EEG at seizure onset, and absence of CNS malformation correlated with seizure remission. Seizures were adequately controlled by anticonvulsants in 42 % and medication was successfully discontinued in patients of normal intelligence who had been seizure free for 3 years. (Noetzel MJ, Blake JN. Seizures in children with congenital hydrocephalus: long-term outcome. Neurology July 1992;42:1277-1281.) (Reprints: Dr. Noetzel, Department of Neurology, Washington University School of Medicine, 400 S. Kingshighway, St. Louis, MO 63110.)

COMMENT. The clinical and neuroradiologic findings in a male infant with congenital hydrocephalus due to intrauterine HTLV-1 infection are reported from the Division of Child Neurology, Institute of Neurological Sciences, Tottori University Faculty of Medicine, Yonago, Japan. A 20 day old male infant was admitted with macrocephaly. The mother developed human T-cell lymphotropic virus type I (HTLV-1) associated myelopathy shortly after the birth of the infant. The infant's serum HTLV-1 antibody was elevated, suggesting an intrauterine route of infection. (Tohyama J et al. Neurology July 1992;42:1406-1408.)

Factors affecting the prognosis of intrauterine hydrocephalus diagnosed in the third trimester are reviewed from the Department of Neurosurgery, Kobe University, School of Medicine, Japan (Oi S. Surg Neurol 1992;37:66-68). Four patients underwent transabdominal or transvaginal cephalocentesis with measurement of intracranial pressure and intrauterine pressure. Another 4 patients had pre- and postnatal CT or MRI measurements of the head performed shortly before and after birth. The results indicated extremely high intracranial pressure in the fetal brain, whereas after birth the macrocephaly was accompanied by a relatively low intracranial pressure. Fetal hydrocephalus is extremely hypertensive and an impairment of neuronal functional development prenatally can be irreversible. The fetal ventricular amniotic shunt was not appropriate for maintaining the decompressive effect and a more reliable drainage system is required.-Editor. *Ped Neur Briefs* Aug 1992.

POST-HAEMORRHAGIC HYDROCEPHALUS

The neuromotor outcome of 33 survivors of grade 3 or 4 neonatal posthaemorrhagic hydrocephalus assessed at a mean age of 4.7 years is reported from the Department of Paediatric Neurology, The Royal Hospital for Sick Children, Edinburgh and the Western General Hospital, Edinburgh. Two-thirds of the children were moderately or severely impaired. Raised intracranial pressure was not significantly different between outcome groups. Of 27 shunted, those with 5 or more operations (10 children) had abnormal neurological outcomes. The rise in morbidity after the 4th shunt was associated with ventriculitis. Outcome was unrelated to the grade of intraventricular hemorrhage or parenchymal changes on ultrasound or CT scanning and was independent of antenatal and perinatal factors. (Lin JP et al. Neurological outcome following neonatal post-haemorrhagic hydrocephalus: the effects of maximum raised intracranial pressure and ventriculo-peritoneal shunting. Child's Nerv Syst June 1992;8:190-197.) (Correspondence: J.P. Lin, M.D., Department of Paediatric Neurology, The Royal Hospital for Sick Children, Sciennes Road, Edinburgh, EH9 2EP, UK.)

COMMENT. This study shows that a rise in intracranial pressure in the acute stage of hydrocephalus does not carry a significant risk of further handicap or visual impairment. An adverse outcome was statistically related to more than 4 shunt procedures and ventriculitis. The authors' criteria for VP shunting were: 1) increasing ventriculomegaly, 2) raised ICP on monitoring, including during sleep, and 3) abnormal cerebral perfusion as shown by repeated Doppler ultrasonography studies of cerebral blood flow velocity.

The surgical management of post-haemorrhagic hydrocephalus is reported in 22 low birth weight infants from the Department of Neurosurgery, Eastern Virginia Medical School, Norfolk, VA (Gurtner P et al. Child's Nerv Syst June 1992;8:198-202). The use of subcutaneous ventricular reservoirs and a low pressure neonatal shunt was associated with a significant reduction in the morbidity and mortality compared to the use of external ventricular drainage devices.

The use of SPECT for the measurement of cerebral blood flow changes in 4 children with hydrocephalus is reported from the Departments of Neurosurgery and Radiology, Tokai University School of Medicine, Bohsei-dai, Isehara, Kanagawa, Japan (Shinoda M et al. Child's Nerv Syst June 1992;8:219-221). A positive reabsorption ratio of radioactivity counted in early and delayed images was correlated with a favorable outcome in 3 patients.

An overview of the surgery of hydrocephalus: past, present and future, by Hirsch JF, Hopital Necker Enfants Malades, Paris, France is published in Acta Neurochir (Wien) 1992;116:155-160. The need for research in the causes and prevention of hydrocephalus is stressed.-Editor. *Ped Neur Briefs* Sept 1992.

OTHER CNS MALFORMATIONS

ENCEPHALOCELES: PROGNOSIS

The outcome of 34 infants with a diagnosis of cephalocele was reviewed at the University of Colorado Health Sciences Center, Denver, and was compared with that of previously published series. Of 22 posterior defects, 5 were meningoceles and of 12 anterior defects, 8 were meningoceles. Additional major abnormalities were present in 15 (44%) of 34 infants, 7 (58%) with anterior defects and 8 (36%) with posterior defects. Those with anterior defects had abnormalities of the cranium, while those with posterior defects had extracranial abnormalities with greater frequency. Mortality was 29% (10/34) and confined to infants with posterior cephaloceles. Microcephaly was noted in 7 children all with posterior defects. Nine had hydrocephalus. Seizures occurred in 14 children, 5 with anterior defects and 9 with posterior defects. Outlook depended on site, operability, and additional major abnormalities. Mortality was confined to posterior defects, inoperability, congenital heart disease, infection, and shunt malfunction. Microcephaly, seizures, and hydrocephalus were associated with a worse outcome. Anterior defects have a better prognosis than posterior defects (Brown MS, Sheridan-Pereira M. Outlook for the child with a cephalocele. Pediatrics Dec 1992;90:914-919). (Reprints: Mark S. Brown, M.D., P/SL Medical Center, 1719 E. 19th Ave., Denver, CO 80218.)

COMMENT. Cephaloceles (cranium bifidum) occur most frequently in the midline. The primary morbidity in children with anterior defects has included facial disfigurement, anosmia and visual problems. Although there were no deaths in infants with anterior defects in this series, significant long-term disability was present in 50% and was associated with severe facial clefting, intracranial abnormalities and visual impairments. In infants with posterior defects, severe long-term disabilities occurred in 25% and mild handicaps in 38% of surviving infants. -Editor. *Ped Neur Briefs* Dec 1992.

CEREBRAL HEMIATROPHY: ETIOLOGY AND PATHOLOGY

Two types of cerebral hemiatrophy are reported from the Institute of Neuropathology at the University of Giessen, Arndtstrafse FRG. A case of "primary cerebral hemiatrophy" is described in a 12 year old boy whose birth was difficult and complicated by perinatal asphyxia. Seizures occurred immediately after birth and the psychomotor development was slow. He had spastic diplegia, asymmetrical, the right side predominating. He died at 12 years of age with cardiac arrest after status epilepticus. At autopsy the left hemisphere was reduced in size, the left lateral ventricle was enlarged and the white matter was decreased, especially on the left. The cerebral peduncles and pyramidal tracts were asymmetrical, and the neurons of the left hippocampus were replaced by glial tissue. Case two, an adult male, had a normal birth and early development and suffered from convulsions at two years of age which were followed by a right hemiparesis and homonymous hemianopsia. CT scan showed cerebral hemiatrophy and skull hypertrophy on the left side. The patient died at the age of 58 from intestinal hemorrhage with liver cirrhosis. The left cerebral hemisphere was atrophied and with crossed cerebellar and pyramidal tract atrophy. There were loss of cortical neurons in the atrophic left hemisphere and replacement by glial cells, a spongy state and abundant corpora amylacea. This was an example of "secondary cerebral hemiatrophy".

The authors propose a classification of primary and secondary cerebral hemiatrophy. The *primary* forms are caused by vascular malformation, perinatal asphyxia and birth trauma and result in ulegyria, lamina necrosis and leukoencephalopathy. The *secondary* forms may be post-ictal with or without fever, or caused by cerebrovascular accident or leukoencephalitis. The pathological findings with the secondary form are sclerosing cortical atrophy and occasionally leukoencephalopathy (Vosskamper M, Schachenmayr W. Cerebral hemiatrophy: a clinical pathological report of two cases with a contribution to pathogenesis and differential diagnosis. Clin Neuropath Sept/Oct 1990;9:244-250).

COMMENT. Cerebral hemiatrophy with homolateral hemihypertrophy of the skull and sinuses was described by Dyke CG, Davidoff L, and Masson C. (Arch Neurol and Psychiat 1933;29:412) and Alpers B J, and Dear R B (J Nerv and Ment Dis 1939;89:653) distinguished the primary and secondary groups of cases. The significance of convulsions in the pathogenesis of cerebral hemiatrophy is emphasized by many authors - the "hemiconvulsion hemiplegia -

epilepsy syndrome." Permanent hemiparesis as a direct result of a febrile convulsion is a rare complication occurring in less than 0.2% (Millichap J. G. Febrile Convulsions, Macmillan, New York, 1968).-Editor. *Ped Neur Briefs* March 1991.

CNS MALFORMATION AND CEREBRAL PALSY

The incidence of minor malformations in a group of 137 adults with cerebral palsy, living in a New York State residential institution, is reported from the Division of Developmental Pediatrics, Robert Warner Rehabilitation Center, State University of New York, Buffalo, NY. Subjects were classified in three etiological groups: (1) prenatal onset, (2) postnatal onset, and (3) perinatal onset. Criteria for enrollment in group 1 included a known prenatal cause (i.e., CNS malformation, chromosomal aberration or congenital infection) or fullterm birth with unremarkable delivery and neonatal course. Of 109 patients with CP of prenatal origin, 82% had unknown causes, 10% CNS malformation, 5% chromosomal aberration and 3% congenital infection. Of 28 patients with postnatal causes, 39% had bacterial meningitis, 32% encephalitis, 11% metabolic disease, 7% cardiopulmonary arrest and 7% trauma. Spastic quadriplegia, profound mental retardation, and seizures occurred in 80-90% of the total sample, and the neurological findings were similar in the two groups. The prenatal group with known etiology and a subgroup with unknown etiology had significantly more minor malformations than the postnatal group. Individuals with CP and multiple minor malformations, in the absence of definitive postnatal or perinatal factors, have CNS developmental dysfunction caused most likely by prenatal influences. (Coorssen EA et al. Multiple minor malformations as a marker for prenatal etiology of cerebral palsy. Dev Med Child Neurol August 1991;33:730-736).

COMMENT. Increased numbers of minor malformations are indicative of aberrant embryonic development of the CNS (Illingworth R. "Why blame the obstetrician? A review." BMJ 1979;1:797-801) Less than 10% of CP is caused by perinatal asphyxia or events related to delivery (Blair E, Stanley F. "Intrapartum asphyxia: a rare cause of cerebral palsy." J Pediatr 1988;112:515-519).-Editor. *Ped Neur Briefs* Aug 1991.

LISSENCEPHALY: CLINICAL AND MRI FINDINGS

Clinical data and MRI scans from 10 patients ages 3 days to 27 years (mean age 4.6 years) with lissencephaly were reviewed in the Departments of Radiology, Neurology and Pediatrics, University of California, San Francisco, CA. The youngest patients had the most severe lissencephaly but no correlation was found between the severity of the malformation as graded by MRI and the severity of clinical disease. One child age 2 1/2 with frontal lobes most severely affected was walking, speaking in 3 to 4 word sentences, and following instructions appropriate to her age, and physical examination revealed only very mild hypotonia. The anatomical deformity in the brain was not associated with any delay in myelination in patients in this study. Seizures occurred in all but one of the patients greater than four months of age; they began with infantile spasms or focal motor seizures and tonic seizures commonly occurred by the end of the second year. Hypsarrhythmia was present in two patients (Barkovich AJ et al. The spectrum of lissencephaly: report of ten patients analyzed by magnetic resonance imaging. Ann Neurol August 1991;30:139-146).

COMMENT. The normal pattern and rate of myelination and the absence of porencephalies or other destructive lesions in 9 of the 10 patients in this report suggests that the arrest of neuronal migration in lissencephaly results from the absence of molecular components of the glial fibers or intracellular matrix. Lissencephaly is described in two types according to clinical, radiological, and pathological characteristics. In *type I lissencephaly,* agyria and pachygyria regions have a molecular layer, an outer cellular layer, a cell-sparse layer, and a deep cellular layer composed of heterotopic incompletely migrated neurons. In *type II lissencephaly,* the thickened cortex is disorganized without evidence of layers, and hydrocephalus and multiple anomalies are usually present.-Editor. *Ped*

Neur Briefs Aug 1991.

LISSENCEPHALY: EEG AND EVOKED POTENTIALS

The EEGs and evoked potentials were studied in 21 Dutch patients with lissencephaly type I at the Departments of Clinical Neurophysiology and Neurology, Juliana Children's Hospital, The Hague, The Netherlands. Compared to patients with atypical cortical dysplasia and to a control group the EEGs in the lissencephaly patients showed the following patterns significantly more often: (a) generalized fast activity (8-18/s) with an amplitude higher than 50 mcV (b) sharp- and slow-wave complexes with high amplitude (range 500 - 3000 mcV and (c) an alternating pattern consisting of bursts of sharp waves alternating with periods of electrocerebral depression. Short latency somatosensory evoked potentials in 10 patients after stimulation of the median nerve were abnormal. (de Rijk-van Andel J.F. et al. EEG and evoked potentials in a series of 21 patients with lissencephaly type I. Neuropediatrics Feb 1992;23:4-9.) (Correspondence: J.F. de Rijk-van Andel, MD, Ignatius Ziekenhuis, Molengracht 21, 4818 CK Breda, The Netherlands.)

COMMENT. Lissencephaly may be differentiated from an atypical cortical dysplasia by CT and/or MRI. In addition, the EEG and evoked potentials may be of diagnostic value. Generalized fast activity and sharp- and slow-wave complexes were noted in 20 of the 21 lissencephaly patients and in only 1 of the 21 patients with atypical cortical dysplasia. An abnormal PET scan suggested the microscopic pathology confirmed at autopsy in an infant with lissencephaly and normal gross cortical structure. The clinical features were intractable seizures and developmental delay but normal head growth (Korobkin R, Sarnat H, Chugani H. Neurology April 1992;4(Suppl 3):354). Radiographic and clinical variability within the 3 subtypes of lissencephaly are reviewed in 19 patients ages 1 day to 6 years (Demos DS et al. Neurology April 1992;42(Suppl 3):286).-Editor. *Ped Neur Briefs* June 1992.

LISSENCEPHALY: CAUSAL HETEROGENEITY

Clinical, cytogenetic and molecular studies in 65 patients with isolated lissencephaly sequence (ILS) are reported from Indiana University School of Medicine, Indianapolis; Tufts New England Medical Center, Boston; Eastern Virginia Medical School, Norfolk; University of Washington School of Medicine, Seattle; and Baylor College of Medicine, Houston. All patients had type I lissencephaly of varying severity and a grossly normal cerebellum; 17% had agenesis of the corpus callosum and 21% had cavum septi pellucidi. The facial appearance was described as essentially normal, but subtle abnormalities were observed, including microcephaly (71%), bitemporal hollowing (70%), abnormal nasal bridge (49%), and small jaw (58%). All were severely mentally retarded, and 76% had a mixed seizure disorder that progressed to infantile spasms in 35% . Seizures were uncommon during the first few months of life, but opisthotonos was often reported. Hypotonia evolved into spasticity, and feeding difficulties usually improved after several days or weeks. During pregnancy, prolonged or heavy vaginal bleeding occurred in 12% and flu-like syndromes in the mothers of 12%. CP and MRI appearances showed a smooth cerebral surface with open sylvian region, a typical "figure-8" appearance on axial images and enlarged posterior lateral ventricles (colpocephaly). Molecular studies showed microdeletions in chromosome band 17p (6 patients). Other causes included autosomal recessive inheritance, intrauterine infection and intrauterine perfusion failure. The calculated risk of recurrence in sibs was 7 % (Dobyns WB et al. Causal heterogeneity in isolated lissencephaly. Neurology July 1992;42:1375-1388). (Reprints: Dr. William B. Dobyns, Division of Pediatric Neurology, University of Minnesota, P.O. Box 380, 420 Delaware Street SE, Minneapolis, MN 55455.)

COMMENT. For further reports on lissencephaly see Ped Neur Briefs August 1991;5:59-60; June 1992;6:48.

The role of human fetal ependyma in the pathogenesis of some cerebral malformations such as lissencephaly/pachygyria and holoprosencephaly is reviewed by Dr. Harvey B. Sarnat in Pediatr Neurol May/June 1992;8:163-78. Lissencephaly is a primary disturbance of neuroblast migration associated with abnormal gyration of the cerebral cortex. Ependymal abnormalities include persistence of the fetal pseudostratified columnar organization and subventricular rosettes of ependymal cells. The author provides an excellent account of the pathogenesis of cerebral dysgenesis. (Correspondence: Dr. Sarnat, Children's Hospital, CH49, 4800 Sand Point Way N.E., Seattle, WA 98105.)-Editor. *Ped Neur Briefs* Aug 1992.

GENERALIZED CORTICAL DYSPLASIA

The clinical and neuropathological findings in three children with diffuse cortical dysplasia are reported from the Departments of Pathology, Neurology and Pediatrics, University of Rochester Medical Center, Rochester, NY. The children had seizures unresponsive to antiepileptic medication throughout life, they were profoundly mentally retarded, and they died after a progressive neurological deterioration at ages 10 months, 3 years and 7 years. Pathologically, the brains showed generalized cortical dysplasia, without any major malformation of the external gyral pattern. The cortical gray matter was thickened and the demarcation of the gray-white matter junction was indistinct. Microscopically, the cortex contained increased numbers of large neurons with disordered cortical lamination and heterotopic neurons scattered throughout the white matter. The cortical involvement was multifocal involving all lobes of the cerebral hemispheres, and the underlying myelin was pale and rarified. (Kazee AM et al. Generalized cortical dysplasia. Clinical and pathologic aspects. Arch Neurol August 1991;48: 850-853).

COMMENT. The authors report these cases as a newly recognized entity of abnormal neuronal migration. In contrast to classic lissencephaly no distinct lamination of the cortical layers was present and the underlying myelin was also involved. The cause of generalized cortical dysplasia is unknown but a genetic etiologic factor is suspected.-Editor. *Ped Neur*

Briefs Aug 1991.

OCCULT CORTICAL DYSPLASLA AND FOCAL STATUS EPILEPTICUS

Four patients, ages 4, 6, 13, and 21 years, with life-threatening focal motor status epilepticus, normal pre-operative MRI, and focal cortical dysplasia defined only in the surgical specimens obtained by corticectomies, are reported from the Montreal Neurological Institute; Austin Hospital, Heidelberg, Australia; University of California, San Francisco; and Royal Children's Hospital, Melbourne, Australia. Seizures began between 3 months and 18 years of age, and therapy-resistant focal status developed after 18 months to 3 years, resulting in persistent motor deficits. A total of 12 MRIs failed to reveal abnormalities. Ictal SPECT was positive in 2 patients. Seizures were controlled after surgery, and 2 patients were seizure-free. (Desbiens R et al. Life-threatening focal status epilepticus due to occult cortical dysplasia. Arch Neurol July 1993;50:695-700). (Reprints: Dr Frederick Andermann, Montreal Neurological Hosp and Institute, 3801 University St, Montreal, Quebec, Canada H3A 2B4).

COMMENT. Neuronal migration disorder as a cause of focal motor status epilepticus or epilepsia partialis continua in a child may not be excluded by the MRI and may require surgical intervention for diagnosis and treatment.-Editor. *Ped Neur Briefs* July 1993.

PERIODIC ALTERNATING GAZE AND CEREBELLAR DYSGENESIS

Two children with periodic alternating gaze deviation, presenting at birth in 1 patient and at 2 months in the other, are reported from the New England Medical Center, Tufts University, Boston, MA. The eyes conjugately drifted from one side to the other. With the head stabilized, a regular nystagmus of low frequency and large amplitude was seen when the patient attempted to direct the eyes away from the gaze bias. Compensatory head turning was noted in both patients. MRI showed multiple congenital abnormalities of the posterior cranial fossa. In 1 patient a left renal aplasia and a right supra-adrenal neuroblastoma were diagnosed by ultrasonography and by resection at 4 weeks of age. (Legge RH et al. Periodic alternating gaze deviation in infancy. Neurology Sept 1992;42:1740-1743.) (Reprints: Dr. Thomas R. Hedges III, 750 Washington Street, Box 381, Boston, MA 02111.)

COMMENT. The periodic alternating gaze phenomenon is rare and points to cerebellar disease, with malformation of the inferior cerebellar vermis as the specific underlying lesion. The association with neuroblastoma in one patient is a coincidence since symptoms of opsoclonus were not described.-Editor. *Ped Neur Briefs* Oct 1992.

SPINA BIFIDA AND CARBAMAZEPINE

The records of all pregnant Medicaid recipients in Michigan who were taking antiepileptic agents during pregnancy were studied at the Center for Drug Evaluation and Research, Food and Drug Administration, Rockville, Maryland. Four cases of spina bifida were identified in infants born to 1,490 women who took anticonvulsants during pregnancy. Among 107 women taking carbamazepine three gave birth with spina bifida; one was taking valproic acid in addition and two were taking phenytoin, barbiturates or primidone in combination with carbamazepine. Among 1,018 infants of mothers taking barbiturates alone only one had spina bifida. Among 444 women taking phenytoin and 50 taking primidone alone, none gave birth to an infant with spina bifida. When the data from approximately 20 published studies were pooled, nine cases of spina bifida occurred among a total of 984 in utero exposures to carbamazepine, and the relative risk was 13.7 times the expected rate (approximately one in 1,500 births). Five cases of spina bifida occurred in infants whose mothers took carbamazepine alone during pregnancy. While exposure to carbamazepine in utero carried a 1% risk of spina bifida the risk with valproic acid was close to 2% but the difference was not significant. The risks with other anticonvulsant drugs was only 0 14% or one in 748 cases. (Rosa, E.W. Spina bifida in infants of women treated with carbamazepine during pregnancy, N Engl J Med March 7, 1991;324:674-677).

COMMENT. The incidence of meningomyelocele has declined steadily from 12 per 10,000 in 1970 to 6 to 8 per 10,000 in 1980 among babies born in the United States. The neural tube closes between 22 and 29 days after conception and exposure to antiepileptic agents such as valproic acid and carbamazepine may interfere with closure. Meningomyelocele may be diagnosed in the fetus with 75 to 80% accuracy by measurements of serum alpha-fetoprotein levels, and ultrasonography can identify the extent and location of these defects. (Hobbins, J.C., Diagnosis and management of neural tube defects today, N Engl J Med, March 7 1991;324:690-691).

The outcome of a neural tube defect may be improved by cesarean section before labor begins (Luthy, D A et al Cesarean section before the onset of labor and subsequent motor function in infants with meningomyelocele diagnosed antenatally, N Engl J Med March 7, 1991;324:662-666). Infants who had been exposed to labor were 2.2 times more likely to have severe paralysis than those delivered by cesarean section without labor. The mean functional motor level was at the second lumbar vertebra in fetuses exposed to labor and at the fourth lumbar vertebra in those delivered before labor began. Cesarean section before onset of labor may result in better subsequent motor function and the ability to walk with minimal mechanical assistance.-Editor. *Ped Neur Briefs* March 1991.

FOLIC ACID AND NEURAL TUBE DEFECTS

The results of a randomized double-blind prevention trial conducted at 33 centers in seven countries to determine the effects of folic acid supplements around the time of conception in the prevention of neural tube defects is reported by the MRC Vitamin Study Research Group, Department of Environmental and Preventive Medicine, Medical

College of St. Bartholomew's Hospital, London EC1, UK. A total of 1,817 women at high risk of having a pregnancy with a neural tube defect were allocated at random to one of four groups - folic acid, other vitamins, both, or neither. Of 27 mothers giving birth to a child with a neural tube defect, six were in the folic acid groups and 21 in the two other groups, a 72% protective effect. Other vitamins showed no significant protective effect. Capsules for those in the folic acid group contained 4 mg of folic acid, one a day until 12 weeks of pregnancy. (Wald N et al. Prevention of neural tube defects: results of the Medical Research Council vitamin study. Lancet July 20, 1991;338:131-137).

COMMENT. This study establishes the specific role of folic acid in the prevention of neural tube defects. Folic acid supplementation in a dose of 4 mg/day is now recommended for all women who have had a previously affected pregnancy, and the diet of all women who may bear children should contain an adequate amount of folic acid. An editorial in this issue of The Lancet comments that this supplement did not prevent all neural tube defects and six unsuccessful cases were not accounted for by unusually low serum folic acid concentrations. A heterogeneous etiology for this group of disorders is suggested. The dosage of folic acid necessary to prevent neural tube defects is not entirely established, and the optimal duration of treatment before conception is uncertain. Can culturally appropriate dietary guidelines be prepared as a matter of urgency for all ethnic groups? Can the requisite folic acid be eaten in food instead of given as a supplement? Providing specific dietary advice about the prevention of malformations to women before pregnancy is a challenging public health problem.- Editor. *Ped Neur Briefs* Sept 1991.

MENTAL RETARDATION SYNDROMES

NEUROANATOMY OF FRAGILE X SYNDROME

Posterior fossa abnormalities measured by magnetic resonance images of the brain were reported in a group of 14 males with fragile X syndrome from the

Division of Child Psychiatry, and the Departments of Psychiatry and Radiology, The Johns Hopkins University School of Medicine, and The Kennedy Institute, Baltimore, MD. The size of the posterior cerebellar vermis was significantly decreased and the fourth ventricle significantly increased in males with fragile X syndrome compared to a group of 17 males with other causes of developmental disability and 18 males with normal IQs. The lack of a significant correlation between age and size of vermis argues against atrophy as the cause but rather a developmental hypoplasia of the posterior vermis. (Reiss AL et al. Neuroanatomy of fragile X syndrome: the posterior fossa. Ann Neurol Jan 1991;29:26-32).

COMMENT. Hypoplasia of the cerebellar vermal lobules VI and VII has also been described in patients with autism (Courchesne E et al. N Engl J Med 1988;318:1349). Autistic-like behavior occurs frequently in males with fragile X syndrome and the posterior vermis hypoplasia may have a causative relation. The cerebellar vermis plays an important role in the modulation and execution of motor behavior, and hyperactivity and repetitive stereotypic movements are common behaviorisms in fragile X patients. Language dysfunction also occurs with fragile X syndrome and the posterior vermis of the cerebellum is involved in auditory processing of language. So-called "cerebellar mutism" may develop after removal of posterior fossa tumors, particularly medulloblastoma, and this complication has been correlated with the amount of the posterior vermis resected. (Platenberg C et al. AJNR 1989;10:891). A seven year old girl with a midline posterior fossa tumor developed mutism postoperatively after removal of an astrocytoma that involved the vermis of the cerebellum. Recovery was slow but speech was regained after a two month period of therapy (Millichap JG, McLone D, unpublished case report).-Editor. *Ped Neur Briefs* Feb 1991.

DIAGNOSIS OF FRAGILE X SYNDROME

Direct diagnosis by DNA analysis of the fragile X syndrome was studied in 511 persons from 63 families with the syndrome at the Institute National de la Sante et de la Recherce Medicale (INSERM), Unite 184, Faculte de Medecine, Strasbourg, France and other laboratories. Analysis of EcoRI and Eagl digests of DNA distinguished between the normal genotype, the permutation and the full mutation. The method was more reliable than cytogenetic testing. All 103 males and 31 of 59 females with full mutations had mental retardation. All mothers of affected children were carriers of either a permutation or a full mutation. Direct diagnosis by DNA analysis is an efficient primary test for the identification of fragile X syndrome after birth and prenatally. (Rousseau F, Mandel JL et al. Direct diagnosis by DNA analysis of the fragile X syndrome of mental retardation. N Engl J Med Dec 12, 1991;321:1673-81).

COMMENT. The authors propose that direct DNA diagnosis may be helpful in the differential diagnosis of mental retardation and in the genetic counseling of families with the fragile X syndrome. The use of a single EcoRI digestion to test for a fragile X mutation in boys or girls with unexplained mental retardation, late onset of speech, or autistic or hyperactive behavior is proposed even if there is no family history of mental retardation. The disease is caused by mutations that increase the size of a specific DNA fragment of the X chromosome. Affected persons have both a full mutation and abnormal DNA methylation. Persons with a smaller increase in the size of this DNA fragment (a permutation) have little or no risk of retardation but are at high risk of having affected children or grandchildren. Among persons with a full mutation, 100% of males and 50% of females will be mentally impaired, whereas the risk of retardation is about 3% in carriers of a permutation. The role of cytogenetic analysis in diagnosis must now be reevaluated.

The prenatal diagnosis of fragile X syndrome by direct detection of the unstable DNA sequence using Southern Blot Analysis is reported from The Department of Cytogenetics and Molecular Genetics, Adelaide Children's Hospital and Queen Victoria

Hospital, Adelaide, Australia (Sutherland GR et al. N Engl J Med Dec 12, 1991;325:1720-22). The carrier status of a cytogenetically normal woman in a family with the fragile X syndrome and the mutation in her male fetus were detected by analysis of a cordocentesis sample and led to the termination of the pregnancy.

Shapiro L from New York Medical College, Valhalla, NY, in an editorial, comments that cytogenetic analysis of fragile X syndrome may be relegated to a secondary role but should be used for index cases to verify that the typical fragile X mutation is present in the family before DNA analyses are performed and genetic counseling undertaken. (N Engl J Med Dec 12,1991;325:1736-37).-Editor. *Ped Neur Briefs* Dec 1991.

FRAGILE X FEMALES AND PSYCHIATRIC DISORDERS

Psychiatric and developmental difficulties in 17 young females with the fragile X mutation were compared with a non-fragile X female group in a controlled study reported from the Department of Psychiatry, Division of Child and Adolescent Psychiatry, The Johns Hopkins University School of Medicine and the Kennedy Institute, Baltimore, MD. Fragile X females showed a greater frequency of avoidant, mood, and stereotypy/habit disorders than controls. They were more withdrawn and depressed and showed greater deficits in interpersonal socialization skills. The frequency of ADHD was not increased. Seven of the subjects in each group had IQs below 70. Size of DNA insertion was correlated with IQ attention problems, and anxiety/withdrawal symptoms. (Freund LS, Reiss AL, Abrams MT. Psychiatric disorders associated with fragile X in the young female. Pediatrics Feb 1993;91:321-329). (Reprints: Dr LS Freund, Behavioral Genetics Ctr, 550 N Broadway, Rm 507, Baltimore, MD 21205).

COMMENT. Contrary to previous reports, the fragile X females did not show a greater frequency of ADHD or undifferentiated attention deficit. The authors comment that the control group may have been biased for attention problems. Similar to other studies, 35% of fragile X females exhibited repetitive behaviors, compared to none of the controls. The absence of retardation among fragile X females does not protect from psychiatric and social difficulties. Sisters of fragile X males should be tested genetically by DNA analysis to provide early diagnosis and allow therapeutic intervention.-Editor. *Ped Neur Briefs* March 1993.

CHARGE SYNDROME

A 12 month old male infant with the CHARGE syndrome (Coloboma, Heart defect, Atresia of the choana, Retarded growth and development, Genital hypoplasia, Ear anomalies or deafness) is reported from the Departments of Pediatrics and Neurology, Loyola University, Chicago. The infant was admitted with repeated cyanotic episodes and generalized seizures. CT revealed agenesis of the cerebellar vermis and a large fourth ventricular cyst. Brain stem auditory evoked responses showed dvsfunction of the distal VIII nerve (Menenzes M, Coker SB. CHARGE and Joubert's syndromes, are they a single disorder? Pediatr Neurol Nov/Dec 1990;6:428-430).

COMMENT. This patient also had Joubert's syndrome (agenesis of the cerebellar vermis, respiratory irregularities, ocular colobomas). Chromosomes were normal. The authors believe that these two syndromes are a single disorder with an overlap of characteristic features.

Various associated abnormalities of brain development may be detected by studies of evoked potentials (Coupland SG, Sarnat HB. Visual and auditory evoked potential correlates of cerebral malformations. Brain Dev 1990;12:466-72). Auditory brain stem responses were abnormal in cases of holoprosencephaly, lissencephaly, pachygyria and generalized megalencephaly. Visual evoked potentials were normal in collosal agenesis, holoprosencephaly and colpocephaly; they were abnormal in septal optic dysplasia and optic nerve hypoplasia.-Editor. *Ped Neur Briefs* March 1991.

SEIZURE ETIOLOGY IN DOWN SYNDROME

The etiology of seizures in 47 infants, children, and young adults with Down syndrome was examined at The Floating Hospital for Infants and Children, Boston, MA; and the Institute for Basic Research in Developmental Disabilities, Staten Island, NY. Of a total of 737 patients with Down syndrome, 47 (6%) had seizures; and 24 had an identifiable etiology usually related to a complication of Down syndrome, including neonatal hypoxia-ischemia, hypoxia from congenital heart disease, or infection. The infections were bacterial meningitis 3, viral meningoencephalitis in 1, brain abscess 1, febrile seizures 2. The patterns of the seizures in those of known etiology were generalized tonic-clonic in 18, infantile spasms in 2, myoclonic 2, absence 1, simple partial 3, and complex partial 1. Mixed partial and generalized seizures occurred in 2. Of 12 patients with seizures related to cardiovascular disease 4 died of complications of acute heart failure. Neonates with hypoxic ischemic injury had relatively poor outcomes. The authors recommend that all Down syndrome patients with seizures be thoroughly evaluated to determine the etiology. (Stafstrom CE et al. Seizures in children with Down syndrome: Etiology, characteristics and outcome. Dev Med Child Neurol March 1991;33:191-200).

COMMENT. Febrile seizures occurred in only two (0.9%) of the authors' patients during the susceptible age range. The relative rarity of febrile seizures in Down syndrome is contrasted with the relatively frequent occurrence of infantile spasms. Wisniewski KE, one of the authors, has previously studied the arrest of neurogenesis and synaptogenesis in brains of patients with Down syndrome. (N Engl J Med 1984;311:1187). Long necked dendritic spines persist after birth suggesting a dysgenetic process, and neuronal membranes in Down syndrome are abnormally hyperexcitable. The mechanism of increased susceptibility to seizures in children with Down syndrome may involve an interplay between hyperexcitable membranes, altered dendritic spines, and reduction of inhibitory interneurons. The present study suggests that seizures in patients with Down syndrome are frequently caused by additional factors, including hypoxia and infection.

The prevalence, onset, and type of seizure disorders and seizure control were studied in 405 individuals with Down syndrome aged six months to 45 years at the Departments of Pediatrics and Neurology, Rhode Island Hospital, Providence, RI. The prevalence of seizures in this group of patients was 8.1%. The onset of seizures occurred before one year of age in 40% and in the third decade of life in another 40%. Infantile spasms and tonic-clonic seizures with myoclonus were most common in the younger age group, and partial simple or partial complex seizures and tonic-clonic seizures occurred in the older patients. A bimodal distribution of seizures in patients with Down syndrome was noted. (Pueschel SM et al. Seizure disorders in Down syndrome. Arch Neurol March 1991;48:318-320).-Editor. *Ped Neur Briefs* April 1991.

WILLIAMS AND DOWN SYNDROMES: BRAIN ANATOMY

The morphological features of the cerebral hemispheres of nine subjects with Williams syndrome (WS) and six with Down syndrome (DS) have been compared using MRIs at the University of California at San Diego, La Jolla, CA. Ages ranged from 10 to 20 years (mean, 15 years). Total cerebral gray matter and total cerebral volume were reduced in both retarded groups when compared to normal controls. Regional analysis of gray matter showed significant differences between WS and DS: frontal cortex and limbic structures of the temporal lobe are disproportionately reduced while the thalamus, putamen, and globus pallidus are normal in volume in DS. Frontal and temporal limbic structures are relatively preserved in WS. (Jernigan TL, Hesselink JR et al. Cerebral morphological distinctions between Williams and Down syndromes. Arch Neurol Feb 1993;50:186-191). (Reprints: Dr Jernigan, Department of Psychiatry, 0631P, University of California at San Diego, 9500 Gilman Dr, La Jolla, CA 92093).

COMMENT. Previous studies in this laboratory showed cerebellar changes in these syndromes: total cerebellar size was reduced in DS and normal in WS. Regional analysis of the cerebellum of WS subjects showed a small vermis and enlarged hemispheres. The relative sparing of frontal and cerebellar structures in WS may explain the relative fluency of speech in subjects with this syndrome. Poor development of cerebellar, limbic, and frontal structures in subjects with DS correlates with their language and social-affective disabilities.

A relationship between Down syndrome and Lewy bodies, a major neuropathological feature of Parkinson's disease, is reported in two middle-aged patients examined at the Department of Neuropathology, Newcastle-upon-Tyne, UK (Raghavan R et al. Detection of Lewy bodies in trisomy 21 (Down's syndrome). Can J Neurol Sci Feb 1993;20:48-51). The substantia nigra was normal in size while the locus coeruleus was small. Alzheimer-type pathology was also present. An etiological connection between Parkinson's and Alzheimer's diseases and trisomy 21 was suggested.-Editor. *Ped Neur Briefs* March 1993.

PENA-SHOKEIR SYNDROME

An infant with Pena-Shokeir syndrome born to a cocaine using mother is reported from the University of Pennsylvania School of Medicine, Philadelphia, PA. The mother had used cocaine on the 1st and 2nd of every month during pregnancy. The Apgars were 2 and 1 and the infant died within minutes after birth. Ultrasound had revealed polyhydramnios in the mother and an autopsy of the infant showed multiple congenital anomalies which included facial anomalies (low-set ears, epicanthic folds, corneal cloudiness, flattened nasal bridge, high-arched cleft palate and micrognathia), skeletal anomalies (arthrogryposis, camptodactyly, ulnar deviation, and bilateral clubfoot), pulmonary hypoplasia, and tetralogy of Fallot with right-sided aortic arch. The brain stem and spinal cord showed diffuse neuronal degeneration and the cerebral cortex showed focal infarction, consistent with acquired intrauterine ischemic damage. The set of anomalies is consistent with the Pena-Shokeir phenotype, also known as the fetal akinesia deformation sequence (Lavi E et al. Fetal akinesia deformation sequence (Pena-Shokeir phenotype) associated with acquired intrauterine brain damage. Neurology Sept 1991;41:1467-1468).

COMMENT. It was concluded that cocaine-induced vasoconstriction caused ischemic-anoxic brain damage, including damage to motor neurons, and resulted in fetal akinesia deformation sequence. There is a heterogeneity of the neuropathology in previously reported Pena-Shokeir phenotype cases, but most present with congenital CNS malformations caused by neuropathic, myopathic or connective tissue abnormalities that lead to decreased fetal motility in utero.-Editor. *Ped Neur Briefs* Dec 1991.

PRADER-WILLI SYNDROME

The clinical and polysomnographic features of 5 patients with Prader-Willi syndrome were studied at the Mayo Clinic, Jacksonville, FL. All patients, including 2 adults, 1 adolescent, and 2 children were obese; they had hypersomnolence and daytime hypoxemia, and they snored. The apnea plus hyponea index was less than 10 episodes per hour of sleep. Polysomnography failed to demonstrate clinically severe obstructive apnea or hypopnea. Sleep architecture and rapid eye movement latency were normal in all patients. Nonapneic reductions in oxyhemoglobin saturation were detected in only 1 adult and in 1 child. Despite the presence of morbid obesity and a history of snoring these patients with Prader-Willi syndrome had only mild sleep-disordered breathing (Kaplan J et al. Sleep and breathing in patients with the Prader-Willi syndrome. Mayo Clin Proc Nov 1991;66:1124-1126).

COMMENT. Prader-Willi syndrome is characterized by infantile hypotonia, early childhood obesity, mental deficiency, short stature, small hands and feet and hypogonadism. Many patients also have hypersomnolence, daytime hypoventilation, and some die prematurely of cardiorespiratory failure. The epidemiology of Prader-Willi syndrome was studied in a rural county in Sweden and reported from the Department of Pediatrics and Child Psychiatry, Child Neuropsychiatry Centre, Goteborg, Sweden (Akefeldt A et al. Dev Med Child Neurol Aug 1991;33:715-721). For the 7-25 year old age group the prevalence of Prader-Willi syndrome was 13 per 100,000 for definite cases, and 20 per 100,000 if borderline cases were included.

Anesthesia and the Prader-Willi syndrome was the subject of a report from the John Radcliffe Hospital, Oxford, England (Mackenzie JW. J Roy Soc Med April 1991;84:239). A 2 year old boy presented for correction of ventral curvature of micropenis and an 18 year old received anesthetic for removal of excess tissue from one thigh. Halothane in nitrous oxide and oxygen were used for induction and isoflurane to maintain anesthesia. Attention to glycaemic control and body temperature is important since glucose intolerance and both hypothermia and hyperthermia have been reported in response to operative stress.-Editor. *Ped Neur Briefs* Dec 1991.

PRADER-WILLI SYNDROME: DIAGNOSTIC CRITERIA

Diagnostic criteria for Prader-Willi syndrome (PWS), developed by consensus of seven clinicians in consultation with experts, are reported from the University of Washington, Seattle, and six additional centers. Three categories evolved, scored on a weighted point system: 1) *Major criteria* (1 point) include neonatal hypotonia, feeding problems, excessive weight gain, characteristic narrow facies with almond-shaped eyes and small, down-turned corners of the mouth, hypogonadism, developmental delay with mild to moderate mental retardation or learning problems, hyperphagia and obsession with food, and chromosomal deletion 5qll-13; 2) *Minor criteria* (one half point) include weak cry, behavioral problems, sleep apnea, short stature, fair skin and hair, small hands and feet, myopia, viscous saliva, and speech defects; and 3)

Supportive criteria (unscored) include high pain threshold, temperature instability, scoliosis, osteoporosis, and expert at jigsaw puzzles. Symptoms change with age: 5 points (4 major) required for diagnosis at birth to 3 years; 8 points (5 major) in the 3 year to adult age groups. (Holm VA et al. Prader-Willi syndrome: consensus diagnostic criteria. Pediatrics Feb 1993;91:398-402). (Reprints: Vanja A Holm MD, Child Development and Mental Retardation Center, WJ-10, University of Washington, Seattle, WA 98195).

COMMENT. Until a biological marker for PWS is available, the diagnosis is more an art than a science. These clinical criteria should ensure uniformity and alert the physician to a suspicion of PWS in hypotonic infants and in obese, mildly retarded and behaviorally disturbed adolescents and adults.-Editor. *Ped Neur Briefs* March 1993.

ACROCALLOSAL SYNDROME

A large highly inbred kindred with 3 definite and 1 possibly affected siblings with acrocallosal syndrome is reported from the Kaplan Hospital, Rehovot and the Emek Central Hospital, Afula, Israel. The family is of Israeli-Arab extraction and the parents are first cousins. The clinical features are divided into three groups: 1) diagnostic/essential findings; 2) frequent findings; and 3) occasional/associated features. The diagnostic findings include macrocephaly, prominent forehead, hypertelorism, epicanthal folds, downslanted palpebral fissures, small nose with wide nasal bridge, polydactyly and absent/hypoplastic corpus callosum. Frequent findings include ear anomalies, short upper lip, high arched palate, tapered fingers, hypotonia, and seizures. Polysyndactyly is the single most variable main sign, both in degree and in presence, even within the same family. A review of 18 published cases and the present family shows that the main manifestations are cranial facial anomalies and the abnormality of the corpus callosum. Most families have been reported from northeastern Switzerland and the Mediterranean basin. The present family supports a chromosomal recessive inheritance (Gelman-Kohan Z et al. Further delineation of the acrocallosal syndrome. Eur J Pediatr Sept 1991;150:797-799).

COMMENT. The acrocallosal syndrome (Schinzel syndrome) and other syndromes which include callosal agenesis are reviewed in Progress in Pediatric Neurology I, Ed. Millichap JG, Chicago, PNB Publishers 1991, 310-312. At least four distinct syndromes include callosal agenesis as a major component: *Aicardi* (with infantile spasms, hypsarrythmia, chorioretinal lacunae and coloboma), *Schinzel* syndrome (with macrocephaly and polysyndactyly), *Andermann* syndrome (with anterial horn cell disease); and *Shapiro* syndrome (with recurrent hypothermia).-Editor. *Ped Neur Briefs* Dec 1991.

CORPUS CALLOSUM AGENESIS AND OSSEOUS LESIONS

A new mental retardation syndrome with agenesis of the corpus callosum and unusual bone changes is reported from the Departments of Radiology and Neurology, Royal Alexandra Hospital for Children, Camperdown, Sydney, NSW, Australia. At 11 months of age, the boy was functioning at a 5 month level, and his head circumference was at the 98th centile. His face was triangular in shape, with a broad frontal region. There was mild hypotonia, and deep tendon reflexes were exaggerated. Skeletal abnormalities included multiple Wormian bones, thin ribs, small iliac bodies, and retarded bone age. (Kozlowski K, Ouvrier RA. Agenesis of the corpus callosum with mental retardation and osseous lesions. Am J Med Genet May 1993;48: 6-9). (Reprints: Dr K Kozlowski, RAHC, Camperdown 2050, NSW, Australia).

COMMENT. Macrocephaly and polydactyly, in Schinzel syndrome, and microcephaly and camptodactyly, in da-Silva syndrome, are additional examples of skeletal abnormalities associated with corpus callosum agenesis or hypoplasia. (see Progress in Pediatric Neurology I, Millichap JG, Ed, Chicago, PNB

Publishers, 1991, pp 310-312).-Editor. *Ped Neur Briefs* May 1993.

ANGELMAN SYNDROME: CHROMOSOME ANOMALY

Clinical, cytogenetic and molecular evidence in 1 patient with paternal uniparental disomy (UPD) for chromosome 15 is reported from the University of Florida College of Medicine, Gainesville, FL. The deletions of chromosome 15 qll-ql3 were demonstrated with DNA probes. Twenty-seven patients with a clinical diagnosis of Angelman syndrome were evaluated in the laboratory by molecular genetic techniques. Twenty had a molecular deletion of 15 qll-ql3, whereas 6 had biparental inheritance for chromosome 15 DNA markers. The 7th patient, who did not have a molecular deletion, had paternal UPD for chromosome 15. This is the first patient in whom UPD involved the critical chromosomal region. The overall frequency of paternal UPD was calculated at 3 7%. The low frequency of UPD in Angelman syndrome contrasts with the high frequency of 25% for maternal UPD in Prader-Willi syndrome (Nicholls RD et al. Paternal uniparental disomy of chromosome 15 in a child with Angelman syndrome. Ann Neurol Oct 1992;32:512-518). (Correspondence: Dr. Nicholls, Department of Neuroscience, Box 100244 JHMHC, University of Florida College of Medicine, Gainesville, FL 32610.)

COMMENT. Angelman syndrome is characterized by severe mental retardation, absence of speech, inappropriate laughter, puppet-like ataxic movements, microbrachycephaly, seizures, an abnormal electroencephalogram, mild hypotonia, hypopigmentation and prognathism with tongue protrusion. Most cases of Angelman syndrome are due to deletions of exclusively maternal origin from a critical region in chromosome 15 qll-ql3. For a review of the diagnostic features of 36 cases of Angelman syndrome see Robb SA et al. Arch Dis Child Jan 1989;64:83; and Progress in Pediatric Neurology I, Millichap JG (ed), Chicago, PNB Publ, 1991, pp 487-88.-Editor. *Ped Neur Briefs* Dec 1992.

ANGELMAN SYNDROME AND EPILEPSY

Characteristic epileptic seizures and EEG abnormalities are reported in three siblings with Angelman syndrome from the Kansai University Otokoyoma Hospital, Kyoto; and the Nagasaki University School of Medicine, Japan. Seizures were generalized, and interictal EEG findings included 2- to 3-Hz high-voltage slow waves bioccipitally and sporadic slow spike wave complexes bifrontally. EEG minor epileptic status occurred in a 38 month old sib and was responsive to clonazepam. The thresholds of wave V in auditory brainstem responses were increased, and the latency of wave I was prolonged in all 3 siblings. Chromosome studies were normal, but DNA deletion of the GABA receptor subunit gene was reported (Saitoh S) in the maternal grandfather, mother, and 3 siblings. (Sugimoto T et al. Angelman syndrome in three siblings: Characteristic epileptic seizures and EEG abnormalities. Epilepsia Nov/Dec 1992;33:1078-1082). (Reprints: Dr T Sugimoto, Department of Pediatrics, Kansai Medical University Otokoyama Hospital, Izumi 19, Otokoyama, Yawatashi, Kyoto, 614 Japan).

COMMENT. Seizures are generalized in 90% of patients with Angelman syndrome. Deafness has been reported previously, but the abnormal auditory brain stem responses recorded in this study appear to be unique.

Eight sporadic cases of Angelman syndrome associated with chromosome 15ql2 deletion are reported from the Central Hospital, and Kobato Gakuen, Aichi Prefectural Colony, Japan (Matsumoto A et al. Epilepsia 1992;33:1083). Angelman syndrome is included in the etiology of West, Lennox-Gastaut and other infantile-onset epileptic syndromes.-Editor. *Ped Neur Briefs* Jan 1993.

POSTERIOR FOSSA MRI IN RETARDED AUTISTIC CHILDREN

Morphological evidence of brain stem but not cerebellar involvement in 12 autistic retarded children is reported from the University of Tokushima School of

Medicine, Japan. Mid-sagittal MRIs showed that the brain stem was significantly smaller in the autistic group compared to 14 controls but not compared to 15 non-autistic retarded children, all groups of mean age 7 years (range, 5-10 years). The cerebellar vermis was not different among the three groups. The ratio of the midbrain to posterior fossa area was significantly smaller only in autistic patients. (Hashimoto T et al. Magnetic resonance imaging of the brain structures in the posterior fossa in retarded autistic children. Acta Paediatr Dec 1992;81:1030-4). (Respond: T Hashimoto MD, Department of Pediatrics, University of Tokushima School of Medicine, 18-15 Kuramoto-cho 3, Tokushima 770, Japan).

COMMENT. The authors suggest that in autism a specific brain stem lesion may be masked by a lesion associated with mental retardation. Further examination of autistic children with normal IQs is planned.-Editor. *Ped Neur Briefs* March 1993.

KALLMANN SYNDROME

The clinical, biological, and molecular genetic aspects of Kallmann syndrome are reported from the Institute of Molecular Genetics, Baylor College of Medicine, Houston, TX. Kallmann syndrome, first described in 1944, is characterized by familial *hypogonadism* and *anosmia* associated with aplasia of olfactory bulbs and tracts. Additional neurologic signs include synkinesia, eye movement abnormalities, horizontal nystagmus, cerebellar ataxia, sensorineural deafness, spastic paraplegia, spatial attention deficits, and mental retardation. Somatic defects including pes cavus, unilateral renal agenesis, and cleft lip and palate are also described. A predominantly X-linked inheritance is reflected in a five-fold excess of male (1 in 10 000) over female (1 in 50 000) patients, and the occurrence of both autosomal dominant and recessive forms indicates genetic heterogeneity. Diagnosis is made at puberty because of a delay in secondary sex characteristics, a eunuchoid habitus, gynecomastia, micropenis, and cryptorchidism. Isolation of the KAL gene responsible for the X-linked form of the disease points to a molecular basis for a neuronal migration defect affecting olfactory axons as the primary cause of Kallmann syndrome . (Rugarli EI, Ballabio A. Kallmann syndrome. From genetics to neurobiology. JAMA Dec 8 1993;270:2713-2716). (Reprints: Dr Rugari, Inst for Molecular Genetics, Baylor College of Med, One Baylor Plaza, Houston, TX 77030).

COMMENT. An adolescent male of eunuchoid build, referred to the neurologist because of attention, coordination and other deficits, should be considered for olfactory tests and an MRI of the olfactory system. For a review of the genetics of Kallmann syndrome, see Martin JB. Ann Neurol Dec 1993.-Editor. *Ped Neur Briefs* Dec 1993.

CHOROIDO-CEREBRAL CALCIFICATION WITH RETARDATION

A family of three children with mental retardation, calcification of the choroid plexus, and increased CSF protein is reported from the Riyadh Armed Forces Hospital, and Maternity and Children's Hospital, Riyadh, Saudi Arabia. A 7-year-old Saudi girl born to nonconsanguinous parents showed delayed development. She sat at 3 years, walked at 5, and spoke two- to three-word phrases at 7 years of age. An 8-year-old brother and 5-year-old-sister were similarly affected. Skull radiographs, CT, and MRI showed calcifications along the distribution of choroid plexuses of the lateral ventricles, and calcification involving the caudate nucleus and septum pellucidum. In one child, these findings at 1 year were unchanged over the next 7 years. CSF protein was 180 mg/dl, while phosphate levels in the CSF were low, with a CSF/serum ratio of 0.25 cf normal of 0.73. (Singh B et al. Choroido-cerebral calcification syndrome with retardation. Neurology Nov 1993;43:2387-2389). (Reprints: Dr B Singh, Div Ped Neurology, Southwestern Medical School, 5323 Harry Hines Blvd, Dallas, TX 75235).

COMMENT. Two previous reports of a family of 6 children with a similar syndrome are cited. An autopsy on one patient had shown multiple small subcortical heterotopias and adrenal atrophy (Lott IT et al. Familial amentia, unusual ventricular calcifications, and increased cerebrospinal fluid protein. Neurology 1979;29:1571). That phosphate metabolism may be involved in the pathogenesis is suggested by Singh and co-authors.-Editor. *Ped Neur Briefs* Dec 1993.

CHAPTER 8

PRENATAL AND PERINATAL DISORDERS

INTRODUCTION

Michael J. Rivkin, M.D.
Department of Neurology, Children's Hospital
Harvard Medical School, Boston, MA

One third the way through the Decade of the Brain, notable progress has been made in the area of prenatal and perinatal diseases. Important contributions have been made to areas as diverse as hypoxic-ischemic brain injury in the newborn, cerebrovascular disease, neonatal intra-ventricular hemorrhage, neurogenetic disease of the newborn, perinatal infectious disease, and developmental anomalies of the nervous system.

Fresh insight has been provided into mechanisms underlying hypoxic-ischemic brain injury that may prove relevant to the newborn. Nitric oxide congeners can be lethal to neurons. Moreover, the neurotoxic nitric oxide species is likely to be endogenously derived within the neuron by nitric oxide synthase following excitatory amino acid activation of NMDA receptors at the plasma membrane. Curiously, nitric oxide may also exert a neuroprotective effect through nitrosylation of the NMDA receptor at the neuron's outer surface. Such a transfer of nitric oxide may lead to disulfide bond formation, thus, down-regulating NMDA-mediated inward calcium currents and providing some measure of neuroprotection. As a result, further investigation into the mechanism of nitrous oxide mediated neuronal toxicity and protection may contribute to an improved understanding of the mechanism of neonatal hypoxic-ischemic brain injury and its treatment.

Recent developments in neuroimaging are yielding important information regarding cerebral hypoxic-ischemic injury of the newborn. The value of cranial ultrasonography to predict the neurodevelopmental outcome of premature infants suffering from periventricular leukomalacia has been established. Transient periventricular echodensities and frank periventricular leukomalacia correlated with a significantly higher incidence of motor handicaps than was found in control infants. Persistent periventricular echodensities also were found to correlate with motor deficits at the age of six years.

Spectroscopy is a new mode of functional imaging that is complementary to more traditional neuroimaging. Near infrared spectroscopy (NIRS) has demonstrated striking decreases in intra-cerebral bloodflow, oxyhemoglobin, and cytochrome oxidase activity in severely asphyxiated neonates, correlating with neurologic handicap at one year of age. Proton and phosphorus magnetic resonance spectroscopy (MRS) have provided functional information about the newborn brain after an hypoxic-ischemic insult, and cerebral MRS is used to evaluate neonates suffering from metabolic disorders such as peroxisomal and mitochondrial disease.

Conventional MR imaging is of value in the diagnosis of developmental anomalies and the determination of stages and patterns of neuroblast migrational arrest that results in various neurodysgenetic disorders. MRI has been of value in elucidating cerebral venous thrombosis in neonates with unexplained seizures and lethargy.

The occurrence and prognosis of intraventricular hemorrhage in the premature infant has been benefited by research concerning the effects of antenatal corticosteroids given to reduce the risk of postnatal respiratory distress syndrome. Corticosteroids administered to mothers about to deliver preterm infants appeared to exert an independent prophylactic effect on the occurrence of postnatal germinal matrix hemorrhage. Prognostically, posthemorrhagic ventricular dilatation sustained early in life is associated with an adverse neurodevelopmental outcome. This observation underscores the importance of improved methods for the evaluation and therapeutic reduction of dilated ventricles in this clinical setting.

Neurogenetic research has elucidated fundamental molecular features of important neonatal disorders, including congenital myotonic dystrophy and infantile spinal muscular atrophy. Several kindreds harboring both adult onset motor neuron disease and SMA 1 have been reported, which suggests a genetic homogeneity between acute and chronic forms of spinal muscular atrophy, both sharing the same domain of the 5q chromosome.

Finally, large strides have been made in the realm of neonatal neurologic infectious disease. Polymerase chain reaction has been established as a valuable but not infallible assay for the early detection of neonatal herpes simplex virus encephalitis, facilitating a speedy diagnosis. Substantial data have been gathered to support prenatal treatment in maternally diagnosed toxoplasmosis. These studies suggest that transmission to the fetus could be minimized with a regimen of pyrimethamine and sulfonamide therapy administered to the mother. - *Michael J. Rivkin, M.D., Children's Hospital, Boston, MA.*

BIBLIOGRAPHY

Dawson, TM, Dawson VL, Snyder SH. A novel neuronal

messenger molecule in brain: the free radical, nitric oxide. Ann Neurol 1992;32:297-311.

Jongmans M et al. Duration of periventricular densities in preterm infants and neurological outcome at 6 years of age. Arch Dis Child 1993;69:9-13.

Moorcraft J et al. Spatially localized magnetic resonance spectroscopy of the brains of normal and asphyxiated newborns. Pediatrics 1991;87:273-282.

Cross JH et al. Proton magnetic resonance spectroscopy studies in lactic acidosis and mitochondrial disorders. J Inher Metab Dis 1993;16:800-811.

Palmini A et al. Stages and patterns of centrifugal arrest of diffuse neuronal migration disorders. Dev Med Child Neurol 1993;35:331-339.

Rivkin MJ et al. Neonatal idiopathic cerebral venous thrombosis: an unrecognized cause of transient seizures or lethargy. Ann Neurol 1992;32:51-56.

Leviton A et al. Antenatal corticosteroids appear to reduce the risk of postnatal germinal matrix hemorrhage in intubated low birth weight newborns. Pediatrics 1993;91:1083-1088.

Gilliam TC et al. Genetic homogeneity between acute and chronic forms of spinal muscular atrophy. Nature 1990;345:823-825.

Uren E et al. Herpes simplex virus encephalitis in pediatrics: diagnosis by detection of antibodies and DNA in cerebrospinal fluid. Pediatr Infect Dis J 1993;12:1001-6.

Ghidini A et al. Results of a preventive program for congenital toxoplasmosis. J Repro Med 1991;36:270-273.

HEAD SIZE AND COGNITION IN VERY LOW BIRTH WEIGHT (VLBW) INFANTS

The effect of VLBW (< 1.5 kg) and subnormal head size at 8 months of age (corrected for prematurity) on neurocognitive abilities at school age was investigated by a longitudinal follow up of 249 children born between 1977 to 1979 and admitted to the neonatal intensive care unit at Rainbow Babies and Children's Hospital, Cleveland, OH. Head size was subnormal at birth in 12%, at term 23%, and at 8 months in 13%. As compared with 216 children with normal head sizes, the 33 children with subnormal head sizes at the age of 8 months had significantly lower mean birth weights and higher neonatal risk scores and at 8 years of age had a higher incidence of neurologic impairment and lower IQ scores. A subnormal head size at 8 months of age was predictive of poor verbal and performance IQ scores at 8 years of age; lower scores for receptive language, speech, reading, mathematics and spelling; and a higher incidence of hyperactivity. (Hack M et al. Effect of very low birth weight and subnormal head size on cognitive abilities at school age. N Engl J Med July 25, 1991;325:231-237)

COMMENT. A relation between subnormal head circumference and cognitive functioning has been reported in many different studies, including children with learning disabilities. Improvements in neonatal growth and development may depend on nutrition of chronically ill neonates and environmental enrichment after discharge from hospital. This study shows that the determination of the head circumference at 8 months of age is a useful means of predicting subsequent cognitive deficits and difficulties in school. Volpe JJ, in an editorial (N Engl J Med 1991;325:276-277), stresses the need for a better method of detection of brain injury in VLBW infants since 77 % of those with normal head circumference at 8 months had IQs below 85 and an academic skill index below 80 in the study by Hack et al. Those infants with a small head circumference at 8 months of age made up only a minority of infants who subsequently had cognitive deficits. Cranial ultrasonography detects overt brain lesions but not the subtle lesions in the periventricular white matter. MRI may detect periventricular injury missed by ultrasound and CT scanning; it is also used to measure the progress and degree of myelination in the human infant in the first months of life. A decreased rate of brain growth in the first months of life might identify a larger proportion of at risk infants and justify further study with the MRI in selected patients.

Collin MF and associates from the Department of Pediatrics, Loyola University Medical Center, Maywood,

IL report that normal infant development is poorly predictive of continued normal development in the extremely low birth weight infant (Pediatrics July 1991;88:115-120). Only 11 (31%) of 36 children had normal development upon ressessment in early childhood. With or without major complications, extremely low birth weight places children at risk for emerging development problems with age. Head circumference was not addressed in this study.-Editor. *Ped Neur Briefs* Aug 1991.

BIRTH ASPHYXIA, CEREBRAL METABOLISM AND HEAD SIZE

Studies of cerebral oxidative metabolism were carried out by phosphorus magnetic resonance spectroscopy during the first week of life in 52 infants with birth asphyxia admitted to the Neonatal Unit at University College Hospital, London. Cerebral phosphocreatine/inorganic phosphate concentration ratio was used as an index of oxidative metabolism and correlated with neurodevelopmental outcome and head growth at 1 year. (Roth SC et al. Relation between cerebral oxidative metabolism following birth asphyxia, and neurodevelopmental outcome and brain growth at one year. Dev Med Child Neurol April 1992;34:285-295.) (Correspondence: Dr. Simon C. Roth, Department of Paediatrics, University College and Middlesex School of Medicine, The Rayne Institute, 5 University Street, London WCIE 6JJ, England.)

COMMENT. The use of these neuroimaging and biochemical techniques should help in the prediction of outcome following neonatal encephalopathy. However, the complexity of the techniques may detract from their value in practice. (Bax M. Editorial. Birth asphyxia. Dev Med Child Neurol 1992;34:283-284.)

Central diabetes insipidus as an unusual complication of hypoxic brain damage is described in 2 children at the Department of Pediatrics, Juntendo University School of Medicine, Tokyo, Japan (Arisaka O et al. Child's Nerv Syst March 1992;8:81-82). Both patients developed cardiopulmonary arrest after choking and both had hypernatremia and low urinary antidiuretic hormone concentrations in the terminal stages. The most common causes of central diabetes insipidus are tumors or trauma in the neurohypophyseal area.-Editor. *Ped Neur Briefs* June 1992.

PREDICTORS OF COGNITIVE AND MOTOR DEVELOPMENT

The relative effects of 4 major areas of adversity on early cognitive and motor development were examined in approximately 1,000 children at age 5 years in the Department of Paediatrics and Child Health, University of Otago Medical School, Dunedin, New Zealand. The 4 areas of adversity examined were perinatal complications, family background, child rearing practices, and physical health. The effects on cognitive ability were measured by IQ, receptive language and expressive language. Girls' cognitive ability and motor ability in early childhood were not related to the number of perinatal complications present during pregnancy or birth but were affected by adverse family background conditions and child rearing practices. Girls' language ability was unrelated to the number of health problems at age 3. In boys, IQ scores, receptive language and motor ability were related to the index of perinatal complications; and family background and child rearing affected IQ, receptive language and motor ability scores. Health index affected motor ability in both boys and girls. (Stanton WR et al. Indices of perinatal complications, family background, child rearing and health as predictors of early cognitive and motor development. Pediatrics Nov 1991;88:954-959.) (Reprints: Dr. Stanton, Dept. Paediatrics, University of Otago Medical School, Box 913, Dunedin, New Zealand.)

COMMENT. In summary, the perinatal complications index was not generally predictive of cognitive ability and motor ability outcomes and the health index was predictive mainly of motor ability. Family background and child rearing were predictive of IQ and receptive language scores. Boys are more susceptible to biological and psychological stress than girls. The results support a concept of a continuum of adversity in the areas of perinatal complications, family background, child rearing, and health during early development of learning and motor ability.-Editor. *Ped Neur Briefs* Jan 1992.

ANTEPARTUM CAUSES OF CEREBRAL PALSY

Six neonates with destructive brain lesions of fetal onset, diagnosed by radiological and neurophysiological studies, are reported from the Departments of Pediatrics, Neurology, Radiology, and Obstetrics and Gynecology, Magee-Womens Hospital, Pittsburgh, PA and Children's Hospital of Pittsburgh. Initial diagnosis of cerebral lesions was made by fetal sonography in 2 patients and CT scan in 4 during the first 30 hours of life. No intrapartum difficulties were noted and 2 patients had definitive evidence of maternal and placental disease that preceded the onset of active labor. The neurological examinations were normal at birth, but 4 presented with isolated seizures at 8-30 hours of life and initial neonatal EEGs showed abnormalities. The authors recommend that cranial imaging and neurophysiological studies should be used during the first days of life for neonates believed to have cerebral lesions based on maternal sonography or isolated seizures. (Scher MS et al. Destructive brain lesions of presumed fetal onset: antepartum causes of cerebral palsy. Pediatrics Nov 1991;88:898-906.) (Reprints: Dr Scher, Develop Neurophysiol, Magee-Womens Hospital, Forbes St, Pittsburgh, PA 15213.)

COMMENT. Cranial ultrasonography and CT studies during the first few days of life may document lesions occurring prenatally. Children with antepartal brain injury may be asymptomatic or exhibit few clinical signs during the neonatal period and may later develop cerebral palsy.-Editor. *Ped Neur Briefs* Jan 1992.

DYSTONIA DUE TO PERINATAL ASPHYXIA

Delayed onset dystonia associated with perinatal asphyxia in two patients and asphyxia in early childhood in two patients is reported from the Neurological Institute of New York. In the perinatal group the mean age of onset was 12.9 years; dystonia progressed for a mean of 7 years and as long as 28 years. The patients had moderate motor disability and none was wheelchair bound. The prognosis was better than that of childhood onset idiopathic torsion dystonias. In the absence of any identifiable cause of dystonia the authors considered the asphyxia as related either directly or indirectly to the development of dystonia. (Saint Hilaire MH et al. Delayed onset dystonia due to perinatal or early childhood asphyxia. Neurology Feb 1991;41:260-222).

COMMENT. Despite the known difficulties in relating adverse perinatal events to static encephalopathies of childhood, the authors claim a relationship between perinatal asphyxia and late onset dystonia based on exclusion of other causes of dystonia and documentation by birth records or a verbal history that asphyxia occurred.-Editor. *Ped Neur Briefs* March 1991.

CLASSIFICATION OF NEWBORN ENCEPHALOPATHY

Investigators from the Department of Neurology, Children's Hospital and Harvard Medical School, Boston and the Neuroepidemiology Branch, Bethesda take issue with the terms hypoxic-ischemic and post-asphyxial encephalopathy when the etiology is frequently in doubt. These authors prefer the simple descriptive terms, neonatal or newborn encephalopathy for infants with a clinically defined syndrome of impaired neurologic function, which includes lethargy, coma, hypotonia, impaired primitive reflexes, depressed or absent respirations and seizures. Difficulties in initiating respiration and maintaining tone and consciousness may be caused by factors that predate birth or onset of labor. Neonatal encephalopathy grading schemes previously described in the literature (Sarnat and Sarnat, Low et al, Levene et al, Amiel-Tilson and Ellison, Fenichel) are considered qualitative rather than quantitative and their potentially correctable limitations are discussed. (Leviton A, Nelson KB.

Problems with definitions and classifications of newborn encephalopathy. Pediatr Neurol March/April 1992;8:85-90.) (Correspondence: Dr. Leviton, Children's Hospital, 300 Longwood Avenue, Boston MA 02115.)

COMMENT. In a previous issue of Pediatric Neurology (1991;7:317-325), Dr. Alan Hill of the University of British Columbia Children's Hospital, Vancouver, reviewed the diagnosis, classification, pathology and management of hypoxic-ischemic cerebral injury in the term newborn. Grade III severe HIE, manifested by coma, hypotonia, seizures, abnormal brain stem and autonomic function, and increased intracranial pressure, is associated invariably with death or severe neurologic sequelae. Grade II moderate HIE, with lethargy/stupor, hypotonia, suppressed reflexes and seizures, has a poor outcome in 20-40% of infants. Grade I mild HIE, characterized by hyper-alertness, jitteriness, exaggerated Moro and stretch reflexes, is transient with duration less than 24 hours and recovery is complete. The author emphasizes that the clinical features of hypoxic-ischemic encephalopathy are not specific and that similar symptoms may be caused by metabolic disorders, infection or cerebral dysgenesis.-Editor. *Ped Neur Briefs* June 1992.

THALAMIC LESIONS IN INFANCY

The clinical, pathologic and etiologic characteristics of thalamic lesions in infancy are reviewed in an editorial. During the past 30 years, two distinct patterns of thalamic hemorrhagic insult in infants have been described, with different etiology, clinical presentation, scan appearance and prognosis. Intrauterine infection with cytomegalovirus, rubella, or toxoplasma and streptococcal and pneumococcal meningitis have also been associated with bilateral thalamic calcification and spastic quadriplegia. Genetic factors have been described occasionally, including a rare autosomal recessive encephalopathy; and chromosomal trisomies 21 and 13 have also been linked with thalamic echogenicity. An asphyxial insult may occur before birth, perinatally or postnatally. Most affected infants were born at term, the thalamic changes were always bilateral, and the MRI was the most sensitive technique in diagnosis.

In one pattern of thalamic hemorrhagic or asphyxial insult, the neurologic abnormalities presented at birth. Many infants died in the neonatal period or early childhood and all survivors were severely handicapped. In another pattern of thalamic lesion, previously healthy term infants with primary thalamic hemorrhage presented acutely at age 11-14 days with seizures, opisthotonos and facial weakness. There was eye deviation to the side of the hemorrhage and a sunsetting phenomenon. In these infants the neurologic outcome was good: 1 child was normal at 20 months and 3 had only mild spastic hemiparesis. In almost 2/3 of term infants with intraventricular hemorrhage the primary lesion is in the thalamus. (Editorial. Thalamic lesions in infancy. The Lancet May 9, 1992;339:1143-1145.)

COMMENT. Thalamic lesions may occur independently of cortical lesions but are always found when cortical or subcortical damage is present. Etat marbre (status marmoratus), characteristically associated with athetoid forms of cerebral palsy, is seen as a hypermyelination in association with striatal marbling or as an isolated phenomenon. Thalamic involvement underlies the severe mental deficiency found in some cases of congenital athetosis. (Norman RM. In Greenfield's Neuropathology, Baltimore, Williams and Wilkins, 1963, 391-393).-Editor. *Ped Neur Briefs* Aug 1992.

INTRAVENTRICULAR HEMORRHAGE: PROGNOSIS

The relationship of periventricular-intraventricular hemorrhage in infants of <32 weeks gestation to the occurrence of disability at 5 years of age was studied in a National Collaborative Survey in the Netherlands. Of 484 infants enrolled, all 304 survivors were examined at age 5 years; 26% of infants with severe hemorrhage and 67% with mild grades I/II survived the neonatal period. Of 85 (28%) survivors with a disability, 27 (9%) had a minor handicap and 23 (8%) a major handicap. The handicap was recorded at the age of 5 but was not present at 2 years in 17 children, while 35 were handicapped at 2 years but not at 5 years. Children with grades I and II as well as III and IV had more disabilities and handicaps than children without hemorrhage. (van de Bor M et al. Outcome of periventricular-intraventricular haemorrhage at five years of age. Dev Med Child Neurol Jan 1993;35:33-41). (Respond: Dr van de Bor, Division of Neonatology, Department of Paediatrics, University Hospital Leiden, PO Box 9600, 2300 RC Leiden, The Netherlands).

COMMENT. The small number of survivors with grades III and IV hemorrhage was attributed to the widely used policy in the Netherlands of withdrawing life-support from infants with severe cerebral damage. Of 65 in this category, 47 died in the neonatal period. At the 5 year evaluation, only 25% of the patients had had severe hemorrhage. Children with only mild hemorrhage had a significantly increased risk of disability at the age of 5 years. Patients with evidence of periventricular leukomalacia were excluded from this study.-Editor. *Ped Neur Briefs* March 1993.

SPASTIC DIPLEGIA AND THE MRI

The MRI findings in 34 children with spastic diplegia examined between 2 and 10 years of age are reported from the Seirei-Hamamatsu General Hospital, Mikatabara, Hamamatsu, Shizuoka; Nagoya City Medical School; and the National Rehabilitation Center for Disabled Children, Tokyo, Japan. There was dilation of the trigone, atrophv of the peritrigonal white matter, and prominent deep cortical sulci. The appearance of cerebral white matter was classified into four patterns: 1) normal; 2) peritrigonal white matter showing a thin contiguous line in one hemisphere; 3) peritrigonal white matter reduced in both hemispheres; and 4) the reduction of the white matter expanded anteriorly from the trigones to the bodies of the lateral ventricles. The degree of cerebral white matter loss correlated with severity of motor disability but not with severity of mental impairment. The distribution of periventricular high intensity T2-weighted images did not correlate with motor or mental disability. (Yokochi K et al. Magnetic resonance imaging in children with spastic diplegia: Correlation with the severity of their motor and mental abnormality. Dev Med Child Neurol Jan 1991;33:18-25).

COMMENT. The MRI findings were similar to those reported with periventricular leukomalacia. In infancy leukomalacia is characterized by delayed myelination and demonstrated as high intensity areas on T2 weighted images. It occurs most commonly in preterm infants and all but three of the children in this study had birth weights lower than 2000 grams. Mild degrees of periventricular white matter reduction are often interpreted as a normal variant in children, but correlations with delay in motor development should be considered.-Editor. *Ped Neur Briefs* Feb 1991.

MRI IN ATHETOTIC CEREBRAL PALSY

The MRI in 22 children with athetotic cerebral palsy was studied in the Department of Pediatric Neurology, Seirei-Mikatabara General Hospital, Hamamatsu, the Department of Pediatrics, National Rehabilitation Center for Disabled Children, Tokyo, and the Department of Pediatrics, Nagoya City University Medical School, Japan. Perinatal asphyxia had been diagnosed in 16, neonatal jaundice in 2, and no predisposing condition in 4. MRI lesions possibly caused by asphyxia were found in the basal ganglia, thalamus, and/or cerebral white matter in 14 of 16 children. No abnormalities were seen in the cerebral cortex of the subjects. Six children with lesions in both the thalamus and putamen had moderate or severe motor abnormality. Children with lesions in the cerebral white matter only had mild motor abnormality. (Yokochi K et al. Magnetic resonance imaging in athetotic cerebral palsied children. Acta Paediatr Scand Sept 1991;80:818-823.) (Corresp: Dr. Yokochi, Seirei-Mikatabara Gen. Hosp., Mikatabara 3453, Hamamatsu, Shizuoka 433, Japan.)

COMMENT. Brain lesions causing athetosis in CP

children may not be revealed by CT scan but high intensity areas in the thalamus, putamen and/or cerebral white matter may be demonstrated in T2 weighted images of the MRI. The evidence of perinatal asphyxia in 16 of the 22 children reported was judged by Apgar scores of 3 and below, generalized hypotonia, and convulsions in the neonatal period. The MR imaging was performed at 2-12 years of age and studies obtained soon after birth might have documented a prenatal timing for the lesions.-Editor. *Ped Neur Briefs* Jan 1992.

NEONATAL CSF CREATINE KINASE AND CP RISK

Creatine kinase brain isoenzyme (CK-BB) was examined in the cerebrospinal fluid of 150 neonates at the Departments of Pediatrics and Neonatal Medicine and Clinical Chemistry, University Hospital, Ghent, Belgium. Indications for lumbar puncture were intraventricular hemorrhage, subarachnoid hemorrhage, postasphyxial encephalopathy, convulsions, birth trauma, periventricular echodensities, or question of sepsis. Newborns with a neurologic disorder showed significantly higher concentrations of immunoreactive CK-BB than did normal newborns or those with subarachnoid hemorrhage. (The median CK-BB for 5 neonates with intraventricular hemorrhage and echodensities was 106 mcg/l and the normal control was 2.14.) An independent effect of seizures on the CK-BB concentration was not documented. High concentrations of CSF CK-BB in the neonatal period were correlated with an adverse outcome - that is death or abnormal neurologic exam at discharge. (De Praeter C et al. Creatine kinase isoenzyme BB concentrations in the cerebrospinal fluid of newborns: relationship to short-term outcome. Pediatrics Dec 1991;8:1204-1210.) (Reprints Dr De Praeter, Dept of Pediatrics, University Hospital, Ghent, De Pintelaan, 185, B-9000, Ghent, Belgium)

COMMENT. Determination of the CK-BB concentration in CSF appears to be a clinically useful test for the prediction of neurologic disorders in high risk neonates. Infants with high CSF CK-BB concentrations should receive careful follow-up. In a previous study (Fernandez F et al. Acta Paediatr Scand 1987;76:914) an elevated serum CPK measured within 4 hours after birth was a sensitive indicator of brain damage in asphyxiated term infants but was of limited prognostic value in assessment of neurological outcome. (See Progress in Pediatric Neurology, Millichap JG ed, 1991, Chicago, PNB Publ, p 333)

Cerebrospinal fluid examination in symptom-free infants with risk factors for infection was evaluated in 284 newborns at the Department of Pediatrics, Rush Presbyterian-St. Luke's Medical Center, Chicago, IL (Fielkow S et al. J Pediatr Dec 1991;119:971-973). Positive cultures without pleocytosis in 5 infants (1.8%) were contaminants and none of the symptom-free infants had meningitis. The authors conclude that CSF examination is not indicated in the diagnostic evaluation of symptom-free infants born to mothers with chorioamnionitis or other risk factors for neonatal infection.-Editor. *Ped Neur Briefs* Jan 1992.

LOCAL ANESTHESIA IN NEONATAL LUMBAR PUNCTURE

The success rate of lumbar punctures was compared in neonates allocated prospectively to 0.2 to 0.5 mL of 1% lidocaine anesthesia (n=48) or a control group (n=52) in a study at the Albany Medical College of Union University, Albany, New York. A struggling motion score increased during the lidocaine injection but decreased at the spinal needle insertion. Despite the decreased motion following lidocaine, the number of attempts per lumbar puncture, failure rate, and traumatic punctures were not different from the controls. The success rate was not dependent on the level of physician training. (Pinheiro JMB et al. Role of local anesthesia during lumbar puncture in neonates. Pediatrics Feb 1993;91:379-382). (Reprints: Dr Pinheiro, Dept of Pediatrics, Albany Medical Center A-101, Albany, NY 12208).

COMMENT. The authors advocate lidocaine anesthesia in neonatal LPs.

NEURODEVELOPMENT AND SERUM BILIRUBIN IN PRETERM INFANTS

The interrelationships of maximal total serum bilirubin concentrations, neonatal cranial ultrasonographic abnormalities, and the occurrence of cerebral palsy and developmental delay were studied in 249 preterm infants of less than 34 weeks gestation at the Departments of Pediatrics, Neurology, and Radiology, Thomas Jefferson University Hospital, Philadelphia, PA. Of 45 children with spastic cerebral palsy, all but 7 had grade III/IV intracranial hemorrhage or moderate to severe periventricular echodensity or both, and ultrasonographic abnormalities. There was no evidence that bilirubinemia (2.3 to 22.5 mg/100 mL total serum bilirubin) was causally related to cerebral palsy, early developmental delay, or periventricular cysts. Large ventricular cysts, moderate to severe periventricular echodensity, and the need for assisted ventilation were associated with the occurrence of cerebral palsy at a statistically significant level (Graziani LJ et al. Neurodevelopment of preterm infants: neonatal neurosonographic and serum bilirubin studies. Pediatrics Feb 1992;89:229-234). (Reprints: Dr. Graziani, Department of Pediatrics, Jefferson Medical College, Thomas Jefferson University, Philadelphia, PA 19107.)

COMMENT. The putative neurotoxic effects of serum bilirubin in the development of spastic cerebral palsy were not supported by this study of preterm infants with neurosonographic abnormalities. The authors note that the significant association between the need for mechanical ventilation and increased risk for CP in preterm infants requires further study .

The effects of neonatal bilirubin exposure on psychoeducational outcome have been studied in a group of grade school children, 9-11 years old, who required neonatal intensive care at the Department of Pediatrics, University of California, Davis, Sacramento, CA. (Hansen RL. J Dev Behav Pediatr Oct 1991;12:287-293) A measure of bilirubin binding, calculated directly from the albumin concentration, correlated significantly with the Kaufman Mental Processing Composite Measure of Psychoeducational Outcome but other more direct measures of bilirubin exposure (maximum total serum bilirubin) did not. It is suggested that the calculated albumin-determined binding value may be more appropriate than the total serum bilirubin in assessing clinical management.-Editor. *Ped Neur Briefs* March 1992.

CEREBRAL ULTRASOUND AND NEURODEVELOPMENT

The relations between lesions detected by ultrasound brain-imaging and neurodevelopmental outcome at 8 years in a cohort of 206 very preterm infants were studied at the Department of Paediatrics, University College and Middlesex School of Medicine, London. Scans were normal at discharge from hospital in 112(54%), and of these, 4% developed major, disabling impairment and 22% had minor impairments. Uncomplicated periventricular hemorrhage (PVH) was diagnosed in 55(27%), ventricular dilatation in 21(10%), hydrocephalus developed in 5, and cerebral atrophy was found in 13(6%). Disabling neurodevelopmental impairments, including epilepsy, mental retardation and cerebral palsy, were documented in 25(12%) children at follow-up. Ventricular dilatation and cerebral atrophy were significant independent predictors of impairment of neurodevelopment, of school performance or achievement, and of the WISC-R Full-scale and Performance subscale IQs. (Roth SC, Reynolds EOR et al. Relation between ultrasound appearance of the brain of very preterm infants and neurodevelopmental impairment at eight years. Dev Med Child Neurol Sept 1993;35:755-768). (Respond: Dr Simon C Roth, Dept Paediatrics, University College and Middlesex School of Medicine, The Rayne Institute, 5 University St, London WClE 6JJ, England).

COMMENT. A normal ultrasound scan or a finding of uncomplicated periventricular hemorrhage in very preterm infants permits reassurance and the likelihood of a favorable developmental outcome. In contrast, infants with ventricular dilatation, hydrocephalus and cerebral atrophy have a poor prognosis. Learning difficulties experienced by some preterm infants may be caused by undetected hypoxic-ischemic injury.

Routine ultrasound screening in a multicenter study involving 15,151 pregnant women did not improve perinatal outcome when compared to the *selective* use of ultrasonography only for medical indications on the basis of clinical judgment (Ewigman BG et al. Effect of prenatal ultrasound screening on perinatal outcome. N Engl J Med Sept 16 1993;329:821-7).-Editor. *Peed Neur Briefs* Oct 1993.

CEREBRAL BLOOD VOLUME AFTER BIRTH ASPHYXIA

Cerebral hemodynamics and oxygenation in 18 perinatally asphyxiated neonates were compared with 13 healthy controls using near-infrared spectroscopy (NIRS) at the Dept of Pediatrics, University Hospital of Leiden, The Netherlands. Cerebral blood volume (CBV) in the first 12 hours of life was decreased in all of 9 severely asphyxiated neonates who subsequently developed neurologic abnormalities. This decrease in CBV was associated with a drop in HbO_2 and cytochrome oxidase. All patients showed stable CBV and enzyme patterns at 12 to 24 hours,. The findings suggest that post-hypoxic-ischemic reperfusion injury of the brain occurs during early neonatal life after severe birth asphyxia. (van Bel F et al. Changes in cerebral hemodynamics and oxygenation in the first 24 hours after birth asphyxia. Pediatrics Sept 1993;92:365-372). (Reprints: Frank van Bel MD,PhD, University Hospital Leiden, Neonatal Unit, Bldg 35, PO Box 9600, 2300 RC Leiden, The Netherlands).

COMMENT. The decrease in cerebral CBV, oxyhemoglobin, and cytochrome oxidase during the first 12 hours of life are indicators of decreased cerebral perfusion and oxygenation. The authors propose a possible relation between a decreased CBV and adverse neurologic outcome, suggesting a relation between cerebral hypoperfusion and brain tissue damage in severely asphyxiated neonates. NIRS may be used to monitor changes in CBV of neonates.-Editor. *Ped Neur Briefs* Oct 1993.

CHAPTER 9

CNS NEOPLASMS

INTRODUCTION

Patricia K. Duffner, M.D., and Michael E, Cohen, M.D.
Department of Neurology, State University of New York at Buffalo, N.Y.

The approach to children with brain tumors is in a state of evolution. Whereas the decades of the 1960's and 70's emphasized improved survivals, pediatric neurooncology in the 1990's has attempted to strike a balance between improved survivals and a reduction in neurotoxicity. The recognition of treatment induced dementia, endocrinopathies, leukoencephalopathy and oncogenesis has lead to a change in the approach to children with low grade tumors and those who are at high risk for treatment induced neurotoxicity. Advances in neuroimaging have allowed the pediatric neurooncologist to safely follow children longitudinally prior to initiating treatment and has lead increasingly to the "watchful waiting" approach to children with low grade supratentorial tumors and those with optic pathway tumors. The recognition of risk factors for neurotoxicity in volume and dose of radiation, young age at time of treatment and concomitant chemotherapy, especially intrathecal methotrexate, has influenced the approach to patients with higher grade tumors. For example concerns over large volume radiation for children with ependymomas lead to a study by the POG to determine whether neuraxis radiation was necessary in the absence of documented metastatic disease. The investigators found that isolated neuraxis failure was exceedingly uncommon in children with ependymomas and therefore local, rather than routine craniospinal radiation, was appropriate. Unlike children with ependymomas, patients with medulloblastomas require neuraxis radiation. The cancer cooperative groups therefore have been attempting to determine the minimal effective dose of neuraxis radiation for patients with medulloblastomas. In the first study, a reduction in radiation to the neuraxis was given to a group of "good risk" children with medulloblastoma and compared to those treated with standard radiation. Unfortunately this approach failed and the study was closed prematurely. Nonetheless, a second study is currently underway in which reduced dose radiation is coupled with chemotherapy in a further attempt to reduce radiation induced neurotoxicity. Young age at time of radiation is perhaps the greatest risk factor for mental retardation, growth failure and leukoencephalopathy. As such, prolonged postoperative chemotherapy was given to a group of children < 3 years of age with malignant brain tumors in an effort to delay radiation and consequently reduce neurotoxicity. The success of that first POG study has lead to subsequent multiinstitutional studies in which increasingly intensive chemotherapy is used with the goal of eliminating radiation entirely. Finally, recognition of the toxicity of intrathecal methotrexate, particularly when given in the context of cranial irradiation, has virtually eliminated this agent from most multiinstitutional studies in the U.S.

Pediatric neurooncology in the 1990's has not solely concentrated on developing regimens to reduce neurotoxicity. Attempts to improve survival have focused on children with high grade, poor prognosis tumors. Most current treatment regimens for children with malignant tumors use intensive adjuvant chemotherapy in addition to radiation. Furthermore the doses of radiation have been increased (although with theoretically less neurotoxicity), by utilizing twice or even three times daily hyperfractionated radiation. In addition, new techniques in radiation therapy including 3D conformal radiation, interstitial radiotherapy, and radiosurgery offer the promise of more focused radiation with less adverse effects on normal tissue. The most aggressive change in the approach to children with brain tumors has come with the advent of autologous bone marrow transplants in highly selected children.

Although higher doses of radiation and new and more toxic chemotherapeutic agents are currently in treatment trials, success rate is still poor in high risk patients. New approaches are needed. Research currently underway incorporates phenotypic and genotypic studies of pediatric brain tumors; molecular techniques to define biologic behavior; and flow cytometry, monoclonal technology and immunocytochemistry to identify neoplastic potential. Knowledge of oncogenes, tumor suppressor genes, antisense technology and gene transfer techniques as well as a host of other biologic advances may become part of the therapeutic armamentarium in the not too distant future. Although advances in neuroimaging, neurosurgery, radiation and chemotherapy have improved both the survivals and quality of life in children with brain tumors, it will be the decade of the 90's and into the 21st century where the most dramatic changes in neurooncology will be made, ie. in the hands of the cellular and molecular biologists. - *Patricia K. Duffner, M. D., and Michael E. Cohen, M.D., State University of New York at Buffalo School of Med.*

PSEUDOTUMOR CEREBRI: EPIDEMIOLOGY

The population-based incidence rates and clinical features of idiopathic intracranial hypertension (IIH) are reported from the Mayo Clinic. Nine patients (8 women, 1 man) were identified among Rochester residents over a 15-year period (1976-1990). The mean age at diagnosis was 28 years (range, 15-40). The annual age-adjusted rates per 100,000 were 0.9 for the total and 1.6 for females. The ratio of female-male age-adjusted rates was 8.4:1.0. For women, the annual incidence rates per 100,000 were 3.3 for the total and 7.7 for those with obesity. Headache was present in all but one and papilledema in all patients when first examined. Mild visual impairment developed in 3 of 18 eyes during a median follow-up of 2.7 years. Visual fields and acuity were normal in 7 of 8 females. (Radhakrishnan K, et al. Idiopathic intracranial hypertension (pseudotumor cerebri). Descriptive epidemiology in Rochester, Minn, 1976 to 1990. Arch Neurol Jan 1993;50:78-80). (Reprints: Dr Kurland, Department of Health Sciences Research, Section of Clinical Epidemiology, Mayo Clinic, Rochester, MN 55905).

COMMENT. Diagnosis of IIH requires the following criteria: IH, normal neuro exam except papilledema and VI nerve paresis, no ventricular enlargement or tumor, normal CSF composition. Frequently reported severe deficits in visual acuity were absent in the present series. Early diagnosis and therapy were cited as the probable explanation for the sanguine prognosis. The absence of pediatric cases was surprising. A review of the literature on "benign intracranial hypertension" showed that 84 (37%) of 224 patients were children; 75 (90%) children were between 5 and 15 years (Millichap JG. Pediatrics 1959;23: 257).-Editor. *Ped Neur Briefs* Feb 1993.

MRI IN PSEUDOTUMOR CEREBRI

The MRI has been used to clarify the pathophysiology of pseudotumor cerebri in seven children, aged between six months and 13 years, reported from British Columbia's Children's Hospital, Vancouver. All had papilledema, three abducens palsies, and six had headache and/or visual impairments. Topical steroid therapy for eczema and mastoiditis were predisposing factors in two. CT head scans were normal. MRIs showed normal signal intensity in the white matter, suggesting that periventricular brain water content was not markedly increased. The authors hypothesize an equilibrium between raised CSF outflow resistance and increased cerebral blood volume and/or mild interstitial cerebral edema. (Connolly MB et al. Magnetic resonance imaging in pseudotumor cerebri. Dev Med Child Neurol Dec 1992;34:1091-1094). (Correspondence: Dr Kevin Farrell, Rm lD14, British Columbia's Children's Hospital, 4480 Oak St, Vancouver, B.C. V6H 3V4).

COMMENT. Increased cerebral blood volume, confirmed by PET, an abnormal CSF dynamics, demonstrated by decreased arachnoid absorption, and cerebral edema, defined by brain biopsy, are some of the hypotheses proposed in pseudotumor cases. Periventricular edema, the expected consequence of a resistance to CSF outflow, was not demonstrated in this MRI study. Predisposing factors in children have included otitis media, venous sinus thrombosis, mastoiditis, mild head trauma, viral infections, vitamin A intoxication, teracyclines, obesity, menstrual irregularities, nutritional disturbances, and steroid therapy or withdrawal.-Editor. *Ped Neur Briefs* Feb 1993.

KNEE-CHEST POSITION: A SIGN OF INCREASED INTRACRANIAL PRESSURE

A preference to lie in the knee-chest position was associated with increased intracranial pressure (ICP) in three children, ages 12 and 20 months and 4 years, reported from the Sackler School of Medicine, Tel Aviv University, Petach Tikvah, Israel. The forehead touched the floor on a level with the chest and knees, and the rest of the trunk was elevated so that the buttocks were uppermost. The 4-year old child had a mass in the pineal area, with obstructive hydrocephalus; the 20 month-old had pseudotumor cerebri that responded to acetazolamide and a return to a normal posture; the 12-month old had a cerebellar astrocytoma and obstructive hydrocephalus. The authors postulate that the knee-chest position favors a reduced pressure in the right heart atrium, thus augmenting the blood flow from the superior vena cava and dural sinuses. (Straussberg R et al. Knee-chest position as a sign of increased intracranial pressure in children. J Pediatr Jan 1993;122:99-100). (Reprints: Rachel Straussberg MD, Dept Pediatrics, Hasharon Hospital, Petach Tikvah, Israel).

COMMENT. In infants and young children with brain tumors and few signs or subjective complaints, the knee-chest posture might be helpful in the clinical suspicion and diagnosis of increased intracranial pressure. This posture is also assumed by children with cyanotic heart disease and is a characteristic sign of acrodynia.-Editor. *Ped Neur Briefs* Feb 1993.

HEADACHE AS FIRST SYMPTOM OF CEREBRAL TUMOR

Five children, ranging in age from 10 months to 4 years, all presenting initially with headache, with or without vomiting, and in whom the final diagnosis was intracranial tumor, are reported from Petah Tiqva, Israel. The initial neurologic examination, including the fundi, was normal in three patients with craniopharyngioma, pinealoma, and cerebellar astrocytoma. Two patients with medulloblastoma and fourth ventricle choroid plexus papilloma had abnormal neurologic findings at presentation. The authors stress the need for neuroimaging studies in children younger than 4 years of age who have headache, especially if accompanied by vomiting, even if the neurologic exam is normal. (Straussberg R, Amir J. Headaches in children younger than 7 years: are they really benign? Arch Neurol Feb 1993;50: 130 [Letter to the Editor]).

COMMENT. In response, Shinnar S and Chu ML emphasize that a presenting complaint of headache, even in young children, is generally associated with a benign clinical syndrome, and a neuroimaging study is not always necessary or advisable. The heavy sedation required for the MRI in this age group and risks of an adverse reaction to contrast medium with CT must be weighed against the benefits of the study. They agree with Honig PJ and Charney E (AJDC 1982;136:121) that headache as the sole manifestation of brain tumor is very uncommon in young children.

Headache in young children is not only a problem in evaluation but also in recognition as a significant isolated symptom. Clinical acumen and careful judgement are required in decisions, 1) to advise a neurologic consultation, and 2) to order sophisticated or invasive tests. The pediatric neurologist usually has the benefit of a pediatrician's knowledge of the child and family and his decision to seek a second opinion. Notwithstanding the relatively rare occurrence of cerebral tumor in children who present with headache, uncomplicated by some other manifestation, the pediatric neurologist's first duty is to exclude the more serious diagnoses. The value of the electroencephalogram as an important preliminary test in the diagnosis and localization of intracranial tumors of children should not be forgotten. (Millichap JG, Backus RE et al. Neurology May 1962;12:329).-Editor. *Ped Neur Briefs* March 1993.

ADVERSE EFFECTS OF RADIATION AND CHEMOTHERAPY

The long-term consequences of radiation and chemotherapy on intellectual and endocrine function in children with brain tumors is reviewed from the Departments of Neurology and Pediatrics, State University of New York, Buffalo, NY. The young age at time of radiation, high doses of radiation, site of the tumor, and use of methotrexate are risk factors for the development of both endocrinopathies and intellectual dysfunction. Delay in the use of radiation and the substitution of post-operative chemotherapy in patients younger than 3 years of age may delay development of intellectual dysfunction in surviving children. The omission of methotrexate from treatment programs may avoid the complications of leukoencephalopathy and dementia, although the influence of other chemotherapeutic agents on intellectual functioning is as yet unknown. All Pediatric Oncology Group protocols currently include base-line neuropsychologic evaluations as well as yearly follow-up exams throughout the course of study. Improved quality of life is a primary goal of treatment regimens. (Duffner PK, Cohen ME. Long-term consequences of CNS treatment for childhood cancer, part II: clinical consequences. Pediatr Neurol July/Aug 1991;7:237-242).

COMMENT. The increase in survival rate of children with brain tumors over the past 20 years has been accompanied by a decrease in intellectual functioning and other serious complications. The recognition of risk factors for long-term adverse consequences of radiation and chemotherapy should lead to modifications of treatment regimens and improvement in academic potential.

In a study at the Children's Hospital and Harvard Medical School, Boston, MA, comparing the effectiveness of thallium-201 SPECT imaging with MRI in tumor assessment, SPECT allowed a more precise assessment of the functional state of the tumor but was less reliable than the MRI in detecting possible radiation injury in some patients (O'Tuama LA et al. SPECT imaging of treated childhood brain tumors. Pediatr Neurol 1991;7:249-257).

Green DM et al, at the Roswell Park Cancer Institute, Buffalo, NY, report that the frequency of congenital anomalies was not increased in children of men or women who had received chemotherapy for cancer during childhood and adolescence, with the possible exception of those treated with dactinomycin, at increased risk for cardiac defects (N Engl J Med July 18, 1991;325:141-6).-Editor. *Ped Neur Briefs* Nov 1991.

COGNITIVE DEFICITS IN BRAIN TUMOR SURVIVORS

The results of studies of cognitive deficits in long-term survivors of childhood brain tumors are summarized from 31 published reports between 1968-1989 in a review paper from the Division of Child Neurology, The Children's Hospital, Philadelphia and the Department of Neurology, Children's National Medical Center, George Washington University, Washington, DC. The increasing use of neuropsychological testing and the development of prospective studies during the first half of the 1980s have shown that from 40% to 100% of long-term survivors have some form of cognitive deficit in various intelligence quotients, visual/perceptual skills, learning abilities, and adaptive behavior. More cognitive deficits are detected the larger the time lapse from treatment to the testing evaluation. Factors predictive of subsequent cognitive deficits included a younger age at diagnosis, radiotherapy, methotrexate chemotherapy, and tumor location. Cognitive deficits occurred more frequently when medulloblastomas adhered to the brain stem, when tumors extended to the hypothalamus, and with hemispheric tumors. Surgery and preoperative hydrocephalus did not appear to modify cognition. (Glauser TA, Packer RJ. Cognitive deficits in long-term survivors of childhood brain tumors. Child's Nerv Syst Feb 1991;7:2-12).

COMMENT. The quality of life for long-term survivors of childhood brain tumors becomes more important as improvements in treatment are developed. Long-term follow-up with neuropsychological tests is necessary since significant progressive deterioration in cognitive function may be demonstrated as the testing interval following treatment increases. (Duffner PK et al. Ann Neurol 1988;23:575).-Editor. *Ped Neur Briefs* May 1991.

STROKE AS LATE SEQUELA OF CRANIAL IRRADIATION

The development of cerebrovascular disease manifested by strokes or transient ischemic attacks six months to four years after treatment of brain tumors in 11 children is reported from the Children's Hospital of Los Angeles, University of Southern California School of Medicine, Los Angeles, CA. All patients had received radiation therapy and seven chemotherapy. One patient, aged 4, with an incompletely resected craniopharyngioma, developed a right hemiparesis two years after treatment followed by left-sided focal motor seizures with quick progression to decerebrate posturing, central hyperventilation, coma, and death. Autopsy revealed bilateral cerebral infarctions as well as diffuse gliosis. Branches of the carotid artery showed severe thickening with subintimal proliferation of connective tissue. Smaller vessels showed cellular intimal proliferation with areas of leukocytic infiltration. (Mitchell WG et al. Stroke as a late sequela of cranial irradiation for childhood brain tumors. J Child Neurol April 1991;6:128-133).

COMMENT. Damage to medium and large intracranial vessels in addition to small vessel damage may result in late onset of stroke or transient ischemic attacks caused by radiation and chemotherapy in children with brain tumors. The combination of methotrexate and cranial irradiation is more likely to produce a leukoencephalopathy than either treatment alone. The addition of chemotherapy may potentiate the damage to endothelial cells produced by radiation (*mineralizing microangiopathy*).-Editor. *Ped Neur Briefs* May 1991.

BRAIN RADIOTHERAPY AND COGNITION

Cognitive function and school achievement were studied prospectively over 3 to 4 years in 19 children treated for brain tumors with whole-brain radiotherapy at the Children's Hospital, Philadelphia, PA. Fourteen children also received adjuvant chemotherapy. A significant drop in IQ was seen among children with non-cortical tumors who received whole-brain radiotherapy with or without chemotherapy and who were treated before age 7. IQ did not decrease significantly in survivors treated after age 7. The IQ fell from a baseline of 104 to 92 at follow-up (Radcliffe J et al. Three- and four-year cognitive outcome in children with noncortical brain tumors treated with whole-brain radiotherapy. Ann Neurol Oct 1992;32:551-554). (Correspondence: Dr. Radcliffe, Division of Child Development and Rehabilitation, Children's Seashore House, 3405 Civic Center Boulevard, Philadelphia, PA 19104.)

COMMENT. All children younger than 7 years in this group were receiving special education at follow-up and 50% of the children over 7 years at diagnosis were receiving supplemental educational services. Increased fatiguability could be another reason for the poor school performance in these children.-Editor. *Ped Neur Briefs* Dec 1992.

POSTOPERATIVE CHEMOTHERAPY, DELAYED RADIATION AND BRAIN TUMORS

To avoid the severe irradiation-related neurotoxic effects of postoperative treatment of malignant brain tumors in infants and children less than 3 years of age, the Pediatric Oncology Group, centered at St Louis, MO, conducted a prospective study of primary postoperative chemotherapy. Treatment consisted of two 28-day cycles of cyclophosphamide plus vincristine, followed by one 28-day cycle of cisplatin plus etoposide. The sequence was repeated 1) until the tumor showed progression or 2) for 2 years in 132 children < 24 months of age at diagnosis and 3) for 1 year in 66 children of 24-36 months of age. Chemotherapy was then followed by radiation. The first two treatment cycles produced complete or partial responses in 39% of 102 patients evaluated. Medulloblastomas, malignant gliomas, and ependymomas were most responsive, whereas brain-stem gliomas or embryonal tumors showed little or no response. The progression-free survival was 40% at the completion of treatment schedules. Cognitive evaluations at base line and after 1 year of chemotherapy showed no deterioration. (Duffner PK et al. Postoperative chemotherapy and delayed radiation in children less than three years of age with malignant brain tumors. N Engl J Med June 17 1993;328:1725-31). (Reprints: Dr Duffner, Pediatric Oncology Group Operations Office (8633, 8634), 4949 W Pine Blvd, St Louis, MO 63108).

COMMENT. Chemotherapy prevents disease progression and permits radiation therapy to be delayed for one to two years in about 40% of infants and very young children with malignant brain tumors. The best results are obtained in those with total surgical resection of localized disease. Chemotherapy is least effective in children with embryonal, primitive neuroectodermal tumors. Dr JC Allen, New York University Medical Center, cautions that delaying cerebral radiotherapy for 1 to 2 years may not spare an infant neurocognitive complications, and that intensive chemotherapy may also prove to have a detrimental effect on brain development. (Editorial. N Engl J Med June 17, 1993;328:1780-1).-Editor. *Ped Neur Briefs* June 1993.

PROGNOSIS OF BRAIN TUMORS WITH EPILEPSY

The prognosis of 560 patients with a clinical and CT diagnosis of intrinsic supratentorial brain tumor was examined retrospectively at the Department of Neurosciences, Walton Hospital, Liverpool, England. Epilepsy was the first symptom in 164 (30%) patients. Patients presenting with epilepsy had a median survival of 37 months compared to 6 months in those presenting with other symptoms; they were more likely to have a normal clinical examination, a non-enhancing low density lesion on CT scan and a low grade tumor. Significant independent variables which adversely affected prognosis were increasing age, focal neurological signs, an enhancing CT lesion at diagnosis, surgical biopsy, and male sex. Primary intracerebral tumors presenting with epilepsy were relatively benign. They were less likely to receive radiotherapy or biopsy, but more likely to undergo resective surgery. No beneficial effects from either early resective surgery or radiotherapy were demonstrated. The average duration of symptoms before CT diagnosis was 28 months (range 2 days - 232 months) in those presenting with epilepsy and 4 months (range 1 day - 175 months) in those with other presentations. Seizures were refractory to antiepileptic drugs, with only 11 of 164 patients ever achieving a 1 year remission (Smith DF et al. The prognosis of primary intracerebral tumours presenting with epilepsy: the outcome of medical and surgical management. J Neurol Neurosurg and Psych Oct 1991;54:915-920).

COMMENT. Backus RE and Millichap JG analyzed

the records of 291 consecutive children treated for intracranial tumor at the Mayo Clinic from 1950-1959 with particular attention to patients with seizures (Pediatrics June 1962;29:978-984). Seizures occurred in 17% of the total group - in 25% of patients with supratentorial tumors and in 12% of those with infratentorial tumors. Seizures were the initial symptoms in 15% of patients with supratentorial tumors and in 1% of those with infratentorial tumors. The average age at onset was 4.9 years in the supratentorial group and 4.8 years in the infratentorial group. The diagnosis of supratentorial tumors was delayed for an average of 2 years, whereas infratentorial tumors were diagnosed within an average time of 3 months of the initial seizure. The electroencephalogram was of localizing value in 92% of tumors that involved the cerebral cortex. The histologic type of tumors was verified in 46 of the 50 patients who had seizures. Seizures were more common in patients with slowly growing astrocytomas grades 1 and 2 (67 % incidence) than in those with rapidly expanding astrocytomas grades 3 and 4 (10% incidence). Symptoms of increased intracranial pressure were present at the time of the first seizure in 20% of patients with supratentorial tumors and in 79% with infratentorial tumors. A delta pattern in the EEG indicative of an expanding lesion occurred in 50% of patients and spike, sharp wave, or spike and wave seizure discharges compatible with a static lesion were recorded in 32% of patients with supratentorial tumors (Millichap JG et al. The electroencephalogram in children with intracranial tumors and seizures. Neurology May 1962;12:329-336).

With the increasing availability of neuroimaging techniques and particularly the MRI, the early diagnosis of tumor in patients with focal epilepsy will be facilitated and may lead to earlier surgical resection. The present study questions the advisability of resective surgery in patients with primary brain tumors presenting with seizures. A prospective, randomized, study of aggressive versus conservative management is required.-Editor. *Ped Neur Briefs* Nov 1991.

LONG-TERM NEUROLOGIC PROBLEMS WITH MEDULLOBLASTOMA

All 11 children who presented since 1976 in Cardiff, Wales with medulloblastoma and who had survived at least 5 years were reviewed neurologically. Current ages ranged from 10 - 24 years. Surgical removal was complete in 6. All received radiotherapy. Nine had additional chemotherapy. Mild cerebellar ataxia was present in 10, and external ocular movement abnormalities in 2. Signs attributable to therapy were optic atrophy in 2, fine motor incoordination in 2, dyspraxia in 7 and dementia in 1. Epilepsy occurred in 2. Only 1 patient who presented at 13 years was free of neurologic consequences of therapy. Only 2 attended grade school, and only 3 are gainfully employed (Wallace SJ, Salaman PF. Long-term neurologic problems of children treated with medulloblastoma. Pediatr Neurol Sept/Oct 1992;8:386-387 (abstract)). (Correspondence: Dr. Sheila J. Wallace, Department of Pediatrics, University Hospital of Wales, Health Park, Cardiff, CF44XN Wales UK.)

COMMENT. Detection of tumor occurrence by surveillance scanning in children with medulloblastoma is reported from the Children's Hospital of Philadelphia. Surveillance brain scans failed to detect recurrent disease in most patients and had virtually no impact on outcome. Follow-up should emphasize parent education and neurologic evaluation to detect relapse and to elicit and remediate late effects of therapy (Torres C et al. Ann Neurol Sept 1992;32:458 (abstract)).

The antineoplastic effects of gallium nitrate on human medulloblastoma in vivo are reported from the Medical College of Wisconsin, Milwaukee, Wl (Whelan HT et al. Pediatr Neurol Sept/Oct 1992;8:323-327). Mice injected intradermally with medulloblastoma Daoy cell line developed tumors. Gallium nitrate treatment reduced tumor growth rate and tumor size, but the animals suffered nephrotoxicity.-Editor. *Ped Neur Briefs* Dec 1992.

SUBARACHNOID METASTATIC TUMORS AND MRI

Subarachnoid metastatic disease was evaluated in 17 children with primary intracranial neoplasms at the Departments of Neurology and Radiology, The Children's Hospital of Philadelphia, PA. The tumors were principally neuroectodermal, ependymomas, and astrocytomas and the majority originated in the posterior fossa. The gadolinium MRI was superior in delineating spinal cord nodules and "sugar coating" whereas myelography and CT more readily revealed nerve root sleeve filling defects. (Kramer ED et al. Comparison of myelography with CT follow-up versus gadolinium MRI for subarachnoid metastatic disease in children. Neurology Jan 1991;41:46-50).

COMMENT. Gadolinium-enhanced MRI appears to be a safe non-invasive test and the technique of choice for the diagnosis of subarachnoid metastatic disease.-Editor. *Ped Neur Briefs* Jan 1991.

INTRACRANIAL ARACHNOIDAL CYSTS

Of 28 cases of intracranial arachnoidal cysts reported from the Clinica Las Condes, Santiago, Chile, 17 were located in the middle cranial fossa, 3 in the quadrigeminal cistern, 2 were parasagital, 3 suprasellar and 3 were in the posterior fossa. Of 23 (82%) treated surgically, 3 received craniotomy with fenestrations, 8 had shunts and 15 were treated by the insertion of cystoperitoneal drainage with excellent results. Twenty-one of the 22 treated cases are asymptomatic and leading a normal life. MRI or CT follow-up showed disappearance of cysts in 14 and marked reduction in size in 7. (Basauri L, Selman JM. Intracranial arachnoidal cysts. Child's Nerv Syst March 1992;8:101-104.) (Reprints: Dr. L. Basauri, Neurosurgical Unit, Clinica Las Condes, Casilla 27014, Santiago, Chile.)

COMMENT. The diagnosis of intracranial arachnoidal cysts and reports in the literature have become more frequent since the routine use of neuroimaging. The danger of intracystic hemorrhage with a high possibility of secondary hydrocephalus following head injury has been quoted as a reason for surgical intervention as a preventive measure in some cases. See Ped Neur Briefs Oct 1991;5:80 for a report of 67 childhood arachnoidal cysts treated surgically and 1 report of spontaneous disappearance of a cyst. Small or medium sized cysts without clinical manifestations are not usually treated but are monitored carefully .

MENINGIOMAS: MRI AND PATHOLOGICAL FINDINGS

MRIs and histopathological studies of five children, aged 3 months to 16 years, with extra-axial meningiomas are reported from the Arkansas Children's Hospital and University of Arkansas for Medical Sciences, Little Rock, AR. Two tumors were supratentorial and three were in the posterior fossa. Two located on the tentorium presented with headache, and one at the foramen magnum caused quadriparesis. All were hyperintense on proton density- and T2-weighted images and showed intense contrast enhancement on T1-weighted images. Two were meningotheliomatous, one transitional, one chordoid, and one hemangiopericytic variant of meningioma. Chromosome 22 deletions were found in two of four tumors studied. (Glasier CM et al. Meningiomas in children: MR and histopathologic findings. AJNR Jan/Feb 1993;14:237-241). (Reprints: Charles M Glasier MD, Department of Radiology, Arkansas Children's Hospital, 800 Marshall Street, Little Rock, AR 72202).

COMMENT. Meningiomas in children are rare (1 to 3% of intracranial tumors) and much less common than in adults (15%). About 25% of meningiomas in children are associated with neurofibromatosis, especially type 2.-Editor. *Ped Neur Briefs* March 1993.

TEMPORAL LOBE TUMOR AND LANDAU-KLEFFNER SYNDROME

A 7-year-old boy with a left temporal lobe tumor and Landau-Kleffner syndrome (acquired aphasia and epilepsy) who improved dramatically after surgery is reported from the New York Hospital-Cornell University Medical Center. A verbal auditory agnosia with mutism had evolved over a 3 month period after onset of refractory partial complex seizures at 5 years. EEG showed left temporal and right occipital spike and S/W discharges. Language comprehension was absent on the Peabody Picture Vocabulary test and Token test. Following removal of a grade 1 astocytoma demonstrated on MRI, seizures stopped, language returned, and after 1 year speech and comprehension were almost normal for age. (Nass R et al. Landau-Kleffner syndrome: Temporal lobe tumor resection results in good outcome. Pediatr Neurol July/Aug 1993;9:303-5). (Respond: Dr Nass, New York Univ Med Ctr, 400 E 34th St RR 212, New York, NY 10021).

COMMENT. The favorable result of surgery in this patient contrasts with the poor outcome of most patients with Landau-Kleffner syndrome treated medically. MRI and ictal SPECT should be considered in all patients with this syndrome to rule out localized structural pathology amenable to surgery.-Editor. *Ped Neur Briefs* Oct 1993.

VON HIPPEL-LINDAU DISEASE AND PHEOCHROMOCYTOMA

Nineteen percent of 82 unselected patients with pheochromocytoma studied at the University of Freiburg, Germany, and the University of California, San Diego, were found to be gene carriers of von Hippel-Lindau disease. Thirty-eight percent of carriers of von-Hippel-Lindau disease had pheochromocytoma as the only manifestation of their syndrome. In 12 of 14 families with von Hippel-Lindau disease, pheochromocytoma, retinal angiomatosis, and hemangioblastoma of the central nervous system occurred in the absence of renal, pancreatic, and epididymal lesions, which suggests a distinct subtype of the disease with unique molecular-genetic characteristics. Hemangioblastoma developed in 17% of carriers. (Neumann HPH et al. Pheochromocytomas, multiple endocrine neoplasia type 2, and von Hippel-Lindau disease. N Engl J Med Nov 18 1993;329:1531-8). (Reprints: Dr Neumann, Division of Nephrology and Hypertension, University of Freiburg, Hugstetterstr. 55, D-79106 Freiburg im Breisgau, Germany).

COMMENT. All patients with pheochromocytomas should be screened for von Hippel-Lindau disease by ophthalmoscopy and MRI of the brain. Retinal angiomas are usually asymptomatic. Hemangioblastoma of the CNS has an excellent prognosis if recognized and removed early.

A three-decade investigation of familial pheochromocytoma involving 619 descendants of 3 siblings of German origin, reported from the University of Pittsburgh (Tisherman SE. Arch Intern Med Nov 22 1993;153:2550-6), showed that education and screening decreased mortality. Symptoms on presentation were the classic triad of sweating, nervousness, and headaches. Weight loss, nausea, vomiting, and abdominal pain were more common in children than in adults with pheochromocytoma. Six had von Hippel-Lindau disease manifested by cerebellar hemangioblastoma or retinal angioma, one becoming blind from bleeding. Regular screening and early diagnosis are important to prevent blindness.- Editor. *Ped Neur Briefs* Dec 1993.

TUBEROUS SCLEROSIS AND NEONATAL ASTROCYTOMA

The relative value of neural imaging studies in the diagnosis of a neonatal astrocytoma associated with tuberous sclerosis is reported from the Departments of Neurosciences, Pediatrics, and Pathology, University of California, San Diego, CA. The infant was hypotonic at birth and had poor respiratory effort. Apgar scores were 3/8. Motor examination revealed decreased tone in proximal upper extremities and neck. Deep tendon reflexes were generally exaggerated and plantar responses were extensor bilaterally. Wood's lamp examination was equivocal. There was no family history of tuberous sclerosis or epilepsy and the parents showed no neurocutaneous stigmata. An echoencephalogram revealed a large mass in the left lateral ventricle arising from the left caudate nucleus and obstructing the foramen of Monroe. The study was consistent with an intraventricular tumor rather than a hematoma. The MRI revealed a large irregular lobulated mass believed to be a tumor arising from the corpus callosum, possibly a lipoma. The CT revealed a nonenhancing, hyperdense mass in the left frontal horn interpreted as an intraventricular hemorrhage. A CT-guided needle biopsy of the mass showed gemistocytic cells resembling large reactive astrocytes. A cardiac echocardiogram revealed multiple nodules in the intraventricular septum, consistent with multiple rhabdomyomas. Funduscopic exam revealed two small retinal hamartomas in the right eye. Ultrasound of the kidneys was negative. At eight weeks of age the infant had developed multiple hypopigmented macules on trunk and extremities. (Hahn JS et al. Neonatal subependymal giant cell astrocytoma associated with tuberous sclerosis: MRI, CT, and ultrasound correlation. Neurology Jan 1991;41:124-128).

COMMENT. The interpretation of the echoencephalogram was closer to the correct diagnosis than that of the MRI and CT. Even without the needle biopsy of the mass the diagnosis of tuberous sclerosis and associated tumor may have been suspected and almost certainly determined bv the echocardiogram and cardiac rhabdomyomas. Echoencephalogram may be the diagnostic study of choice in newborns. The MRI picture is atypical showing decreased signal intensity on T2-weighted imaging and increased signal intensity on Tl-weighted studies.-Editor. *Ped Neur Briefs* Feb 1991.

MANAGEMENT OF INTRACRANIAL NEOPLASMS IN NEUROFIBROMATOSIS

Recommendations are proposed for the diagnosis and management of CNS neoplasms with NF-1 and NF-2 at the Department of Neurology, Section of Pediatric Neurology, Cleveland Clinic Foundation, Cleveland, Ohio; Phoenix Children's Hospital, Phoenix, AZ; and Children's National Medical Center, George Washington University, Washington, D.C.: (1) MRI is indicated in most childhood patients with NF-1 to screen for visual pathway astrocytomas with substantial visual loss or progressive disease. Treatment should include surgery, irradiation or chemotherapy. (2) Focal areas of signal intensity identified in asymptomatic patients should not be treated as neoplastic unless there is pathologic confirmation. (3) Specific CNS neoplasms (i.e., astrocytomas, ependymomas, meningiomas) should be treated with standard management protocols. (4) Intrinsic brainstem tumors with NF-1 should be observed for progressive disease and considered for biopsy and/or resection. (5) Gadolinium-enhanced MRI for acoustic neuromas is indicated in children at risk for NF-2. (6) Formal protocols to clarify the incidence, natural history, and management of intracranial neoplasms in NF-1 and NF-2 should be developed in collaborative national studies (Cohen BH, Kaplan AM, Packer RJ for the Children's Cancer Study Group. Management of intracranial neoplasms in children with neurofibromatosis type 1 and 2. Pediatr Neurosurg Nov 1991;16:66-72).

COMMENT. Optic nerve and tract astrocytomas are the most common intracranial neoplasms in NF-1 with an incidence of 5-15%. They may present with proptosis, extraocular nerve palsies or nystagmus. Some patients have MRI appearance of "tumor streaking" without mass effect, from the chiasm along the optic tracts and optic radiations. The significance of this streaking is not known. The guidelines for the treatment of visual pathway tumors is controversial, especially for asymptomatic patients or patients with non-progressive defects. For an overview of CNS tumors and neurofibromatosis see Progress in Pediatric Neurology I, Millichap ed. 1991, Chicago, PNB Publ, pp. 374-379.-Editor. *Ped Neur Briefs* Feb 1992.

POST-SURGICAL CEREBELLAR MUTISM

Mutism immediately following removal of a large midline posterior fossa medulluloblastoma and a cerebellar arteriovenous malformation is reported in 2 children from the Department of Neurosurgery, University of Florida, Gainsville, FL. The 7 year old boy with medulluloblastoma showed only a mild dysarthria and truncal ataxia at 3 month follow up and a 15 year old girl with acute posterior fossa bleed and obstructive hydrocephalus was similarly affected by a dysarthria and truncal ataxia when examined at 3 months. A review of the literature disclosed 19 cases of transient mutism after surgical removal of posterior fossa tumors. The more widespread the injury to the midportion of the cerebellum with dentate nuclear involvement, the greater the risk of developing postoperative mutism (Dietze DD Jr., Mickle JP. Cerebellar mutism after posterior fossa surgery. Pediatr Neurosurg, Oct 1991;16:25-31). (Reprints: Donald D. Dietze, Jr., M.D., Department of Neurosurgery, University of Florida, Box J-265, J. Hillis Miller Health Center, Gainesville, FL 32610.)

COMMENT. The authors advise that this possible complication of posterior fossa surgery should be discussed with patient and parents as part of the preoperative planning. Mutism is not restricted to tumor pathology but may be associated with any acute pathological insult to the midportion of the cerebellum. Fortunately, the mutism resolves completely or to a mild cerebellar dysarthria over a 3 month period. Surgery of midline medulloblastomas is particularly at risk for the development of postoperative mutism.-Editor. *Ped Neur Briefs* Feb 1992.

CHAPTER 10

NEUROCUTANEOUS SYNDROMES

INTRODUCTION

Manuel R. Gomez, M.D.
Section of Pediatric Neurology, Mayo Clinic
Rochester, MN

Advances in molecular biology have culminated in the triple cloning of the gene of the following three *Neurohamartomatoses:* Neurofibromatosis 1 (NF-1), Neurofibromatosis 2 (NF-2) and Tuberous Sclerosis Complex (TSC).

NF-1 with a prevalence rate of 1:3000 is the commonest genetically transmitted disorder affecting the nervous system. The gene locus for NF-1 was found by positional cloning (linkage analysis) to be in the chromosomal region 17q11.2. It was already known by the year 1990 that the NF-1 gene locus is in the pericentromeric region of chromosome 17q. Finding patients with a reciprocal chromosomal translocation that had fractured the region 17q11.2 causing them to lose the NF1 gene provided the key for precisely locating, cloning and characterizing the NF1 gene. The protein-coding region of NF-1 spans some 400 kb of genomic DNA, and has 51 exons that codify 11 to 13 kb of mRNA. It has been found in all tissues examined. Its product, a protein with 2818 aminoacids was named *Neurofibromin* (White 1991). Evidence indicates that NF1 is a tumor-suppressor gene. The product of the NF1 mutations that cause NF-1 is an inactive neurofibromin that disrupts the mechanism to signal for growth-inhibition. NF-1 and the failed function of the mutant NF1 can be best explained with the Knudson's "double hit" hypothesis: First, a mutation of the NF1 gene in germline cells alters the antioncogene protein *Neurofibromin*. Second, a random somatic mutation, occurring only in clones of somatic cells, results in a double dose of damaged growth-inhibiting protein in those cells, allowing or promoting tumor growth only in those clones of cells with loss of heterogeneity by chance deletion or random point mutation.

□Bilateral Acoustic Neuromas Neurofibromatosis, BANF, Central Neurofibromatosis, Neurofibromatosis 2 or simply NF-2 is an uncommon hamartomatosis with a prevalence of 1:1000,000. It is now well established that NF-2 is due to a mutation in the chromosomal region 22q12 and genetically, clinically, and pathologically, NF-2 is different from NF-1, although also of autosomal dominance inheritance, and NF-2 patients may have a few cafe-au-lait spots on their skin. The clinical expression of NF-2 usually begins after the first decade of life and is characterized chiefly by the development of bilateral tumors in the vestibular branch of cranial nerve VIII, and on other cranial nerves such as the VII and XII, and spinal roots. The patients often develop intracranial or spinal meningiomas.

The gene product of the normal NF-2 gene is a protein that has been named *Merlin,* an acronym formed with the initials of a family of proteins known as *Moesin, Ezrin, Radixin* _and from the words *like potein*. It is now possible to determine by positional cloning if an asymptomatic individual at risk of suffering this disease indeed carries the NF2 gene mutation (Trufatter, 1993).

The diagnosis of TSC may be made in children who present with seizures and whose MRI demonstrates subcortical areas of high intensity signals in T-2 sequences. The hypomyelination indicates the presence of cortical tubers. The MRI may also reveal radial lines of increased signal spanning from the periventricular region to the cerebral cortex. This sign points out the site where neuroblasts, having failed to migrate and differentiate, have formed nests of heterotopic atypical neurons along migration paths for construction of the cerebral cortex. The presence of only white spots in an infant with complex partial or generalized seizures is very suggestive, though not pathognomonic of the disease.

In 1993 a European group of researchers identified five TSC-associated deletions at region 16p13.3 and isolated four genes in a 120 kb region that was cloned. One gene interrupted by five deletions and several intragenic mutations including one *de novo* deletion was designated TSC-2. The investigators proposed that the product of the normal gene is a protein with regions similar to GAP, a GTP-ase activating protein. They have named this protein *Tuberin*. (The European Chromosome 16 Tuberous Sclerosis Consortium, 1993). Another gene previously found by positional cloning is now known as TS-1 (Fryer, 1987). Its product remains unknown but is probably another antioncogene. TSC is both phenotypically and genetically heterogeneous. *-Manuel R. Gomez, M.D., Section of Pediatric Neurology, Mayo Clinic, Rochester, Minnesota.*

BIBLIOGRAPHY

White R. Identification of the neurofibromatosis gene. In: J Brugge, T Curran, E Harlow et al. (eds). Origins of Human Cancer. A Comprehensive Review. 1991, Cold Spring Harbor, NY; Cold Spring Harbor Laboratory Press, pp 623-632.

Trufatter JA et al. A novel moesin-, ezrin-, radixin-like

gene is a candidate for the neurofibromatosis 2 tumor suppressor. Cell 1993;72:1-20.

The European Chromosome 16 Consortium. Identification and characterization of the tuberous sclerosis gene on chromosome 16. Cell 1993;75:1305-1315.

Fryer AE et al. Evidence that the gene for tuberous sclerosis is on chromosome 9. Lancet 1987;1:659-661.

TUBEROUS SCLEROSIS

MRI AND EEG IN TUBEROUS SCLEROSIS

The relationship between MRI cortical lesion sites and the topographic distribution of EEG spike-and-wave foci was studied in 34 children with tuberous sclerosis at the Service de Neuropediatrie, Hopital Saint Vincent de Paul, Paris, France and the Instituto di Neuropsichiatria Infantile, Roma, Italy. Seizures had appeared in the first year of life in 30 patients, they were partial in ten and infantile spasms in 11, or both in nine. MRI revealed localized cortical areas of high intensity signal, or tubers, in all but two patients. EEG performed at the same age as MRI showed focal spikes and slow waves in all but three patients. Of 34 patients 26 (76%) had both MRI cortical large or intermediate tubers and EEG foci. There was a significant correlation between the number of large tubers and the number of EEG foci. Patients with frontal lobe involvement on MRI showed frontal EEG foci after age two. Secondary bilateral synchrony in the EEG was associated with frontal tubers. (Cusmai R et a;. Topographic comparative study of magnetic resonance imaging and electroencephalography in 34 children with tuberous sclerosis. Epilepsia Nov/Dec 1990;31:747-755).

COMMENT. The MRI is more efficient than CT in detecting and localizing tubers of tuberous sclerosis which appear as high intensity signal areas in T2-weighted sequence. The cortical tubers shown on MRI are epileptogenic whereas subependymal calcifications as detected by CT are non-epileptogenic. Frontal lesions present from the first year of life often have a delayed

EEG expression, in keeping with the posteroanterior migration of epileptic foci in childhood, the result of maturational changes.-Editor. *Ped Neur Briefs* Jan 1991.

TUBEROUS SCLEROSIS AND NEONATAL ASTROCYTOMA

See Chapter 9: Hahn JS et al. Neonatal subependymal giant cell astrocytoma associated with tuberous sclerosis: MRI, CT, and ultraound correlation. Neurology Jan 1991;41:124-128. The relative value of neural imaging studies in the diagnosis of a neonatal astrocytoma associated with tuberous sclerosis is reported from the Departments of Neurosciences, Pediatrics, and Pathology, University of California, San Diego, CA.

VISUAL LOSS IN TUBEROUS SCLEROSIS

Visual loss in 4 patients with tuberous sclerosis complicated by subependymal giant-cell astrocytoma is reported from the Departments of Ophthalmology, Neurology, and Radiology, University of Michigan Medical Center, Ann Arbor, MI. The patients presented at 12-20 years of age with obstructive hydrocephalus. Surgery relieved elevated pressure in all cases but 2 patients became blind and 1 has severe visual field loss from the effects of chronic papilledema on the optic nerves . Early surgical decompression prevented visual loss in the fourth patient whose tumor was removed at 12 years of age and who required further resection of a giant-cell astrocytoma at 20 years. (Dotan, SA et al. Visual loss in tuberous sclerosis. Neurology Dec 1991;41:1915-1917.) (Reprints: Dr. J.D. Trobe, W.K. Kellogg Eye Center, 1000 Wall St, Ann Arbor, MI 48105.)

COMMENT. Periodic ophthalmologic examination and brain imaging are advisable in tuberous sclerosis patients with subependymal nodules. The timely relief of increased intracranial pressure may arrest or prevent loss of vision.-Editor. *Ped Neur Briefs* Jan 1992.

TUBEROUS SCLEROSIS: DIAGNOSTIC CRITERIA

The Diagnostic Criteria Committee of the National Tuberous Sclerosis Association reports primary, secondary, and tertiary features of the disease complex and considers the specificity and reliability of the various lesions. The histological pattern of a lesion when available is generally more reliable than visual or radiographic appearances. Definite, probable and suspect diagnoses are categorized. (Roach ES et al. Report of the Diagnostic Criteria Committee of the National Tuberous Sclerosis Association. J Child Neurol April 1992;7:221-224.) (Correspondence: Dr. ES Roach, University of Texas Southwestern Medical School, Department of Neurology, 5323 Harry Hines Blvd., Dallas, TX 75235)

COMMENT. In an editorial, Dr. Robert M. Shuman notes that assumptions about the specificity of lesions will need to be tested. The Committee intends these criteria to be adaptable and modified as data are collected.-Editor. *Ped Neur Briefs* June 1992.

SEIZURES AND IQ IN TUBEROUS SCLEROSIS

The relationship of seizures to intellectual disability was examined in 104 patients with tuberous sclerosis ascertained from the total population of the West of Scotland and reported from the Royal Hospital for Sick Children, Yorkhill, Glasgow, Scotland. Of 48 patients with seizures, 18 (35%) had normal intelligence, 6 (12%) had moderate intellectual disability, and 24 (45%) had severe intellectual disability. Seizures were significantly associated with intellectual disability. No patient who developed seizures after the age of 5 years was intellectually impaired. Most individuals with intellectual disability presented with infantile spasms or other seizures under 1 year of age, or had multiple seizure types. A higher incidence of intellectual disability was found among individuals who had more than 1 seizure type. Also, children with TS whose first seizure is febrile have a high risk of developing intellectual disability (Shepherd CW, Stephenson JBP. Seizures and intellectual disability associated with tuberous sclerosis in the West of Scotland. Dev Med Child Neurol Sept 1992;34:766-774). (Correspondence: Dr. C.W. Shepherd, Craigavon Area Hospital, Portadown, Northern Ireland BT63

5QQ.)

COMMENT. Several papers on tuberous sclerosis were presented at the 6th Congress of the International Child Neurology Association, November, 1992, Buenos Aires, Argentina. Laan LA et al. Rotterdam, found vigabatrin in therapy of resistant epilepsy with tuberous sclerosis to be valuable, if given early in childhood. Calderon-Gonzalez R et al. of Monterrey, Mexico, found 7 (26%) of 27 children with TS had infantile autism evident by 3.5 years of age. Rett syndrome was associated with tuberous sclerosis in 2 patients reported by Philippart M of Pomona, California. Curatolo P et al. of Rome, Italy reported topographic spike mapping of the EEG in TS which showed that "generalized" spike-and-wave discharges were of focal origin (Pediatr Neurol Sept/Oct 1992;8:344-411). See Chapter 1 for reports of seizures and TS.-Editor. *Ped Neur Briefs* Nov 1992.

EPILEPSY SURGERY AND TUBEROUS SCLEROSIS

The results of operation for treatment of epilepsy in 5 male and 4 female patients with tuberous sclerosis in a 5-year period from 1986-1990 are reported from the Mayo Clinic. Pathological examination of resected lesions demonstrated 7 cortical tubers and 2 astocytic hamartomas. MRIs correlated with clinical and focal EEG findings. Seven patients are free from seizures and 2 are partially controlled. In selected TS patients with single or multiple cerebral lesions, both the primary and secondary epileptogenic lesions were modified by removal of the primary ictal focus. (Bebin EM, Kelly PJ, Gomez MR. Surgical treatment for epilepsy in cerebral tuberous sclerosis. Epilepsia July/Aug 1993;34:651-657). (Reprints: Dr MR Gomez, Dept of Neurology, Mayo Clinic, 200 First St, SW, Rochester, MN 55905).

COMMENTS. See Chapter 1 for reports of surgery for epilepsy due to cortical dysplasia. The use of MRI and PET should improve the identification of patients amenable to surgery.-Editor. *Ped Neur Briefs* Sept 1993.

NEUROFIBROMATOSIS

SEIZURES AND NEUROFIBROMATOSIS I

Twenty-two (6%) patients, ages 5 to 57 years, had developed seizures among 359 attending a neurofibromatosis clinic at the Dept of Neurology, Children's Hospital, Harvard Med School, Boston. The majority of seizures could be attributed to causes unrelated to NF1: 6 had febrile seizures and 3 had primary generalized epilepsy with onset before 5 years. Complex partial seizures in 9 (41%), infantile spasms in 1, and seizures with aqueductal stenosis in 2 may have been caused by NF1, but no specific brain lesions were detected. None of the seizures was a symptom of brain tumor, and neuroimaging failed to uncover a seizure focus. Routine EEG of all patients with NF1 was considered unproductive. (Korf BR, Carrazana E, Holmes GL Patterns of seizures observed in association with neurofibromatosis 1. Epilepsia July/Aug 1993;34:616-620). (Reprints: Dr BR Korf, Children's Hospital, 300 Longwood Ave, Boston, MA 02115).

COMMENT. Seizures appear to be relatively uncommon in association with NF1. A possible increased frequency of infantile spasms in NF1 patients was suggested in two previous reports (Huson SM et al. Brain 1988;111:1355; (see Progress in Pediatric Neurology I, Millichap JG, ed, Chicago, PNB Publ, 1991. -Editor. *Ped Neur Briefs* Sept 1993.

LISCH NODULES IN NEUROFIBROMATOSIS TYPE 1

The prevalence of Lisch nodules among 167 patients with neurofibromatosis 1 is reported from the Department of Pediatrics, Genetics Division, Miami Children's Hospital, Miami, FL. Lisch nodules are dome-shaped hamartomatous lesions with a clear, yellow or brown appearance. The overall prevalence of Lisch nodules was 73.7% and similar to that of neurofibromas (68.3%). The prevalence varied directly with the age of the patients: 5% in children less than 3 years of age, 42% in those 3 to 4 years old, 55% at 5 to 6 years; and 100% in adults of 21 years of age or older. Lisch nodules appeared more frequently than neurofibromas in all but the youngest age group. Of 145 patients having radiological studies, 17 had optic gliomas (12%), 9 had other types of CNS tumor, and one had both optic glioma and another CNS tumor. The proportion of Lisch nodules was similar in those with or without CNS tumors. If Lisch nodules do not appear with increasing age, the risk of having the gene for neurofibromatosis 1 is reduced from 50% at birth to 31% at 5 to 6 years of age, 15% at 9 to 14 years of age, 8% at 15 to 20 years of age, and 0% in those over the age of 20. (Lubs MLE, Bauer MS et al. Lisch nodules in neurofibromatosis type 1. N Engl J Med May 2, 1991;324:1264-1266).

COMMENT. Multiple Lisch nodules, unlike cafe-au-lait spots and neurofibromas, are specific for the diagnosis of neurofibromatosis 1. Except for one case they have been absent in central neurofibromatosis 2. Lisch nodules are useful in the early diagnosis of neurofibromatosis 1 and slit-lamp examination is important in suspected cases.-Editor. *Ped Neur Briefs* June 1991.

FAMILIAL SPINAL NEUROFIBROMATOSIS

The clinical features and genetic linkage analysis of two pedigrees with familial spinal neurofibromatosis (NF) are described from the Divisions of Neurology and Medical Genetics, Cedars-Sinai Medical Center, UCLA School of Medicine, Los Angeles, CA; the Neurofibromatosis Institute, Pasadena, CA; and Department of Medical Informatics, University of Utah, Salt Lake City, UT. On clinical grounds, it was difficult to assign the two families to NF1 or NF2 based on the criteria established by the National Institutes of Health. Cutaneous tumors, Lisch nodules or acoustic tumors were absent. Cafe-au-lait spots were present in 1 family and absent in the other. The inheritance pattern was autosomal dominant in both pedigrees. Genetic linkage analysis was performed with markers linked to the NF1 gene on chromosome 17 and markers linked to the NF2 gene on chromosome 22. The location for the mutation in the first family was in the NFl gene, whereas that in the second family was excluded from the NF1 locus, although the phenotype was similar to that of family 1. (Pulst SM, Riccardi VM et al. Familial spinal neurofibromatosis: clinical and DNA linkage analysis. Neurology Dec 1991;41:1923-1927.) (Reprints: Dr. Pulst, Div Neurol, Cedars-Sinai Medical Center, 8700 Beverly Blvd, Los Angeles, CA 90048.)

COMMENT. Studies of families in which all affected individuals express the same subset of the NF phenotype allow a correlation between the mutation and its clinical characteristics. Symptomatic spinal neurofibromas occur in less than 5% of patients with NF1, but are commonly found in NF2. This may be the first report of familial spinal neurofibromatosis in families with NF1. One individual in each pedigree developed a neurofibrosarcoma and died of its complications. This is a rare complication in NF1, explained by the authors as a familial predisposition related to the mutations.-Editor. *Ped Neur Briefs* Jan 1992.

MANAGEMENT OF INTRACRANIAL NEOPLASMS IN NEUROFIBROMATOSIS

See Chapter 9 for article on recommendations proposed for the diagnosis and management of CNS neoplasms with NF-1 and NF-2 from the Department of Neurology, Section of Pediatric Neurology, Cleveland Clinic Foundation, Cleveland, Ohio, and other centers. (Cohen BH, Kaplan AM, Packer RJ for the Children's Cancer Study Group. Management of intracranial neoplasms in children with neurofibromatosis type 1 and 2. Pediatr Neurosurg Nov 1991;16:66-72).

COMMENT. Optic nerve and tract astrocytomas are the most common intracranial neoplasms in NF-1 with an incidence of 5-15%. They may present with proptosis, extraocular nerve palsies or nystagmus. For an overview of CNS tumors and neurofibromatosis see Progress in Pediatric Neurology I, Millichap ed. Chicago, PNB Publ, 1991, pp. 374-379.-Editor. *Ped Neur Briefs* Feb 1992.

CVA WITH NEUROFIBROMATOSIS TYPE I

A two year old developmentally delayed girl with neurofibromatosis type I and a sudden onset of left sided hemiparesis is reported from the Children's National Medical Center and George Washington University School of Medicine, Washington, D.C. There was no history of sickle cell disease or hypertension. The hemiparesis gradually improved and the patient received aspirin, 80 mg. daily. Four months later there was a left focal seizure and an acute progression of the left hemiparesis. At 5 years of age the patient presented with sudden right-sided weakness and right focal seizure. Cerebral angiography revealed bilateral distal internal carotid arterial occlusion. (Gorelick MH et al. Progressive occlusive cerebrovascular disease in a patient with neurofibromatosis type 1. Clin Pediat May 1992;31:313-315.) (Correspondence: Kenneth N. Rosenbaum, M.D., Department of Medical Genetics, Children's National Medical Center, 111 Michigan Avenue NW, Washington, D.C. 20010.)

COMMENT. Moyamoya may be seen in association with a number of systemic conditions including NF-1 or as a distinct disease entity of unclear etiology. Occlusion of the intracranial arteries is a rare complication of NF-1 and the progressive occlusion noted in this case appears to be unique.

The gene for NF-1 has been mapped to chromosome 17, and closely linked DNA markers have made accurate diagnosis by linkage analysis possible in most cases of familial NF-1. DNA testing by linkage analysis on 24 individuals with a family history of NF-1 and on 9 couples who requested testing for prenatal diagnosis was found useful as an adjunct to the clinical diagnosis: 1) in children less than 6 years of age with incomplete clinical signs, 2) in NF-1 families for prenatal testing, and 3) when complete clinical examination is impractical. (Hofman KJ, Boehm CD. J Pediatr March 1992;120:394-398.)-Editor. *Ped Neur Briefs* July 1992.

VON HIPPEL-LINDAU DISEASE

VON HIPPEL-LINDAU DISEASE AND GADOLINIUM MRI

Gadolinium-enhanced MRI was used to determine the frequency and distribution of CNS lesions in 50 patients with Von Hippel-Lindau Disease (VHL) at the National Institutes of Health, Bethesda, MD; University of Louisville, KY; and the Massachusetts General Hospital, Boston, MA. CNS hemangioblastomas were found in 36 (72%). The cerebellum was affected in 52%, spinal cord in 44%, and the brainstem in 18%. One-half of these tumors were asymptomatic and without clinical signs. The youngest patient was 11 years old and asymptomatic. The youngest synptomatic patient with VHL was 2 years of age with symptoms of ocular lesions. The mean age of all VHL patients was 34 years with a range of 11-62 years. (Filling-Katz MR et al. Central nervous system involvement in Von Hippel-Lindau disease. Neurology Jan 1991;41:41-46).

COMMENT Hemangioblastomas and VHL may be detected by 11 years of age and the screening of patients at risk for VHL should begin at 11 years using gadolinium-enhanced MRI. Ophthalmic examination should be initiated within the first two years of life. Diagnosis of VHL is important for genetic counseling as well as early detection of unsuspected ocular and visceral tumors which may lead to blindness or early death unless treated.-Editor. *Ped Neur Briefs* Jan 1991.

VON HIPPEL-LINDAU DISEASE: FAMILIAL SYMPTOM CLUSTERS

The clinical manifestations and prevalence of von Hippel-Lindau syndrome (HLS) were reported from the Department of Medicine, Albert-Ludwigs-Universitat, Freiburg im Breisgau, Germany, and Department of Pathology, University of Zurich, Switzerland. A striking familial clustering of HLS lesions was discovered: angiomatosis retinae in 51% (47/92), haemangioblastoma of the CNS in 46% (42/92), renal lesions in 33% (30/92) and phaeochromocytoma in 24% (22/92). Of the 92 patients, 52 had 1, 31 had 2, and

9 had 3 of the 4 HLS lesions. Of 29 evaluated kindreds, 18 had renal lesions. Some features of HLS were frequently combined whereas others seemed to be almost exclusive. The patterns of lesions within individual kindreds were stable. Vascular lesions of the syndrome (angiomatosis retinae and haemangioblastoma of the CNS) occurred in most families and represented core features whereas phaeochromocytoma at one end of the scale, and renal lesions, pancreatic cysts and epididymal cystadenoma at the other end of the scale, were unlikely to develop in the same family and were mutually exclusive. The authors suggest that HLS is caused from different mutations within a complex genetic locus, or additional genetic lesions, which cooperate with the HLS gene on chromosome 3p. The data point to a linear sequence of features. The calculated prevalence of the disease in the district of Freiburg, Germany, with a population of 1.909 million, was 1/38951. (Neumann HPH, Wiestler OD. Clustering of features of von Hippel-Lindau syndrome: evidence for a complex genetic locus. Lancet May 4, 1991;337:1052-54).

COMMENT. These familial patterns of lesions are important in prognosis and the clinical management of HLS gene carriers. Patients with renal lesions are at a high risk for hemangioblastoma of the CNS, the principal cause of death in HLS patients. Patients presenting with renal disorders should be carefully monitored for the development of CNS lesions. Patients with pheochromocytoma are likely to develop angiomatosis retinae but are usually spared the CNS complication.

Von Hippel-Lindau disease has been associated with loss of a region of chromosome 3 that is often deleted in renal cell carcinoma. This region contains a tumor suppressor gene whose absence is associated with the development of renal cell carcinoma, hemangioblastoma and other tumors of von Hippel-Lindau disease. Deletion of the tumor suppressor gene may allow ectopic production of erythropoietin by the intracranial hemangioblastoma. Production of erythropoietin by a recurrent intracranial hemangioblastoma in a 59 year old woman was thought to explain the erythrocytosis in this patient with von Hippel-Lindau disease. (Horton JC et al. Von Hippel-Lindau disease and erythrocytosis: Radioimmunoassay of erythropoietin in cyst fluid from a brainstem hemangioblastoma. Neurology May 1991;41:753-754).-Editor. *Ped Neur Briefs* June 1991.

CNS LESIONS IN VON HIPPEL-LINDAU SYNDROME

Ninety-seven gene carriers of von Hippel-Lindau syndrome (HLS) were studied at the University of Freiburg, Germany, to evaluate the prevalence and location of CNS lesions. Hemangioblastomas of the CNS were found in 43 patients (44%); 74% were intracranial and 26% were in the spinal cord. Seventy-five percent were cystic and 25% solid. Multiple lesions occurred in 42% of HLS hemangioblastomas but in none of 51 CNS hemangioblastomas without HLS. Cerebellar hemangioblastomas were the major cause of death in 82% of the patients with HLS (Neumann HPH et al. Central nervous system lesions in von Hippel-Lindau syndrome. J Neurol Neurosurg Psychiatry Oct 1992;55:898-901) (Correspondence: Dr Neumann, Medizinische Klinik, Hugstetter Str 55, D-7800 Freiburg, Germany)

COMMENT. Other manifestations of von Hippel-Lindau syndrome were as follows: retinal angiomatosis (44%), renal cysts (47%), pheochromocytoma (5%), pancreatic cysts (30%), and epididymal cystadenoma (15%). The MRI and gadolinium-enhanced MRI have improved the detection of small CNS lesions which are the initial manifestations of the syndrome and the largest percentage of patients. Multifocal tumor development and recurrence are serious problems in management and prognosis.-Editor. *Ped Neur Briefs* Nov 1992.

CUTANEOUS GRANULOMAS AND ATAXIA-TELANGIECTASIA

Development of cutaneous granulomas in 8 patients with ataxia-telangiectasia is reported from the Departments of Pediatrics and Dermatology,

Northwestern University Medical School, Chicago, IL; the Hospital for Sick Children, Toronto, Canada; Henry Ford Hospital, Detroit, MI; and University of North Carolina, Chapel Hill. The granulomas were atrophic lesions that frequently became encrusted and ulcerative. Their appearance differed significantly from the well circumscribed annular plaques or skin colored subcutaneous nodules of typical granuloma annulare. The lesions were persistent rather than self-limited and no infectious organisms were demonstrated. Treatment with intravenous immune globulin, topical antibiotic therapy and topical corticosteroid therapy were unsuccessful. The authors postulate that the granulomas were an attempt to localize antigen in patients with a dysfunctional immune system. (Paller AS et al. Cutaneous granulomatous lesions in patients with ataxia-telangiectasia. J Pediatr Dec 1991;119:917-922.) (Reprints: Dr Paller, Division of Dermatology, Children's Memorial Hospital, 2300 Children's Plaza, Chicago, IL 60614)

COMMENT. Patients with ataxia-telangiectasia have dysfunction of humoral and cell-mediated immunity as demonstrated by an immature thymus; absent or small tonsils; low levels of immunoglobulins A, E, G2 and G4; and a poor response to antigenic stimulation.-Editor. *Ped Neur Briefs* Jan 1992.

LHERMITTE-DUCLOS-COWDEN DISEASE

Two unrelated patients with clinical characteristics of both Lhermitte-Duclos disease and the autosomal dominant Cowden disease are reported from the Department of Neurology, University Hospital, Leiden, The Netherlands. Patient 1 was a mentally retarded woman with a large head, a high arched palate, dysarthria, mild cerebellar signs, and a single seizure at the age of 37 years. She also exhibited multiple papules on her nose, cheek, forehead and ears and on the oral mucosa. CT scan showed a nonenhancing mass in the cerebellar vermis and left cerebellar hemisphere, enlarged third and lateral ventricles, and a hypodense lesion in the centrum semiovale of the left cerebral hemisphere. A dysplastic gangliocytoma of the left cerebellar hemisphere was diagnosed at surgical resection of the tumor. Microscopic examination of skin biopsies showed trichilemmomas. Bilateral nonmalignant breast tumors were diagnosed at follow-up. The second patient had a history of tonic-clonic seizures in childhood, thyroid surgery at age 38 and he presented with cerebellar signs at 48 years of age. A dysplastic gangliocytoma was removed from the left cerebellar hemisphere. Skin lesions included papules on the face, limbs, and on the gingiva and tongue. Siblings of both patients showed the mucocutaneous lesions, thyroid disease, breast tumors, ovarian tumors, and also neurological signs including macrocephaly, mental retardation, seizures, tremor, and dysdiadochokinesia. The authors propose that Lhermitte-Duclos disease and Cowden disease are manifestations of a single phakomatosis. (Padberg GW et al. Lhermitte-Duclos disease and Cowden disease: A single phakomatosis. Ann Neurol May 1991;29:517-523).

COMMENT. Lhermitte-Duclos disease (dysplastic gangliocytoma of the cerebellum) may present in infancy or childhood but the onset of symptoms is more usually delayed until adulthood when a slowly progressive cerebellar syndrome with hydrocephalus is a frequent complication. The characteristic skin lesions of Cowden disease are multiple facial trichilemmomas; hamartomas of other organs, including breast and ovary, occur frequently. Macrocephaly may be an early finding, and the present report suggests that neurological complications of Cowden disease may be under-reported.-Editor. *Ped Neur Briefs* June 1991.

CHAPTER 11

VASCULAR DISORDERS AND MALFORMATIONS

INTRODUCTION

E. S. Roach, M.D.
Division of Pediatric Neurology
University of Texas Southwestern Medical School
Dallas, Texas

Ischemic stroke in children is most often due to congenital heart disease, hemoglobinopathy, or various inflammatory disorders; the number of other conditions known to promote stroke in children continues to expand. A thorough evaluation will discover the cause of an ischemic stroke about two thirds of the time. The origin of intracranial hemorrhage is even more likely to be confirmed. Common causes of hemorrhage include trauma, coagulation or platelet disorders, hemoglobinopathy, and structural vascular lesions. In some pediatric series, intracranial hemorrhage is recorded more often than cerebral infarction.

New diagnostic techniques make it easier to define the nature and extent of cerebrovascular lesions in children with minimal risk. Magnetic resonance angiography and other tests have made diagnosis easier and safer, particularly in very young children and in patients with sickle cell disease. Magnetic resonance imaging and magnetic resonance angiography can sometimes confirm a cerebrovascular lesion even in children with only non-specific findings such as lethargy or seizures. In some children magnetic resonance angiography provides enough information that standard arteriography is unnecessary. However, standard cerebral angiography is still more reliable for demonstrating lesions such as small aneurysms and arteriovenous malformations, and for this reason will not soon be replaced by magnetic resonance angiography. Small arteriovenous malformations or cavernous malformations may not be evident with magnetic resonance imaging, computed tomography, or angiography, particularly if the lesions is surrounded by acute hemorrhage and edema.

Magnetic resonance angiography is particularly useful in the evaluation of dural sinus and venous thrombosis, because the clinical features of these lesions are sometimes subtle. Magnetic resonance contrast studies can demonstrate the abnormal intracranial veins of Sturge-Weber syndrome, often before an infant becomes symptomatic and sometimes before other studies become abnormal. This is an important advance because most neonates with an upper facial cutaneous angioma do not have abnormal intracranial vessels (and thus little chance of subsequent neurologic problems), yet other studies do not reliably identify the infants at risk for neurologic complications of Sturge-Weber syndrome.

Concern that standard radiographic contrast agents might promote thrombosis in sickle cell patients led many of us to recommend against standard arteriography in these children unless the percent of sickle hemoglobin had been reduced by transfusion. Two recent developments make it easier to assess the cerebrovascular system without standard angiography. First, magnetic resonance angiography often shows widespread vasculopathy in sickle cell patients (similar to the pattern seen with moyamoya syndrome); small asymptomatic cerebral lesions are often visible with magnetic resonance imaging, although the significance of these areas is still uncertain. Second, transcranial Doppler studies make it easier to predict which patients with sickle cell disease have the highest risk of stroke. Recent studies have shown that transcranial Doppler is both sensitive and specific for detecting cranial vasculopathy due to sickle cell disease, and it may eventually be possible to use this technique to select patients for treatment <u>before</u> their first stroke, instead of the current method of starting periodic transfusions after the first stroke to prevent additional infarctions.

About half of the sickle cell disease patients who survive an initial stroke have another stroke later, and this high recurrence risk is the reason for starting a chronic transfusion program despite concern about eventual iron toxicity. The risk of recurrent stroke persists even after several years of periodic transfusion, although recent evidence suggests that less aggressive transfusion (maintaining the hemoglobin S near 50% instead of 30%) may effectively lower the risk of stroke with fewer transfusions and lower long-term risk of iron toxicity. Complete cessation of transfusion after a stroke-free interval reintroduces the higher risk for stroke, but, if effective, reduction of the amount of transfused blood would reduce the risk of iron toxicity.

Moyamoya is a radiographic syndrome with progressive stenosis and occlusion of the carotid arteries. Collateral channels develop distal to the carotid stenosis to form a telangiectatic network visible angiographically as the "puff of smoke" for which the syndrome is named. The external carotid arteries and the vertebrobasilar system can also be affected. Moyamoya is usually idiopathic, but the same radiographic pattern is seen in some patients with sickle cell disease, neurofibromatosis, cranial irradiation, and other conditions. Thus moyamoya is more appropriately designated a syndrome than a disease. Children usually present with hemiplegia or other focal deficit, headache, or epileptic seizures; adults are prone to intracranial hemorrhage (probably from rupture of a telangiectatic vessel). Magnetic resonance angiography is good for initial screening of moyamoya and for followup studies, but tends to overestimate the extent of carotid stenosis and is less effective than angiography for demonstrating collateral vessels.

Various surgical treatments have been touted for moyamoya syndrome. Most of these reports are as enthusiastic as they are uncontrolled, and some patients eventually do well without surgery. Despite these reservations, the procedure that seems to be the most logical is superficial temporal artery to middle cerebral artery bypass. There was also great enthusiasm for this bypass procedure for atherosclerosis a few years ago until a controlled trial was stopped before completion because of poor results. More evidence is needed before the procedure can be wholeheartedly endorsed for moyamoya syndrome.

In MELAS syndrome, characterized by mitochondrial myopathy, encephalopathy, lactic acidosis, and stroke-like episodes, the radiographic lesions seldom conform to the territory of a specific named artery, and individual radiographic lesions may resolve. Angiography is usually normal, but both carotid occlusion and dilatation of cerebral arteries and veins have been noted. Several groups have confirmed a mitochondrial tRNA $^{LEU(UUR)}$ mutation in most patients with MELAS syndrome. Patients without the mutation are clinically and pathologically identical to those who have it, and others with the mutation do not have all of the classical features of MELAS. (see Chapter 15 for abstracts and further commentary).

This section summarizes some of the exciting recent progress in our understanding of pediatric cerebrovascular disorders. Although interest in cerebrovascular disease in children has increased markedly, the actual incidence has changed little. What has changed is our willingness to consider the diagnosis of cerebrovascular disease in children and our ability to confirm the diagnosis once it is made. - *E. S. Roach, M.D., Division of Pediatric Neurology, University of Texas Southwestern Medical School, Dallas, Texas.*

STROKE

STROKE AS LATE SEQUELA OF CRANIAL IRRADIATION

The development of cerebrovascular disease manifested by strokes or transient ischemic attacks six months to four years after treatment of brain tumors in 11 children is reported from the Children's Hospital of Los Angeles, University of Southern California School of Medicine, Los Angeles, CA. All patients had received radiation therapy and seven chemotherapy. One patient, aged 4, with an incompletely resected craniopharyngioma, developed a right hemiparesis two years after treatment followed by left-sided focal motor seizures with quick progression to decerebrate posturing, central hyperventilation, coma, and death. Autopsy revealed bilateral cerebral infarctions as well as diffuse gliosis. Branches of the carotid artery showed severe thickening with subintimal proliferation of connective tissue. Smaller vessels showed cellular intimal proliferation with areas of leukocytic infiltration. (Mitchell WG et al. Stroke as a late sequela of cranial irradiation for childhood brain tumors. J Child Neurol April 1991;6:128-133).

COMMENT. Damage to medium and large intracranial vessels in addition to small vessel damage may result in late onset of stroke or transient ischemic attacks caused by radiation and chemotherapy in children with brain tumors. The cambination of methotrexate and cranial irradiation is more likely to produce a leukoencephalopathy than either treatment alone. The addition of chemotherapy may potentiate the damage to endothelial cells produced by radiation (*mineralizing microangiopathy*).-Editor. *Ped Neur Briefs* May 1991.

IDIOPATHIC STROKE

Of 4 children with idiopathic stroke syndrome examined at the Department of Neurosciences and Pediatrics, UMD-New Jersey Medical School and the University of Rochester Medical Center, all 4 were heterozygous for human leukocyte antigen (HLA-B51). Control samples from 3 patients with non-idiopathic stroke syndrome failed to reveal the HAL-B51 marker. (Mintz M, Epstein LG, Koenigsberger MR. Idiopathic childhood stroke is associated with human leukocyte antigen (HLA)-B51. Ann Neurol June 1992;31:675-677.) (Correspondence: Dr. Mintz, Department of Neurosciences, UMD-New Jersey Medical School, MSB-H506, 185 South Orange Avenue, Newark, NJ 07103.)

COMMENT. The finding of a common immunogenetic marker in children with idiopathic stroke syndrome suggests a genetic predisposition and susceptibility. The authors suggest that host factors, possibly triggered by transient viral precipitants, may contribute causally to these vascular occlusions.

Delayed onset hemiparesis and vascular thrombosis may occur approximately 6 weeks after primary varicella zoster virus infection and may explain some cases of misdiagnosed idiopathic stroke in children. (Bodensteiner JB, et al. Clinical features of vascular thrombosis following varicella. AJDC Jan 1992;146:100-102.) The importance of this clinical entity is emphasized in an editorial (Lancet June 13, 1992;339:1449-1450). The prognosis was good regardless of therapy and all patients recovered completely or nearly completely. The MRI was more sensitive than CT or angiography in demonstrating infarction of the basal ganglia and/or internal capsule. The delay in onset of the hemiparesis may result from the time taken for the vascular media to be infected with the virus.-Editor. *Ped Neur Briefs* July 1992.

CVA WITH NEUROFIBROMATOSIS TYPE I

A two year old developmentally delayed girl with neurofibromatosis type I and a sudden onset of left sided hemiparesis is reported from the Children's National Medical Center and George Washington University School of Medicine, Washington, D.C. There was no history of sickle cell disease or hypertension. The hemiparesis gradually improved and the patient received aspirin, 80 mg. daily. Four months later there was a left focal seizure and an acute progression of the left hemiparesis. At 5 years of age the patient presented with sudden right-sided weakness and right focal seizure. Cerebral angiography revealed bilateral distal internal carotid arterial occlusion. (Gorelick MH et al. Progressive occlusive cerebrovascular disease in a patient with neurofibromatosis type 1. Clin Pediat May 1992;31:313-315.) (Correspondence: Kenneth N. Rosenbaum, M.D., Department of Medical Genetics, Children's National Medical Center, 111 Michigan Avenue NW, Washington, D.C. 20010.)

COMMENT. Moyamoya may be seen in association with a number of systemic conditions including NF-1 or as a distinct disease entity of unclear etiology. Occlusion of the intracranial arteries is a rare complication of NF-1 and the progressive occlusion noted in this case appears to be unique.-Editor. *Ped Neur Briefs* July 1992.

ANTIPHOSPHOLIPID IMMUNOREACTIVITY AND TIAs

Clinical features that may predict the presence of antiphospholipid antibodies (aPL) in young patients with transient focal neurological events were determined in a study at the Henry Ford Hospital, Detroit, MI. Among 68 patients 29 were aPL-positive and 39 aPL-negative. The aPL-positive group was distinguished by a greater frequency of monocular visual symptoms, hemisensory symptoms, and systemic lupus erythematosus and less common binocular visual symptoms, accompanying headache, and personal and family history of migraine. Amaurosis fugax, unilateral paresthesias, and absence of a family history of migraine may predict aPL positivity (lupus anticoagulants and/or anticardiolipin antibodies) in young persons with transient focal neurologic deficits. (Tietjen GE, Levine SR, Welch KMA et al. Factors that predict antiphospholipid immunoreactivity in young people with transient focal neurological events. Arch Neurol Aug 1993;50:833-836). (Reprints: Dr Tietjen, Neurology, K-ll, Henry Ford Hospital, 2799 W Grand Blvd, Detroit, MI 48202).

COMMENT. Cerebral infarction, transient ischemic attacks (TIAs), and migraine have been associated with aPL positivity. Immune-mediated thrombotic tendency conferred by the antibodies has been postulated. Monocular visual loss, hemiparesthesia, and no family history of migraine in young patients with transient focal neurological events should prompt examination for aPL antibodies and further determination of risk of stroke.-Editor. *Ped Neur Briefs* Sept 1993.

PROGNOSIS OF VENTRICULAR HEMORRHAGE

The relationship of periventricular-intraventricular hemorrhage in infants of <32 weeks gestation to the occurrence of disability at 5 years of age was studied in a National Collaborative Survey in the Netherlands. Of 484 infants enrolled, all 304 survivors were examined at age 5 years; 26% of infants with severe hemorrhage and 67% with mild grades I/II survived the neonatal period. Of 85 (28%) survivors with a disability, 27 (9%) had a minor handicap and 23 (8%) a major handicap. The handicap was recorded at the age of 5 but was not present at 2 years in 17 children, while 35 were handicapped at 2 years but not at 5 years. Children with grades I and II as well as III and IV had more disabilities and handicaps than children without hemorrhage. (van de Bor M et al. Outcome of periventricular-intraventricular haemorrhage at five years of age. Dev Med Child Neurol Jan 1993;35:33-41). (Respond: Dr van de Bor, Division of Neonatology, Department of Paediatrics, University Hospital Leiden, PO Box 9600, 2300 RC Leiden, The Netherlands).

COMMENT. The small number of survivors with grades III and IV hemorrhage was attributed to the widely used policy in the Netherlands of withdrawing life-support from infants with severe cerebral damage.

Of 65 in this category, 47 died in the neonatal period. At the 5 year evaluation, only 25% of the patients had had severe hemorrhage. Children with only mild hemorrhage had a significantly increased risk of disability at the age of 5 years. Patients with evidence of periventricular leukomalacia were excluded from this study.-Editor. *Ped Neur Briefs* March 1993.

HEMORRHAGIC STROKE IN INFANTS AND CHILDREN

Medical and autopsy records, and brain imaging studies of 178 children with possible stroke within the Greater Cincinnati metropolitan area child population of almost 300,000 during 1988 and 1989 were reviewed in the Departments of Neurology and Neuroradiology, University of Cincinnati and Children's Hospital Medical Centers. Stroke occurred in 16 cases (13 whites and 3 blacks), with an overall yearly incidence rate of 2.7 strokes per 100,000 children. The rate was similar for blacks and whites and for boys and girls. The combined incidence rate for intracerebral and subarachnoid hemorrhage of 1.5 per 100,000 was slightly greater than the rate for cerebral infarction of 1.2 per 100,000. Hemorrhagic stroke was related to arteriovenous malformation in 3 cases, cavernous hemangioma in 2, hypothalamic glioma in 2, and aneurysm in one. Mortality for hemorrhagic stroke was 22% as compared to 14% for cerebral infarction. (Broderick J et al. Stroke in children within a major metropolitan area: the surprising importance of intracerebral hemorrhage. J Child Neurol July 1993;8:250-255). (Respond: Dr Joseph Broderick, University of Cincinnati, Dept of Neurology, 231 Bethesda Ave, Cincinnati, OH 45267).

COMMENT. In 81 children <17 yrs of age evaluated for stroke at the Medical College of Georgia, hemorrhagic stroke occurred in only 16 (20%), of whom 12 had intracerebral and 4 subarachnoid hemorrhage. Seizures occurred in 47%, and were recurrent in 26%. A late onset of seizures and cortical infarction were risk factors for recurrent seizures.(Yang JS, Park YD, Hartlage P. Ann Neurol Sept

1993;34:445, abstr).-Editor. *Ped Neur Briefs* Sept 1993.

MOYAMOYA

MOYAMOYA DISEASE: RESULTS OF SURGERY

An angiographic study of the effects of encephalo-duro-arteriosynangiosis (EDAS) in 27 children with moyamoya disease is reported from the Departments of Radiology and Neurosurgery, Tokyo Medical and Dental University, Tokyo, Japan. Comparing pre- and post-operative angiograms, the development of collaterals from the external carotid arterial system into the middle cerebral artery territory was excellent in 16 of 54 cerebral hemispheres after EDAS, good in 25 and poor in 13. The development of collateral vessels from the ECA to the MCA territory increased with the severity of the stenosis of the ICA on preoperative angiograms, but in most advanced stages the development of collateral supply was less marked. The development of collateral vessels was associated with a decrease of abnormal net-like vessels. Stenosis in the ICA had progressed on 12 of the 54 cerebral hemispheres as compared with preoperative angiograms. (Yamada I, Matsushima Y, Suzuki S. Childhood moyamoya disease before and after encephalo-duro-arteriosynangiosis: an angiographic study. Neuroradiology Aug 1992;34:318-322.) (Correspondence: Dr. Yamada or Dr. Matsushima, Departments of Radiology and Neurosurgery, School of Medicine, Tokyo Medical and Dental University, Tokyo, Japan.)

COMMENT. This study suggests that EDAS for childhood moyamoya disease should be performed as early as possible so that the development of irreversible ischemia and permanent neurological defects may possibly be prevented.

Cerebral blood flow (CBF) reactivity to hyperventilation in children with moyamoya disease was studied at the Department of Neurosurgery, Hokkaido University School of Medicine, Sapporo, Japan

(Isobe M et al. Neurol Surg April 1992;20:407). CBF was measured by single photon emission CT (SPECT) in 11 children divided into bypass and non-bypass groups. There was some hemodynamic insufficiency in the frontal lobes of the non-bypass group who underwent procedures such as EDAS. The reduction of CBF was less after hyperventilation, especially in the frontal lobes of the bypass group in which a much better collateral blood flow occurs.-Editor. *Ped Neur Briefs* Sept 1992.

MOYAMOYA DISEASE AND HEMIPLEGIC MIGRAINE

A 6-year-old girl presenting with a 6-month history of classical familial migraine, complicated by transitory hemiparesis and moyamoya disease diagnosed by MRI, is reported from the Kaiser Permanente Medical Center, Hayward, CA. Headaches occurred each week and were associated with nausea, vomiting, and photophobia. She awoke on 3 occasions with right-sided weakness, numbness, and garbled speech. All symptoms resolved after two hours of sleep. Neurologic exam was normal between attacks. MRI showed bilateral occlusion of the carotid arteries and increased vascularity of collateral vessels in the basal ganglia, consistent with moyamoya. (Bernstein AL Hemiplegic migraine and moyamoya disease. AJDC July 1993;147:718-719). (Respond: Dr Bernstein, Dept of Neurology, Kaiser Permanente Medical Center, 27400 Hesperian Blvd, Hayward, CA 94545).

COMMENT. Children with a diagnosis of hemiplegic migraine may have a vascular malformation or moyamoya disease as the underlying pathology. The clinical course depends on the rapidity and extent of vascular occlusion and the ability to develop a collateral circulation. Early diagnosis and surgical revascularization have been advocated because of the risk of permanent neurologic deficits. (See Ped Neur Briefs July 1987, and Progress in Pediatric Neurology, Chicago, PNB Publ, 1991, pp389-391).-Editor. *Ped Neur Briefs* July 1993.

VENOUS THROMBOSIS

NEONATAL CEREBRAL VENOUS THROMBOSIS

The clinical presentation and management of 7 neonates with idiopathic cerebral venous thrombosis (CVT) are reported from the Floating Hospital for Infants and Children, New England Medical Center Hospitals, Tufts University School of Medicine, Boston, MA. Unexplained seizures in 3 infants and unexplained lethargy in 4 led to neurological evaluation and the diagnosis of CVT. Follow-up neurological evaluation through 6 months of age showed normal development. Conventional magnetic resonance images indicated more extensive thrombosis than was suggested by cranial CT. MR phase imaging confirmed thrombosis and established absence of blood flow in cerebral veins or sinuses. No infant received treatment with anticoagulants. (Rivkin MJ et al. Neonatal idiopathic cerebral venous thrombosis: an unrecognized cause of transient seizures or lethargy. Ann Neurol July 1992;32:51-56.) (Correspondence: Dr. Rivkin, New England Medical Center Hospitals, Box 330, Division of Pediatric Neurology, 750 Washington St., Boston, MA 02111.)

COMMENT. Cerebral venous thrombosis may explain transient neonatal seizures or lethargy in newborn infants and may be diagnosed by MR and MR phase imaging.-Editor. *Ped Neur Briefs* Sept 1992.

HEMIPLEGIA WITH SUPERIOR SAGITTAL SINUS THROMBOSIS

A 2-year-old boy who developed a thrombosis of the superior sagittal sinus due to inherited protein S deficiency is reported from the Hospital de Cruces, Vizcaya, Spain. While recovering from pneumonia, the patient had symptoms of an acute disseminated intravascular coagulation disorder associated with sinus thrombosis, left hemiparesis, focal seizures, and thrombosis of the left femoral vein. The paresis resolved within two months. (Prats JM et al. Superior sagittal sinus thrombosis in a child with protein S deficiency. Neurology Dec 1992;42:2303-5). (Reprints: Dr

Jose Maria Prats, Neuropediatric Unit, Hospital de Cruces, 48903 Baracaldo, Vizcaya, Spain).

COMMENT. Homozygous protein S deficiency, an autosomal dominant trait with partial penetrance, usually presents with purpura fulminans in the newborn period. Heterozygous cases are responsible for recurrent peripheral thromboembolisms mainly in adults. Cerebral venous thrombosis is a rare complication of protein S deficiency, but should be considered in the etiology of acute hemiparesis in children.-Editor. *Ped Neur Briefs* Jan 1993.

ANEURYSMS

OCULOMOTOR PARESIS AND BASILAR ANEURYSM The clinical and pathologic findings in a 10 month old girl with congenital heart disease who died after rupture of a congenital distal basilar artery aneurysm are reported from the University of Connecticut Health Center, Farmington, CT and the Children's Hospital of Philadelphia, PA. She was hospitalized at 10 months of age after having had 4 syncopal episodes within a 6 week interval. Twenty-four hours after cardiac catherization the infant developed an adduction deficit of the left eye which resolved over the next 36 hours. Five days after surgical correction of the cardiac defect she had a massive subarachnoid hemorrhage. (DiMario FJ Jr., Rorke LB. Transient oculomotor nerve paresis in congenital distal basilar artery aneurysm. Pediatr Neurol July/Aug 1992;8:303-306.) (Communications: Dr. DiMario, Division of Neurology, University of Connecticut Health Center, 263 Farmington Avenue, Farmington, CT 06030.)

COMMENT. Transient third nerve paresis in an infant with a history of recurrent syncope and congenital heart disease should suggest a possible intracranial arterial aneurysm. The authors found 6 previous reports of basilar aneurysm preceded by a transient third nerve dysfunction. A migraine variant is another explanation (Shevell MI et al. Ann Neurol Sept 1992;32:484 (abstr)).-Editor. *Ped Neur Briefs* Oct

1992.

ASYMPTOMATIC ANEURYSMS AND HIV INFECTION

Aneurysms of major cerebral arteries in two children, aged 11 and 12 years, infected with human immunodeficiency virus from blood transfusions are reported from the National Institutes of Health, Bethesda, MD, and Georgetown University Hospital, Washington, DC. The incidence among 250 children treated and monitored with MRI was 0.8 percent. The aneurysms developed and progressed during therapy and follow-up but were asymptomatic. The role of HIV infection in these lesions was undetermined. (Husson RN et al. Cerebral artery aneurysms in children infected with human immunodeficiency virus. J Pediatr Dec 1992;121: 927-930). (Reprints: Philip A Pizzo MD, Pediatric Branch, National Cancer Institute, Bldg 10, Rm 13N240, 900 Rockville Pike, Bethesda, MD 20892).

COMMENT. CNS involvement in children with HIV infection is common and is frequently manifested with cognitive dysfunction or regression of developmental milestones. Calcifications in the basal ganglia and frontal lobes, white matter changes, and cerebral atrophy are the usual MRI findings. Cerebrovascular disease is an uncommon but potentially hazardous complication. (See Ped Neur Briefs Aug 1991;5:57-58, for further discussion of CNS involvement in HIV infection).-Editor. *Ped Neur Briefs* Feb 1993.

LATERAL MEDULLARY SYNDROME FOLLOWING VARICELLA

The acute onset of lateral medullary (Wallenberg's) syndrome in a 6-year-old boy 32 days after varicella infection is reported from the Children's Hospital, Harvard Med Sch, Boston. He presented with headache, dizziness, nausea and vomiting, blurred vision, and a tendency to fall to the right. Signs included anisocoria (ipsilateral Horner's sign), right ptosis, nystagmus, dysmetria, Romberg's sign, ataxia, and hypalgesia in left leg. CT was normal but MRI showed high T2 signal in right medulla. Sequelae at 5 months were bilateral exophoria, head tilt, rotary nystagmus, and hypoesthesia of right face. (Kovacs SO et al. Lateral medullary syndrome following varicella infection. AJDC Aug 1993;147:823-825). (Reprints: Dr Karl Kuban, Dept Neurology, Children's Hospital, 300 Longwood Ave, Boston, MA 02115).

COMMENT. The signs and symptoms together with MRI findings point to lateral medullary infarction in the distribution of the posterior inferior cerebellar artery. Vasculitis was the most likely pathology.-Editor. *Ped Neur Briefs* Sept 1993.

MULTIPLE ARTERIOVENOUS SHUNTS

Symptoms, management, and outcome of 13 cases of multiple cerebral arteriovenous malformations (MAVMs) are reported from the Centre Hospitalier de Bicetre, France. The age ranged from 6 months to 15 years. The incidence of MAVM among the pediatric population with brain AVMs was 16.9%. Congenital and acquired types were distinguished. Hemorrhage was the presenting symptom in 31%. Spontaneous regression occurred in 15%. Angiogenesis, or sprouting around a true AVM following hemorrhage, may account for some acquired MAVMs. Embolization was the most successful mode of treatment, but anatomical cure was rarely obtained. (Iizuka Y et al. Multiple cerebral arteriovenous shunts in children: report of 13 cases. Child's Nerv Syst Dec 1992;8:437-444). (Correspondence: P Lasjaunias MD, Service de Neuroradiologie, Centre Hospitalier de Bicetre, 78, Rue du General Leclerc, F-94275 Le Kremlin Bicetre Cedex, France).

COMMENT. The rate of serious morbidity following a hemorrhage from an AVM is about 30% and the mortality is about 10%. AVMs in children are more apt to bleed than those in adults. Total excision seems the treatment of choice when feasible. (See Progress in Pediatric Neurology, Ed Millichap JG, Chicago, PNB Publishers, 1991). With multiple AVMs in the present study, embolization was preferred.-Editor. *Ped Neur Briefs* Feb 1993.

CARDIAC SURGERY AND BRAIN INJURY

The incidence of perioperative brain injury after deep hypothermia with circulatory arrest was compared to that associated with low-flow cardiopulmonary bypass during repair of D-transposition of the great arteries in 171 patients operated within the first three months of age at the Children's Hospital, Boston. Circulatory arrest was associated with a higher likelihood of clinical and EEG seizures, a longer time to the recovery of normal EEG activity, and a greater release of the brain isoenzyme of creatine kinase in the first 6 hours after surgery. The duration of total circulatory arrest was of equal importance to the method of support treatment in predicting the neurologic outcomes. Clinical seizures occurred in 11% of infants with circulatory arrest, but EEG seizure activity was detected in 26%. At time of discharge, the two treatment groups were similar in overall incidence of neurologic abnormalities. (Newburger JW et al. A comparison of the perioperative neurologic effects of hypothermic circulatory arrest versus low-flow cardiopulmonary bypass in infant heart surgery. N Engl J Med Oct 7 1993;329:1057-64). (Reprints: Richard A Jonas MD, Dept of Cardiovascular Surgery, Children's Hospital, 300 Longwood Ave, Boston, MA 02115).

COMMENT. The assessment of the effect of total circulatory arrest on later neurologic and developmental outcome awaits further follow-up by the neurologists who collaborated in this large prospective, randomized clinical study. In an editorial, Dr Julie A Swain of the University of Nevada outlines three mechanisms of neurologic injury in infants undergoing cardiac surgery: 1) mechanical injury from microemboli; 2) alterations in blood flow, distribution, and pressure; and 3) neuropsychological effects of neuroleptic drugs, anxiety, pain, and postoperative isolation. Some protection from cerebral injury is provided by hypothermia and drugs that decrease cerebral metabolism.-Editor. *Ped Neur Briefs* Oct 1993.

CHAPTER 12

CNS TRAUMA

INTRODUCTION

J. Keith Brown, M.D., F.R.C.P.
Paediatric Neurology Department
Royal Hospital for Sick Children
Edinburgh, Scotland, UK

Head injury in children is either due to a) birth trauma (compression head injury), b) accidental injury (penetrating, impact, either acceleration or deceleration) and c) non accidental injury (penetrating, shaking or impact injuries).

Neonatal compression head injury caused distortion, traction and compression of intracranial structures. This resulted in venous tears and bleeding, causing in turn, subdural hematomas, transtentorial bleeds and cerebral edema. Such birth trauma (but not asphyxia) has responded dramatically to preventative measures of "the new obstetrics," ie never let the sun set twice on the same labor (less 24 hours), a one hour second stage and avoid postmaturity. One has a degree of renewed anxiety as these obstetric criteria are now being relaxed again. In the past our own figures showed that severe compression birth injury carried a reasonable prognosis, with 64/82 normal, 7/82 dead and 10/82 surviving with definite handicap.

Road traffic accidents are still the commonest cause of head injury in children (Fig 1). Prevention of accidental injury is the ideal.

Figure 1.

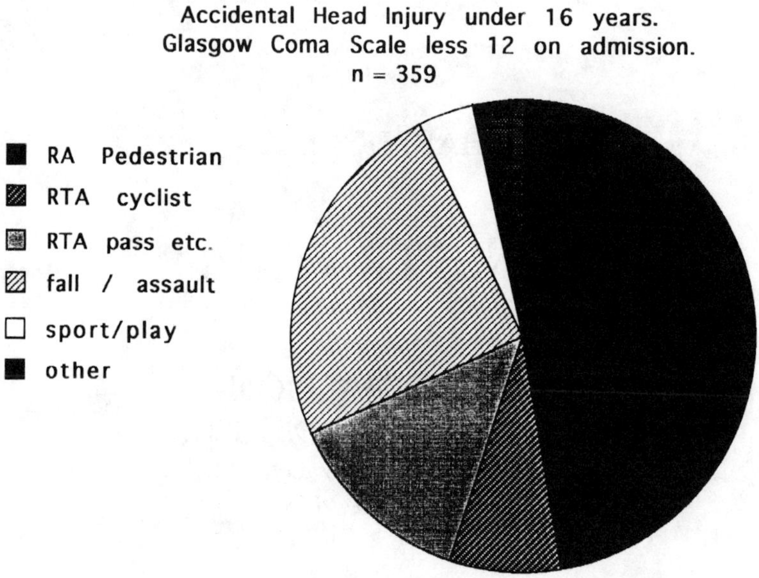

The newer methods of detecting speeding, by the use of speed cameras together with stiffer fines, tighter control of drink and drive by spot breathalyser checks, and the compulsory use of rear as well as front seat belts, do appear to be making a definite impact on the number of children seriously injured. It is known that the majority of head injury patients who die do so, not from traumatic injury to the brain or compression from blood clot, but because of extensive hypoxic ischemic damage. Up to 40% of patients who die actually speak after the accident, which emphasizes that it is not necessarily the impact which kills but rather the secondary effects of hypotensive shock, loss of airway, brain swelling and raised intracranial pressure causing hypoxic ischemic damage. The idea of a therapeutic window, ie a short period of time after the actual accident during which one has a chance to prevent further damage, is the basis of most intensive care unit management. The need for immediate stabilization of airway and management of shock at the site of the accident is therefore strongly supported. Although surgical removal of extradural clot is imperative, this is more easily diagnosed early with the use of modern imaging. If one closes ones eyes at any meeting on head injury, one might be excused for being unsure whether the meeting was about perinatal asphyxia, problems of cardiac bypass surgery or status epilepticus. Glutamate toxicity and the place of brain protective agents are heatedly discussed at all three, having as the basic aim the prevention of secondary neuronal necrosis from ischemia. The continuous monitoring of intracranial pressure, blood pressure, arterio-venous oxygen differentials, with controlled ventilation, barbiturate protection, mannitol etc, are recommended to achieve this goal.

The severity of a head injury was judged retrospectively in the past by the duration of retrograde and post-traumatic amnesia. Now, this evaluation is aided prospectively by the Glasgow coma scale, although the scale needs modification for use in very young children or those with facial lacerations, swelling, or in patients already intubated when first examined. The prevalence of accidental head injury appears to be falling, and secondary prevention is succeeding in reducing some long term handicaps. An overall low mortality of less than 10% may be expected in moderate and severely head injured children less than 16 years of age with a GCS on admission of <12; the expected mortality is only 1 in 1000 in children with minor head injuries and a normal or near normal GCS.(Table 1).

Table 1.- Head Injury in Children < 16 years. n = 1442.

Severity / n	*G. C. S.*	*No. / deaths*
Severe / 188	< 8	41/ 22%
Moderate/184	9 - 12	1/ 0.5%
Mild / 1070	13 - 15	1/ 0.09%

Over 80% should show a very good recovery, but this hides the need for good rehabilitation facilities (Fig. 2). Claims of "complete" recovery, ie walk, talk and normal intelligence, and a good outcome in terms of residual behavior, psychiatric and schooling problems, especially spelling, epilepsy, and unemployment in up to 33% of cases of head injury, have been doubted (Klonoff et al. 1993).

Figure 2.

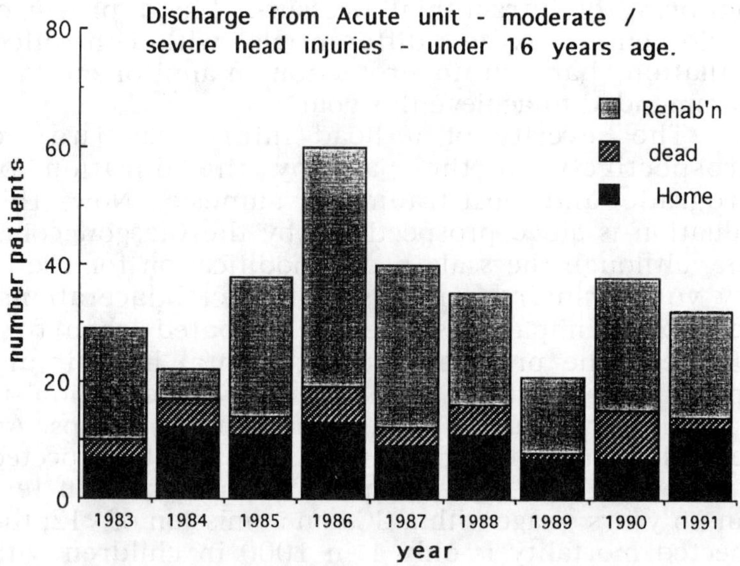

We are not seeing any reduction in numbers of non-accidental head injuries, possibly an increase. These injuries are associated with massive cerebral edema and vascular damage (intracerebral and extracerebral) which do not respond well to secondary preventative measures. The acute cerebral edema causes brain necrosis, and attempts at surgery may necessitate amputation of brain tissue to obtain closure, Mannitol and hyperventilation are not as successful in these cases as in children with accidental injuries. It would appear that the mechanism of damage by shaking (21 cases) and repeated rotational injury plus impact (15 cases) causes more vascular damage to the brain than simple accidental impact. Impact as well as shaking - the impact shaking injury - may be more common than appreciated because of lack of local bruising or fractures. Compression of the chest, causing a high central venous pressure with venous rupture in the eye (Purtcher retinopathy), may also make the differential rotational inertia between skull and brain or grey and white matter more likely to rupture engorged veins. Penetrating injuries from shooting or knife wounds are very rare in the U.K.

The subdural hematoma present in 21 / 37 cases usually resolves, and hydrocephalus requiring shunting develops in 33%. Diffuse ischemic necrosis is seen on CT, with subsequent cerebral atrophy and failure of brain growth causing microencephaly. Tears in brain substance can be identified on ultrasound. The number of children dying (12 / 37) is approximately the same as those who are normal (13 / 37); 12 have mental handicap, epilepsy or cerebral palsy. (Brown and Minns, 1993). These figures of 1/3 dead, 1/3 normal and 1/3 handicapped are much worse than those for birth trauma or accidental injury. Non-accidental injury in children is near exceeding accidental trauma as a cause of long-term handicap. - *J. Keith Brown, M.D., F.R.C.P., Paediatric Neurology Department, Royal Hospital for Sick Children, Edinburgh, Scotland, U.K.*

BIBLIOGRAPHY

Brown JK, Minns RA. Non-accidental head injury with particular reference to whiplash shaking injury. Dev Med Child Neurol 1993;35:849-869; Ped Neur Briefs Dec 1993.

Klonoff H, Clark C, Klonoff PS. Long-term outcome of head injuries: a 23 year follow up study of children with head injuries. J Neurol Neurosurg Psychiatry 1993;56:410-415.

Miller D. Edinburgh Head injury statistics bank (access gratefully acknowledged).

DELAYED COGNITIVE ABNORMALITIES AND FRONTAL LOBE DAMAGE

The consequences of early frontal lobe damage, restricted to the polar and mesial portion of the left prefrontal cortex and deep white matter, on higher cognitive and psychologic development are reported in a 33-year-old woman who sustained injury at 7 years of age and was evaluated at the Division of Behavioral Neurology and Cognitive Neuroscience, University of Iowa College of Medicine, Iowa City. The birth and milestones of development were normal, and academic achievement was average before she sustained a spontaneous intraparenchymal cerebral hemorrhage at 7 years. Her neurological exam was normal and generalized tonic clonic seizures were controlled with medication. MRI revealed the lesion in the left prefrontal cortex and deep white matter, and cerebral blood flow studies were abnormal in left and right frontal regions. Defects in higher cognition were noted especially in self regulation of emotion and affect and in social behavior. These were of delayed onset and were followed by a period of progression and finally an arrest of development in adolescence. The progressive impairment resulted from a discrepancy between the demands of adolescent development and the altered maturation of frontal lobe neural and cognitive systems. The patient failed to acquire the executive and self regulatory processes associated with frontal lobe function. (Eslinger PJ et al. Developmental consequences of childhood frontal lobe damage. Arch Neurol July 1992;49:764-769.) (Reprints- Dr. Eslinger, Division of Neurology, The Milton S. Hershey Medical Center, 500 University Drive, Hershey, PA 17033.)

COMMENT. In this patient, the brain damage syndrome was the result of an intraparenchymal cerebral hemorrhage and injury sustained in childhood. A variety of neuropsychological syndromes including Gerstmann's Syndrome are described as a consequence of lesions or stimulation to the left posterior perisylvian territory (Benton AL. Gerstmann's syndrome. Arch Neurol May 1992;49:445-447). A cortical stimulation study in a 17-year-old epileptic boy had shown that repeated stimulation of different loci in the posterior perisylvian region had elicited diverse cognitive syndromes (i.e. acalculia, agraphia, alexia, anomia, constructional apraxia, finger agnosia, and right-left disorientation). Stimulation of adjacent loci, between the angular and supra-marginal gyri, had produced a complete Gerstmann syndrome without accompanying deficits.-Editor. *Ped Neur Briefs* Aug 1992.

HEAD INJURY IN VERY YOUNG CHILDREN

A prospective study of 100 children aged 24 months or younger who were admitted with a diagnosis of head injury is reported from the Children's Hospital of Philadelphia and Rhode Island Hospital, Providence. Falls accounted for the majority of injuries (73) and motor vehicle accidents occurred in 9, the child being unrestrained in 6. Thirty-two children had a soft tissue injury and/or concussion only. Twenty-seven had a linear skull fracture with or without loss of consciousness. There were 8 depressed fractures, 3 children had epidural hematomas and 22 had intradural hemorrhages. Twenty-four children had inflicted injuries and an additional 32 had child maltreatment consults because of social problems and suspicion of neglect. Most household falls were neurologically benign. Intradural hemorrhage was more likely to occur from motor vehicle accidents and inflicted injury. Retinal hemorrhages found in 10 patients were related to inflicted injuries in 9 and all had subdural hemorrhage, the majority complicated by seizures. Of 4 deaths in the series, 1 was accidental and 3 were inflicted; all had subdural hemorrhage. These more serious injuries were related to rotational rather than translational forces. (Duhaime, AC et al. Head injury in very young children: mechanisms, injury types, and ophthalmologic findings in 100 hospitalized patients younger than 2 years of age. Pediatrics Aug 1992;90:179-185.) (Reprints: A.C. Duhaime, M.D., Department of Neurosurgery, Children's Hospital, 34th and Civic Center Blvd., Philadelphia, PA 19104.)

COMMENT. Accidental head injuries in very

young children are common and inflicted injury accounts for nearly 1/4 of admissions. The occurrence of retinal hemorrhages and more severe brain damage should arouse suspicion of an inflicted injury. Social or family problems are a major risk factor for the occurrence of severe head injuries in the very young.

Serial head circumference determinations may help in the diagnosis of subdural hemorrhage following head injury in young children. A study which limits the value of the head circumference test is reported from the Bnai Zion Medical Center, Haifa, Israel (Jaffe M et al. Variability in head circumference growth rate during the first 2 years of life. Pediatrics Aug 1992;90:190-192). Of 415 healthy children studied, 51% demonstrated variable HC tracking of which 19% showed acceleration in head growth. This so-called "physiological variability" in HC can involve more than 2 centile lines and the fluctuations stabilized usually by the age of 13 months. The authors suggest a period of clinical observation rather than imaging procedures in a baby whose HC crosses centile curves but whose general health, psychomotor development and neurological status are all within normal limits.-Editor. *Ped Neur Briefs* Sept 1992.

BRAIN DAMAGE AND VIOLENCE

The neurologist's role in understanding violence and brain damage as a neurological defense of violent crime are reviewed by neurologists at Georgetown University, Washington, DC. Pincus stresses the role of biological factors as contributory to aggressive behavior and notes that cognitive impairment, lapses of attention, and psychotic symptoms are more common among violent compared to nonviolent criminals. He concludes that programs of research targeting brain damage and child abuse as causes of violence might lead to more effective preventive methods of management than prisonexpansion. Resnak points out that the majority of violent criminals have no history or evidence of brain damage and concludes that neurology will not solve the mystery of violent behavior and murder. Admitting that many murderers have a higher incidence of epilepsy, head injury, child abuse, malnutrition, and learning disabilities, but the majority of epileptics, abused, and mentally retarded do not commit violence. Both experts agree that brain damage can decrease the threshold for violent, impulsive behavior, and serve as a mitigating factor in determining responsibility and defense for some crimes. (Pincus JH. Neurologist's role in understanding violence. Arch Neurol Aug 1993;50:867-869. Restak R. The neurological defense of violent crime. 'Insanity defense' retooled. Arch Neurol Aug 1993;50:869-871). (Reprints: Dr Resnak, Neurology Associates, 1800 R St NW C-3, Washington, DC; Dr Pincus, Georgetown University Hospital, 3800 Reservoir Rd NW, Washington, DC 20007).

COMMENT. Three criteria are required by law for alleged brain damage to serve as a mitigating factor in determining responsibility. 1) Is there evidence of *brain damage* (deviation from normal brain structure) and is it reponsible for a *deficit* (impairment or loss or alteration of intelligence and emotion, and behavioral abnormality)?; 2) Is the deficit a contributing cause of the defendant's crime?; 3) Without the deficit and resulting behavior, would the crime not have happened? Of 14 death row juveniles who had committed capital crimes, 11 had suffered head trauma, 9 had abnormal EEGs or neurologic examinations, and 12 gave a history of physical or sexual abuse (Lewis DO, Pincus JH et al. Am J Psychiatry 1988;145:584). Brain damage may unleash violence, but it does not explain it, according to Hachinski V. (Arch Neurol Aug 1993;50:871).

A study of frontal lobe-subcortical circuits in the mediation of a wide range of human behavioral disorders, reported from the Departments of Neurology, Psychiatry and Biobehavioral Sciences, UCLA School of Medicine, Los Angeles, CA (Cummings JL. Arch Neurol Aug 1993;50:873-880) demonstrates that we should not entirely dismiss a possible role of brain damage in crimes of violence.-Editor. *Ped Neur Briefs* Aug 1993.

SHAKEN BABY SYNDROME

Non-accidental head injury, with particular reference to whiplash shaking injury, is reviewed by pediatric neurologists at the Royal Hospital for Sick Children, Edinburgh. Of 30 children with non-accidental head injury followed by the authors, 17 were due to shaking and 13 to impact. Subdural hematoma was diagnosed in 16 (53%), subarachnoid hemorrhage in 3, and intracerebral hemorrhage in 4. Eleven (37%) developed post-hemorrhagic hydrocephalus. Velocity, the number of shakes per second, and duration are important components of degree of injury. The most common age for whiplash abuse is 5 months, when the head is large in relation to the body, and the neck muscles and head control are weak. Shaking injuries are rare after the second year. Vascular, midbrain, and white matter shearing injuries, cerebral edema, and retinal and subdural hemorrhages result. The clinical diagnosis and medico-legal aspects of non-accidental head injury are discussed in detail. (Brown JK, Minns RA. Non-accidental head injury, with particular reference to whiplash shaking injury and medico-legal aspects. Dev Med Child Neurol Oct 1993;35:849-869). (Respond: Dr JK Brown, Royal Hospital for Sick Children, Sciennes Road, Edinburgh EH9 1LF, Scotland).

COMMENT. Despite an increase in support services and media publicity, non-accidental head injury remains the leading cause of death or long-term disability among child abuse cases in Scotland and in the USA. The American Academy of Pediatrics Committee on Child Abuse and Neglect review the "Shaken baby syndrome: Inflicted cerebral trauma" in the current issue of Pediatrics Dec 1993;92:872-875. Subtle or mild trauma is particularly difficult to diagnose, often mistaken for viral illness, feeding problems, or infant colic.-Editor. *Ped Neur Briefs* Dec 1993.

CHAPTER 13

INFECTIOUS DISEASES

AIDS and the NERVOUS SYSTEM

INTRODUCTION

Anita L. Belman, M.D.
Department of Neurology, SUNY at Stony Brook, NY

Central nervous system [CNS] involvement frequently complicates the course of HIV-1 infection and AIDS in infants and children. The CNS may be affected by: 1) HIV-1 itself, due to either the direct or indirect effects of HIV-1 on the CNS, HIV-1 associated CNS disease, or 2) secondary complications associated with immunodeficiency.

Early in the AIDS epidemic, CNS involvement was recognized as a frequent complication in infants and children. It was noted that by the time HIV-1 infection had advanced to "full blown" AIDS, cognitive and motor impairments of varying duration, progression and severity were extremely common. It was also noted that in the majority of these children, CNS dysfunction was not due to opportunistic infections or neoplasms. Neurologic, neuropathologic, and virologic investigations from various clinical and laboratory studies indicated that the CNS was infected by HIV-1. A recent consensus report on nomenclature suggested that the term "HIV associated progressive encephalopathy of childhood" be adopted to replace AIDS encephalopathy and other terms found in the literature to describe the CNS abnormalities directly related to HIV-1 infection.

NOMENCLATURE. Initially two forms of encephalopathy were described, "progressive" and "static." As children were followed longitudinally several patterns of disease were recognized. Based on progression and severity of neurologic deficits, the terms "subacute progressive" and "plateau" were introduced to allow further clinical characterization. The spectrum and diversity of "HIV-1 encephalopathy" is much wider than previously appreciated, and the term "HIV-1 associated CNS disease" is used by this investigator to refer to a syndrome complex or complexes with a constellation of cognitive, motor and behavioral manifestations. The prevalence of "encephalopathy" in children with advanced HIV-1 disease ranged from 31%-83% in various cohorts studied.

DIAGNOSIS. The diagnosis of HIV-1 associated progressive encephalopathy is relatively straight forward if the patient has been followed prospectively. Examination will reveal *progressive* motor involvement. The infant may lose head control, develop axial hypotonia, and upper motor neuron signs. The toddler or older child may have a change in gait, become hyperreflexic, refuse to walk and over time, develop progressive corticospinal tract signs, or less frequently, ataxia. Concomitant cognitive problems with a decline in psychometric test scores may also occur.

Diagnostic difficulties often arise when an HIV-1 infected youngster is found, at the initial neurologic evaluation, to have neurologic deficits or "delays" in mental or motor development or both. A psychological assessment and reevaluation by the neurologist and psychologist in 2-4 months are advised. Neuroimaging studies and head circumference measurements are very helpful; evidence of atrophy accompanied by acquired microcephaly strengthens the diagnosis.

Secondary CNS complications must be considered in the differential diagnosis of the child with HIV-1 infection who presents with the new onset of neurologic deficits, headache, seizures, or mental status changes. Cytomegalovirus encephalitis and *C. albicans* meningitis and microabscesses are the most frequent opportunistic infections reported. Neoplasms (mainly lymphoma) and strokes may also complicate the course of HIV-1 infection in children.

THERAPY. Clinical trials in progress are investigating various antiretroviral agents, different dosage regimens, combination therapies, and immunomodulating agents. New "targets" for therapy are in investigation and new protocols are in development. In parallel are rehabilitation programs, including infant stimulation programs, therapeutic nursery schools, and special educational classes, as well as physical and occupational therapy programs.

FUTURE RESEARCH. In order to care for these children and to design rational approaches for treatment and prevention, it is now critical to develop a better understanding of how HIV-1 affects the developing nervous system. Areas of research to be addressed include: prevention of maternal HIV-1 infection and maternal-fetal transmission, timing of congenital HIV-1 infection and route of CNS invasion, pathophysiologic mechanisms of HIV-1 associated CNS diseases, correlation with neuroimaging, staging of syndromes, and evaluation of therapies. - *Anita L. Belman, M.D., Departments of Neurology and Pediatrics, School of Medicine, State University of New York at Stony Brook, NY.*

BIBLIOGRAPHY

American Academy of Neurology AIDS Task Force. Nomenclature and research case definitions for neurologic manifestations of human immunodeficiency virus type 1. Neurology 1991;41:778-785.

Belman, AL. AIDS and the child's central nervous system. Pediatric Neurology. Pediatr Clin North Am 1992;39:691-714.

Belman AL. Central nervous system involvement in pediatric HIV-1 infection, an overview. Int Pediatr 1992;7:126-135.

Belman AL et al. Neurologic status of infants born to HIV-1 infected mothers and their controls: a prospective study from birth to 24 months of age. Neurology 1993;43:A347.

CNS INVOLVEMENT IN HIV INFECTION

The neurological findings in 41 HIV-seropositive children are described from the Departments of Paediatric Neurology and Hematology and Oncology, Zentrum der Kinderheilkunde, Goethe Universitat, Frankfurt, Germany. 23 children were symptomatic. HIV encephalopathy was manifested by acquired microcephaly, developmental regression and progressive motor deterioration. Progressive pyramidal signs, ankle clonus and generalized muscle weakness were documented for 6 children, 4 had extrapyramidal and cerebellar symptoms, and 5 infants of drug-addicted HIV infected mothers had seizures during the neonatal period. Behavioral changes consisting of aggression, anxiety and depression were noted in 5 children. Autistic behavior combined with deterioration in play and loss of language skills developed in one child. 4 patients had recurrent headaches which disappeared in 3 cases after treatment with azidothymidine (AZT). 8 children treated with immunoglobulin therapy (IVIG) and 7 treated with IVIG and AZT have not deteriorated neurologically since therapy began (Schmidt B et al. Central nervous system involvement of children with HIV infection. Dev Med Child Neurol June 1991;33:535-540).

COMMENT. The differentiation of static and progressive encephalopathy is sometimes difficult. The majority of HIV infected children have developmental delay and deficits in cognitive functions, language and motor skills. Seizures are an uncommon feature and usually an isolated event associated with fever or opportunistic CNS infection. Opportunistic CNS infections are uncommon with childhood HIV infection. Isolated cases of cerebrovascular involvement including intracranial hemorrhage and ischemic infarctions have occurred among children with immune thrombocytopenia or arteritis. Acute hemiplegia secondary to a large infarct is described in a 16-month-old infant with congenitally acquired HIV infection (Kugler SL et al. Ped. Neurol May/June 1991;7:207-10). School achievement and tasks requiring motor speed, attention and concentration were impaired at 4-8 years of age in 15 HIV-1 seropositive children infected through neonatal blood transfusion (Cohen SE et al. Pediatrics July 1991;88:58-68).

CT scans may demonstrate enlarged CSF spaces and bilateral symmetrical calcification of the basal ganglia and frontal white matter in 17-61% (Belman A L et al. A J D C 1988;142:29-35). Wiley C A et al. report neocortical damage during HIV infection in an autopsy study of adults (Ann Neurol June 1991;29:651-657). Wizdicks E F M et al. report a fatal disseminated hemorrhagic toxoplasmotic encephalopathy as the initial manifestation of AIDS in a 28 year-old woman (Ann Neurol June 1991;29:683-686).-Editor. *Ped Neur Briefs* Aug 1991.

MYOPATHY IN ZIDOVUDINE TREATED HIV INFECTION

Elevations in serum CK levels in 80% of 87 children enrolled in a multi-centered trial of oral zidovudine treatment for symptomatic HIV infection are reported from the Department of Pediatrics, University Medical Center, Durham, NC. A myopathy developed in a 3 year old girl with acquired HIV infection who received long-term zidovudine therapy. Muscle biopsy was consistent with a non-inflammatory myopathy but a beneficial response to prednisone suggested an inflammatory component. Severe neurologic impairment related to HIV encephalopathy masked the early signs of proximal muscle weakness. Electron microscopy revealed no mitochondrial changes. She had received zidovudine (180 mg/m^2 every 6 hours) for two years. Therapy was discontinued because of fever and neutropenia. The CK level fell from a peak of 25,945 IU/L to 185 IU/L at the time of discharge. (Walter E B et al. Myopathy in human immunodeficiency virus-infected children receiving long-term zidovudine therapy. J Pediatr July 1991;119:152-155).

COMMENT. Myopathy associated with HIV infection is usually an inflammatory polymyositis with proximal muscle weakness and an elevated CK level. It may also be non-inflammatory or linked to treatment with antiretroviral agents such as zidovudine. Myopathy associated with zidovudine is characterized by reversible changes in muscle mitochondria, whereas mitochondrial features are normal in specimens from HIV infected patients not receiving zidovudine.

Low-dose zidovudine in 65 children with HIV-l infection acquired in the perinatal period was well tolerated in a study reported from the Pediatric Neurology Division, Bicetre Hospital, Institut National de la Sante et de la Recherce Medicale, France (Blanche S et al. Pediatrics Aug 1991;88:364-370). The dosage (400 mg/m^2 per day) was lower than that used in the above myopathy case report (720 mg/m^2 daily). Moderate elevations in CK levels are to be expected with zidovudine therapy, and muscle biopsy and EMG may be reserved for children with clinical myopathy or markedly elevated CK levels.-Editor. *Ped Neur Briefs* Aug 1991.

ASYMPTOMATIC ANEURYSMS AND HIV INFECTION

Aneurysms of major cerebral arteries in two children, aged 11 and 12 years, infected with human immunodeficiency virus from blood transfusions are reported from the National Institutes of Health, Bethesda, MD, and Georgetown University Hospital, Washington, DC. The incidence among 250 children treated and monitored with MRI was 0.8 percent. The aneurysms developed and progressed during therapy and follow-up but were asymptomatic. The role of HIV infection in these lesions was undetermined. (Husson RN et al. Cerebral artery aneurysms in children infected with human immunodeficiency virus. J Pediatr Dec 1992;121: 927-930). (Reprints: Philip A Pizzo MD, Pediatric Branch, National Cancer Institute, Bldg 10, Rm 13N240, 900 Rockville Pike, Bethesda, MD 20892).

COMMENT. CNS involvement in children with HIV infection is common and is frequently manifested with cognitive dysfunction or regression of developmental milestones. Calcifications in the basal ganglia and frontal lobes, white matter changes, and cerebral atrophy are the usual MRI findings. Cerebrovascular disease is an uncommon but potentially hazardous complication. (See Ped Neur Briefs Aug 1991;5:57-58, for further discussion of CNS involvement in HIV infection).

A recent neuropsychologic study of HIV-infected children with hemophilia at the University of North Carolina, Chapel Hill, suggested an overall trend toward lower motor, attentional, memory, and sensory perceptual functioning. When the results were contrasted to those in a control group of children who also had hemophilia, no significant differences were apparent. The early, subtle psychological deficits could not be attributed solely to CNS effects of HIV infection. (Whitt JK et al. Neuropsychologic functioning of human immunodeficiency virus-infected children with hemophilia. J PediatrJan 1993;122:52-59). (Reprints: JK Whitt MD, Dept of Psychiatry, Campus Box No 7160, University of North Carolina, Chapel Hill, NC 27599).-Editor. *Ped Neur Briefs* Feb 1993.

HIV CNS COMPLICATIONS AND HEMOPHILIA

A multicenter prospective study of the growth and neuropsychological function of 207 boys (mean age 12 years) with hemophilia and seropositive for human immunodeficiency virus type 1 (HIV-l) is reported from the University of Iowa College of Medicine, Iowa City. Head trauma was sustained in 40%, intracranial hemorrhage occurred in 10%, and seizures in 9%. Behavioral disorders in 15% and intracranial infections in 4% of the total were most frequent in the HIV positive group. Neurologic abnormalities involving cranial nerves (11%), deep tendon reflexes (17%), coordination (25%), muscle strength (23%), and tone (31%) were more common in children of 12 years and older. They were similar in frequency in HIV-seronegative and seropositive subjects, except for deep tendon reflexes and muscle tone and bulk, which were more frequently abnormal in seropositive individuals. Substantial neurological dysfunction could be attributed to hemophilia, but HIV-l contributes to the neurologic morbidity of hemophiliacs.(Bale JF Jr et al. Neurologic history and examination results and their relationship to human immunodeficiency virus type 1 serostatus in hemophilic subjects: Results from the hemophilia growth and development study. Pediatrics April 1993;91:736-741). (Reprints: James F Bale Jr MD, Division of Pediatric Neurology, Dept of Pediatrics, University of Iowa Hospitals and Clinics, Iowa City, IA 52242).

COMMENT. The effect of HIV-1 or its treatment on muscle and peripheral nerve was reflected by non-hemophilia-related reductions in muscle tone and bulk, identified only in HIV-1 seropositive subjects. HIV-1 was also responsible for the majority of behavioral disorders and intracranial infections observed in hemophilic children.

Of multiple MRI abnormalities, including arachnoid cysts, focal lesions, and multifocal white-matter lesions, found in 80 of 310 hemophilic boys, only diffuse cerebral atrophy was associated with HIV infection, and only in subjects with compromised immunologic function. (Mitchell WG et al. Pediatrics April 1993;91:742-746). Cerebral atrophy is the most consistent neuroradiological abnormality among children with HIV infection, reported in 85%.(Mintz M, Epstein LG. Neurologic manifestations of pediatric acquired immunodeficiency syndrome: Clinical features and therapeutic approaches. Seminars in Neurology March 1992;12: 51-56).-Editor. *Ped Neur*

Briefs April 1993.

CT ABNORMALITIES WITH HIV ENCEPHALOPATHY

Qualitative analysis of 100 consecutive computed tomographic (CT) studies of the brain in children with symptomatic but untreated acquired immunodeficiency syndrome is reported from the National Institutes of Health, Bethesda, MD, and the Children's National Medical Center, Washington, DC. Evidence of CNS damage from HIV, as expressed by abnormalities on CT, was seen in 86% of patients. Ventricular enlargement was the most frequent abnormality, found in 65 (78%), followed by cortical atrophy in 57 (68%). Less common abnormalities were leukoaraiosis (26%), cerebral calcification (19%), and cerebellar atrophy (12%). Children with encephalopathy (65%) were younger and had more CT abnormalities than nonencephalopathic children. (DeCarli C et al. The prevalence of computed tomographic abnormalities of the cerebrum in 100 consecutive children symptomatic with the human immune deficiency virus. Ann Neurol Aug 1993;34:198-205). (Respond: P Brouwers PhD, Bldg 10, Rm 13N240, National Inst of Health, 9000 Rockville Pike, Bethesda, MD 20892).

COMMENT. Routine use of CT in children with HIV infection may uncover evidence of presymptomatic brain disease. The authors stress the need for early assessment of possible brain involvement and modification of therapy regimens to prevent or ameliorate the onset of encephalopathy. Pathogenetic mechanisms of HIV-type 1 infection of the CNS are discussed by Epstein LG and Gendelman HE (Ann Neurol 1993;33:429). Infected macrophages initiate neurotoxicity, which is then amplified through cell-to-cell interactions with astrocytes.

Low serum vitamin B_{12} levels, often noted in patients with HIV-1 infection, showed no significant relation to neurological abnormalities in 153 HIV-1-positive adults studied at the AIDS Neurological Center, Univ of North Carolina at Chapel Hill, NC. (Robertson KR et al. Arch Neurol 1993;50:807).

In a prospective evaluation of 181 children at risk for perinatal HIV infection, hypotonia at 6 months was related to symptomatic infection whereas hypertonia was not associated with infection at this age. In older HIV-infected children, hypertonia reflects involvement of the brain. Antiretroviral therapy altered progression of HIV encephalopathy (Chiriboga CA, Hauser WA et al. Ann Neurol Sept 1993;34:500, abstract).-Editor. *Ped Neur Briefs* Oct 1993.

ENCEPHALITIS

EPIDEMIOLOGY OF ENCEPHALITIS

The incidence and epidemiology of encephalitis in children have been analyzed in a 20 year survey at the Department of Virology and the Children's Hospital, University of Helsinki, Finland. There were 405 patients with an overall male to female ratio of 1.4:1. Patients were grouped according to age: One to 11 months (33), one to four years (139), five to nine years (159), and ten to 16 years (74). The etiology was determined in 69%; it was unknown among one-half of the youngest children and in only one-fourth of those at least ten years of age. The incidence was highest in children younger than two years (16.7/100,000 child years) and was very low in those 14 to 16 years of age (1/100,000 child years). After the introduction of vaccination against mumps, measles and rubella in 1983, the major encephalitides have been varicella-zoster, Mycoplasma pneumoniae, and respiratory and enteroviruses. Enteroviruses and Herpes simplex were most common in the infants younger than one year of age whereas respiratory viruses and Mycoplasma pneumoniae as well as varicella-zoster dominated in older children. Mumps and varicella were more common in boys, and adenovirus and Mycoplasma pneumoniae were more common in girls. Seasonal accumulation appeared in February and March and the incidence was lower in July and August. (Koskiniemi M et al. Epidemiology of encephalitis in children: a 20-year survey. Ann Neurol May 1991;29:492-497).

COMMENT. This study is important in emphasizing a greater interest in childhood encephalitis and the need for early diagnosis and treatment especially in young infants. The Mayo Clinic study in 1984 had shown that encephalitis in young children is often diagnosed late. The authors suggest that convulsions of unknown origin may be due to ill-defined encephalitis caused by respiratory viruses and adenovirus in winter months and enteroviruses in autumn. The etiology is often difficult to establish but antigen tests for respiratory viruses, adenoviruses, Herpes virus, and Mycobacterium pneumoniae are available and will provide the diagnosis within a few hours.-Editor. *Ped Neur Briefs* June 1991.

POSTENCEPHALITIC TOURETTE SYNDROME

A six year old girl who developed a Tourette-like syndrome following herpes encephalitis is reported from the Division of Child Neurology, Walter Reed Army Medical Center, Washington, DC and Departments of Neurology and Pediatrics, Johns Hopkins University School of Medicine, Baltimore, MD. A three day prodrome of headaches, malaise, nausea and vomiting was followed by fever and focal motor seizures involving the left side of the face and the left arm. Lumbar puncture showed 122 WBCs (80% lymphocytes) and a protein of 31 mg/dl. A repeat lumbar puncture within 24 hours showed 750 WBCs, 43 RBCs, and protein 85 mg/dl. CT on hospital day three and subsequent MRIs showed a small hemorrhagic lesion in the right mesial temporal region and progressive edematous changes in the right temporal lobe, basal ganglia and thalamus. EEG showed focal slowing over the right temporal and frontal lobes. A presumptive diagnosis of herpes encephalitis was made and Acyclovir was given for ten days. At two weeks after discharge she developed eye blinking and sudden rapid recurrent purposeless nonrhythmic stereotyped motor movements and vocalizations. The tics were characterized by facial grimacing, head twitching, and shoulder shrugging plus eye rolling, facial contorsions, jumping, touching objects and body parts and making obscene gestures. Vocal tics included grunting, sniffing, and snorting sounds. The tics were suppressed after several weeks on Pimozide (Orap 1 mg b.i.d.). (Northam RS, Singer HS. Postencephalitic acquired Tourette-like syndrome in a child. Neurology April 1991;41:592-593).

COMMENT. The authors refer to reports of acquired Tourette syndrome in adults. Tics followed withdrawal from neuroleptic medications or in association with herpes and other encephalitides, toxic and metabolic encephalopathies, strokes, cerebral tumors, trauma, multiple sclerosis, syphilis, Huntington's, Alzheimer's, and Creutzfeldt-Jakob diseases.-Editor. *Ped Neur Briefs* June 1991.

RELAPSING HERPES SIMPLEX ENCEPHALITIS WITH CHOREA

Herpes simplex encephalitis (HSE) followed a biphasic course with relapse in 3 children aged 11 years, 9 months, and 11 months reported from the Hospital for Sick Children, London and South Hampton General Hospital, England. All 3 presented with fever and seizures and relapse was accompanied by generalized or hemi-chorea in 2 patients. All patients received repeat courses of acyclovir, antibiotics and anticonvulsants. Dexamethasone was added in the older patient and the acyclovir course was followed by vidarabine in 2 patients. All patients had residual sequelae at discharge: 1 had a mild right facial weakness and persisting dysphasia, another was severely handicapped with persisting chorea and a third was visually inattentive and had a right hemiplegia and left hemichorea. The cause of the relapse was not definitely determined. A possible resistant organism might indicate a longer initial course of high dose acyclovir or alternatively, a post-infectious neuroallergic process might suggest the substitution of immunomodulatory treatment in place of further antiviral treatment (Pike MG et al, Herpes simplex encephalitis with relapse. Arch Dis Child Oct 1991;66:1242-4).

COMMENT. Relapsing herpes simplex encephalitis is not uncommon in adults but is rare in children.

Chorea in association with HSE relapse is of interest. The authors refer to 7 additional patients reported in the literature.

Autism is another unusual sequel to herpes simplex encephalitis described in a 31 year old adult at the University of Goteborg, Sweden. (Gillberg IC. Autistic syndrome with onset at age 31 years: Herpes encephalitis as a possible model for childhood autism. Dev Med Child Neurol Oct 1991;33:920-924). Other cases in the literature have occurred in pre-adolescence. Autism is not necessarily a developmental disorder and temporal lobe damage caused by herpes encephalitis may explain some cases. The Kluver-Bucy syndrome, characterized by emotional instability, hypersexuality and hyperorality, has also been described as a complication of herpes encephalitis when both temporal lobes have been involved.-Editor. *Ped Neur Briefs* Nov 1991.

HERPES SIMPLEX VIRUS ENCEPHALITIS

The difficulties in diagnosis in 6 children aged 13 days to 9 years with herpes simplex encephalitis (HSE) are stressed in a report from the Departments of Child Health and Pathology, University Hospital of Wales, Cardiff. The original diagnoses in 3 cases were post-traumatic epilepsy, bacterial meningitis and febrile convulsion. Fever was absent in 2 cases and the CT was normal in 2. All cases had abnormal EEG findings with encephalitic changes in 5. Brain biopsy was diagnostic in 2. The outcome was poor in all 6. The authors stress that the absence of fever at presentation and a normal CT scan should not discourage the use of acyclovir for children presenting with focal seizures and altered consciousness (Cameron PD et al. Herpes simplex virus encephalitis: problems in diagnosis. Dev Med Child Neurol Feb 1992;34:134-140). (Correspondence: Dr S.J. Wallace, Department of Child Health, University Hospital of Wales, Heath Park, Cardiff CF4 4XW, Wales.)

COMMENT. Mikati MA and colleagues at the Children's Hospital and Massachusetts General Hospital, Boston have shown that the EEG is a sensitive test that may be superior to radiologic procedures in the early diagnosis of neonatal herpes simplex encephalitis. The multifocal periodic pattern in the presence of CSF pleocytosis is highly suggestive of the diagnosis. The CT and ultrasound studies may be normal when the EEG is abnormal during the first few days of the infection. An MRI with T2 weighted images may be more revealing than the CT and will show multiple small disseminated lesions (see Progress in Pediatric Neurology, Chicago, PNB Publishers, 1991, p 423).-Editor. *Ped Neur Briefs* April 1992.

HUMAN HERPESVIRUS-6 AND ROSEOLA INFANTUM MENINGITIS

Two infants with roseola infantum and meningitis caused by human herpesvirus-6 infection are reported from the Department of Pediatrics, College of Medicine, National Taiwan University, Taipei, Taiwan. A 7 month old girl presented with fever, bulging anterior fontanelle and mild hepatomegaly. Lumbar puncture showed 18 mononuclear and 2 polymorphonuclear cells/mm^3 and CFS protein of 0.35 g/l and glucose 3.05 mmol/l. The first serum on the 4th day of the illness was positive for IgM anti-HHV-6 (titre 1:10), and the second serum taken 11 days later was positive for both IgG and IgM anti-HHV-6 (1:160 and 1:80 respectively). A maculopapular rash appeared on the face, scalp and neck on the 4th day of illness. Case 2. A 4 month old boy presented with cough and high fever and 4 episodes of generalized seizures in the next 2 days. CSF examination on the third day revealed 8 polymorphonuclear cells and 1 mononuclear cell/mm^3. CSF protein and glucose were normal. A blood smear revealed lymphocytosis. Liver function tests were abnormal. A rash appeared on the 4th day and fever subsided. The first serum was negative for both IgG and IgM anti-HHV-6 and the second serum taken 12 days later was positive for both (1:160 and 1:40 respectively). The boy recovered without sequela. (Huang Li-Min et al. Meningitis caused by human herpesvirus-6. Arch Dis Child; Dec 1991;66:1443-1444). (Reprints: Dr. Li-Min Huang, Laboratory of Molecular Microbiology, 9000 Rockville

Pike, Building 4, Room 306, NIAID, National Institutes of Health, Bethesda, MD 20892.)

COMMENT. The illnesses linked to human herpesvirus-6 infection have included roseola infantum, hepatitis, lymphadenitis and mononucleosis. Roseola infantum is the infectious fever most commonly associated with febrile convulsions. In a review of the literature over 3 decades (1934-64) of 3,168 patients reported in 13 publications, roseola infantum was the cause of febrile convulsions in 4% (range 0.6-7.6%). The average incidence of convulsions among 581 patients with roseola infantum reported in 11 publications was 22%. The evidence for an encephalitic process such as CSF pleocytosis was lacking except for a rare case and the height of the body temperature that usually accompanies roseola infantum was considered sufficient to explain the frequent complication of convulsions (Millichap JG, Febrile Convulsions, New York, Macmillan, 1968). The present report of HHV-6 infection associated with roseola infantum supports the theory of an encephalitic illness in the etiology of the seizure. Inclusion of roseola infantum as a cause of simple febrile seizures must be reevaluated in the light of this report.-Editor. *Ped Neur Briefs* April 1992.

PROGNOSIS OF ENCEPHALITIS

A population based, controlled follow-up study of the general outcome of 73 children followed for 2 to 12 years after the acute phase of childhood encephalitis is reported from the University of Oulu, Finland. Varicella accounted for 23% of cases, mumps 11%, herpes simplex 8%, measles 5%, and the etiology was unknown for 44%. The mean age at onset was 5.9 years (range 5 days to 14 years). The 61 school-age children had lower performance and full-scale IQs than their randomly selected, age- and sex-matched controls. Visual acuity was more often reduced and EEG and ENG abnormalities were more frequent. A poor prognosis was infrequent, the incidence being 3.5 per million children at risk annually. Dysarthria was the most frequent sequel of HSV encephalitis. Ataxia, seen most commonly with varicella encephalitis in the acute phase, persisted in only 1 of 17 children at follow-up examination. The prognosis for childhood encephalitis in this study is much better than anticipated on the basis of earlier follow-up studles that included a greater number of HSV cases (Rantala H et al. Outcome after childhood encephalitis. Dev Med Child Neurol Oct 1991;33:858-867).

COMMENT. A case of severe macrocephaly and brain damage is reported in association with second trimester congenital varicella infection from the Departments of Neurology and Clinical Genetics, The Hospital for Sick Children, Great Ormond Street, London, England (Scheffer IE, Baraitser M, Brett EM. Dev Med Child Neurol Oct 1991;33 :916-920).-Editor. *Ped Neur Briefs* Nov 1991.

CYTOMEGALOVIRUS IN PRETERM INFANTS

The clinical, radiological and neuropathological findings in 15 premature infants with lethal congenital cytomegalovirus infection were studied at the Departments of Pediatrics and Pathology, University of Texas Southwestern Medical Center, Dallas, TX. Six infants were stillborn and 9 were live born, but died at a postnatal age of 18+/-21 days. Clinical findings included microcephaly (77%), seizures (55%), hypotonia (33%), multiple contractures (18%), chorioretinitis, optic atrophy and corneal opacities. CT scan in 2 infants showed periventricular calcification; MRI in 1 infant demonstrated cerebellar hypoplasia and diffuse cortical atrophy. Sonograms were normal in 4 infants and 2 had ventriculomegaly and periventricular calcification. Neuropathological findings included periventricular necrosis and calcification, cerebellar hypoplasia, leukomalacia, intraventricular hemorrhage, hydrocephalus and porencephalic cyst. Systemic inclusion bodies were present in all infants and intranuclear bodies within the brain in 4 infants. The atypical findings in preterm infants which are rarely reported in term infants included hypotonia, multiple contractures, periventricular leukomalacia and optic atrophy (Perlman JM, Argyle C. Lethal cytomegalovirus infection in preterm infants: clinical, radiological, and neuropathological findings. Ann Neurol Jan 1992;31:64-68). (Reprints: Dr. Perlman, Department of Pediatrics, University of Texas Southwestern Medical Center, 5323 Harry Hines Blvd., Dallas, TX 75235.)

COMMENT. These findings indicate that cytomegalovirus infection should be considered in the differential diagnosis of unexplained hypotonia and arthrogryposis multiplex congenita in premature infants. Newer antiviral agents such as ganciclovir may modify the prognosis and may be indicated in treatment of some preterm infants with congenital CMV infection.

Fowler KB and colleagues at the University of Alabama, Birmingham, AL, compared the outcomes of CMV-infected infants born to mothers who acquired primary CMV during pregnancy (primary-infection group) with those born to mothers with immunity (recurrent-infection group). Infants in the primary-infection group had symptomatic CMV infection at birth in 18%, sequelae in 25% including sensorineural hearing loss in 15%, and mental impairment in 13%. Infants born to mothers with recurrent infection and having antibody to CMV before conception had no symptoms at birth, sequelae in only 8%, and none became mentally impaired at early childhood follow-up. The presence of maternal antibody to CMV before conception provides protection against sequelae to congenital CMV in the newborn. (N Engl J Med March 5, 1992;326:663-7).

CMV was the most common viral infection complication in 100 children who underwent liver transplantation at Addenbrooke's Hospital, Cambridge, England. Of 23 infected, 13 had primary infections and one died of encephalitis. Of 9 receiving ganciclovir, 8 recovered fully. (Salt A, Barnes ND et al. BMJ Feb 15, 1992;304:416-421.-Editor. *Ped Neur Briefs* April 1992.

PRE-ERUPTIVE VARICELLA ENCEPHALITIS AND CEREBELLAR ATAXIA

A 2 year old boy who developed varicella encephalitis with cerebellar ataxia 16 days before the appearance of the exanthem is reported from the Department of Neurology, Children's Hospital, Harvard Medical School, Boston, MA. The child was previously healthy, but had been exposed to his 5 year old brother who had developed varicella 4 days previously. The serum varicella-zoster IgG was absent on admission and 69.6 ELISA units/ml 5 weeks later (Liu GT, Urion DK. Pre-eruptive varicella encephalitis and cerebellar ataxia. Pediatr Neurol Jan/Feb 1992;8:69-70). (Correspondence: Dr. Urion, Department of Neurology, Children's Hospital, 3010 Longwood Ave., Boston, MA 02115.)

COMMENT. Pre-eruptive neurologic complications of varicella are rare but the diagnosis should be considered in children presenting with cerebellar ataxia. The authors cite a reference to my case-report from the Mayo Clinic of a 5 year old boy presenting with symptoms and signs of intracranial hypertension and cerebellar ataxia which antedated the exanthema by 11 days (Goldston AS, Millichap JG, Miller RH. Cerebellar ataxia with pre-eruptive varicella. Am J Dis Child 1963;106:197-200). In our patient the fundoscopic examination disclosed bilateral papilledema and a right sixth nerve palsy that led to ventriculography to exclude a space occupying lesion. In 15 previous reports of pre-eruptive neurologic complications of varicella, cerebellar ataxia was mentioned only in 1.-Editor. *Ped Neur Briefs* April 1992.

ACUTE ENCEPHALOPATHY OF OBSCURE ORIGIN

Six previously healthy children who developed an acute encephalopathy several days after a prodromal illness are reported from the Hopital Bicetre, and Hopital Necker-Enfants Malades, Paris, France. Prodromal illnesses consisted of upper respiratory infection with fever, and headache and vomiting. Coma was the initial symptom in 4 patients. Abnormal movements included gesticulation, chewing, swallowing, orofacial dyskinesia, limb dystonia, and

choreoathetosis. Rigidity was constant in 5 patients and intermittent in one. Seizures occurred in 2 patients. Recovery extended for several weeks and was characterized by a rapid return of motor function and persistent behavioral and cognitive disturbances. Four patients recovered fully, and two had mild sequelae. (Sebire G et al. Coma associated with intense bursts of abnormal movements and long-lasting cognitive disturbances: An acute encephalopathy of obscure origin. J Pediatr Dec 1992;121:845-51).
(Reprints: G Sebire MD, Service de Neurologie, Departement de Pediatre, Hopital Bicetre, 78 rue du general Leclerc, 94275, Le Kremlin Bicetre Cedex, France).

COMMENT. These cases with a favorable outcome were thought to represent a different syndrome from that described by Lyon, Dodge, and Adams, whose 16 patients died from an acute encephalopathy of obscure origin. Attempts at viral isolation and antibody detection were negative.-Editor. *Ped Neur Briefs* Jan 1993.

EXANTHEM SUBITUM CNS COMPLICATIONS

Central nervous system (CNS) complications of exanthem subitum were analyzed in 21 infants examined at the Departments of Pediatrics and Neurology, Fujita Health University School of Medicine, Toyoake, Japan. The primary infection with human herpesvirus 6 was confirmed by isolation of the virus from the blood and/or a rise in antibody titers, and the virus DNA was detected in the cerebrospinal fluid of 6 infants, including 3 with encephalitis/encephalopathy (E/E). Convulsive seizures (15 generalized and 6 focal) occurred during the pre-eruptive stage of the illness, and persisted for more than 45 minutes in 7 infants. Four patients with E/E had prolonged focal seizures and loss of consciousness, abnormal EEGs and CT scans; 3 had a pleocytosis and elevated protein in the CSF. One developed epilepsy and one died. Infants without E/E recovered with no sequelae. (Suga S et al. Clinical and virological analyses of 21 infants with exanthem subitum(roseola infantum) and central nervous system complications. Ann Neurol June 1993;33:597-603). (Respond: Yoshizo Asano MD, Department of Pediatrics, Fujita Health University School of Medicine, Toyoake, Aichi 470-11, Japan).

COMMENT. Exanthem subitum is a common, usually benign, infectious disease of infants, characterized by a four day fever and a rash that appears after the fever subsides. Seizures may complicate the illness during the febrile stage and before the rash erupts. Human herpesvirus 6, recently identified as the causative agent, may rarely invade the CNS and cause encephalitis.

A febrile seizure has long been recognized as the most common complication of exanthem subitum, occurring in 22 percent of 581 patients reported in 11 publications (Millichap JG. Febrile Convulsions. New York, Macmillan, 1968). Evidence for an encephalitic process and a direct involvement of the brain was lacking, and the degree of fever was considered sufficient to explain the frequent complication of convulsions. The present report demonstrates that seizures associated with exanthem subitum and fever are not always simple in type. They are occasionally prolonged and complex and a manifestation of encephalitis or encephalopathy.-Editor. *Ped Neur Briefs* June 1993.

SEVERE REACTIONS TO DTP VACCINE

Severe reactions experienced by 60 children within 48 hours of DTP immunization were reported from the UCLA School of Medicine, Los Angeles, CA. These included seizures in 40 or 66% (6 with fever >40.5°C), collapse episodes in 14, and persistent crying in 6. Subjects with encephalopathy were not included in the study. Those with seizures had a high rate of personal and family histories of seizures, and 10% were afebrile. Chinese hamster ovary cell assays failed to reveal active pertussis toxin in acute sera. Long-term follow-up for possible neurologic sequelae was not performed. (Blumberg DA, Cherry JD et al. Severe reactions associated with diphtheria-tetanus-pertussis vaccine: Detailed study of children with seizures, hypotonic-hyporesponsive episodes, high fevers, and persistent crying. Pediatrics June 1993;91:1158-1165). (Reprints: Dean A Blumberg MD, Dept of Pediatrics, UCLA School of Medicine, 10833 Le Conte Ave, Los Angeles, CA 90024).

COMMENT. Seizures induced by pertussis immunization and fever are more severe than simple febrile seizures. Cherry JD and associates report that a first febrile convulsion within 3 or 7 days of pertussis immunization is more likely to last longer than 10 minutes, to be recurrent, and to have a focal pattern when compared to first seizures occurring more than 7 days after immunization (J Pediatr June 1993;122:900-3). They have estimated that one in a 1000 children immunized will have a seizure, and 6% of first febrile seizures are associated with pertussis immunization. The use of acellular DTP vaccines, recently approved by the FDA, may hopefully reduce the frequency and severity of neurological complications.-Editor. *Ped Neur Briefs* June 1993.

SENSORINEURAL DEAFNESS AND MMR IMMUNIZATION

Nine reports of sensorineural hearing loss after measles, mumps, and rubella (MMR) immunization were evaluated at the Radcliffe Infirmary, Oxford, England. In 6 cases, the MMR was possibly related and in 3, the immunization was not the cause. In those affected by the MMR, the deafness was bilateral in 2 and unilateral in 4. (Stewart BJA, Prabhu PU. Reports of sensorineural deafness after measles, mumps, and rubella immunization. Arch Dis Child July 1993;69:153-154). (Respond: Dr Stewart, Community Health Offices, Radcliffe Infirmary, Oxford OX2 6HE, England).

COMMENT. Deafness is reported with all components of MMR.-Editor. *Ped Neur Briefs* Aug 1993.

SPINAL CORD SCHISTOSOMIASIS

A seven year old girl with Schistosoma mansoni infection of the spinal cord mimicking cord neoplasm is reported from the Department of Neurology, University of Michigan, Ann Arbor, MI. Exposure to Schistosomal parasites occurred while bathing in a river in Sierra Leone, Southern Africa. The illness presented with back and leg pain and a low-grade fever. Within 24 hours she had weakness of the leg and four days later she was unable to walk, to urinate or defecate. Sensation was diminished below the low thoracic area. CSF showed 2 RBCs, 250 WBCs with 78% lymphocytes, protein 584 mg/dl and glucose 55 mg/dl. Myelography revealed a large intramedullary mass at thoracic levels 11 and 12. MRI with Gadolinium demonstrated enhancement of the cord at T10 level through the conus. Decompressive laminectomy was performed with resection of a yellow gliotic appearing cord of neoplastic appearance. Histologic examination revealed eggs characteristic of S. mansoni. After treatment with praziquantel, lower extremity strength gradually improved and six months later, she was walking well with braces. (Selwa IM, Garofalo EA et al. Spinal cord schistosomiasis: A pediatric case mimicking intrinsic cord neoplasm. Neurology May 1991;41:755-757).

COMMENT. In patients with acute or subacute paraparesis who have been exposed to endemic areas (South Africa, South America, Caribbean or the Middle East), schistosomiasis must be suspected. Spinal cord involvement can be delayed for up to six years after exposure, and findings on MRI and myelography may mimic spinal cord neoplasms. Patients with mild or early involvement of the spinal cord may be benefited by antiparasitic medications alone and surgery may be unnecessary.-Editor. *Ped Neur Briefs* June 1991.

CNS COMPLICATIONS OF RHEUMATOID ARTHRITIS

Mass lesions in the basal ganglia bilaterally and mainly involving the globus pallidus are reported in a two year old boy with juvenile rheumatoid arthritis from the Department of Pediatrics, Hokushin General Hospital, Nishi, Nagano, Japan. At ten months after the onset of the arthritis he developed a relapse with fever, heart murmur, vomiting, hypotonia, dystonia, and aphasia. Deep tendon reflexes were exaggerated and plantar responses extensor. The abnormal neurologic signs and basal ganglia lesions gradually improved with corticosteroid treatment and almost disappeared after one year. The right optic fundus showed chorioretinitis. A stereotactic brain biopsy performed to exclude a neoplasm revealed proliferation of astrocytes of undetermined origin, either reactive or low-grade astrocytoma. The dystonia subsided after one year but peculiar mouthing behavior persisted. A CNS primary lymphoma could not be excluded. (Hirabayashi S et al. Basal ganglia mass lesions in juvenile rheumatoid arthritis. Pediatr Neurol March/April 1991;7:141-3).

COMMENT. A chronic inflammatory process involving cerebral vessels was suspected in this patient but angiography failed to demonstrate a cerebral vasculitis. Other rheumatic diseases with CNS complications include lupus erythematosus, polyarteritis nodosa and rheumatic fever. Seizures are a common presenting sign of lupus erythematosus.- Editor. *Ped Neur Briefs* June 1991.

CRITICAL-ILLNESS POLYNEUROPATHY

A review of the neurological complications of sepsis from the University of Western Ontario, London, and Queen's University, Kingston, Ontario, Canada, draws attention to "critical-illness polyneuropathy" as a cause of difficulty in weaning from the ventilator. Patients with major medical, surgical, or traumatic illnesses who are in the recovery phase of septic encephalopathy may develop respiratory difficulties as an early sign of polyneuropathy. Electrophysiological studies, showing reduction of diaphragmatic action potential and denervation of chest wall muscles, may be diagnostic of the neuropathy before weakness of limbs and areflexia develop. In contrast to the central nervous system, damage to the peripheral nervous system is more severe and sometimes persistent in the septic syndrome. (Bolton CF et al. The neurological complications of sepsis. Ann Neurol Jan 1993;33:94-100). (Correspondence: Dr Bolton, Victoria Hospital, 375 South

Street, London, Ontario N6A 4G5, Canada).

COMMENT. In addition to encephalopathy and polyneuropathy, patients with sepsis may develop myositis or myopathy and an elevated CPK. The EEG and EMG are sensitive indicators of these complications of the selptic syndrome.-Editor. *Ped Neur Briefs* Feb 1993.

LYME NEUROBORRELIOSIS

The clinical and epidemiological features of 187 consecutive patients with neuroborreliosis recognized in Denmark over a 6-year period, 1985-1990, are reported from the Department of Infection-Immunology, Statens Seruminstitut, Copenhagen, Denmark. The most common manifestation was a painful lymphocytic meningoradiculitis (Bannwarth's syndrome), and CNS involvement in early cases was rare. Neuroborreliosis in children showed a different course compared to adults. Headache was considerably more frequent (70%) compared to adults (35%) whereas radicular pain was significantly less common and less severe in children. Clinical signs of meningitis were reported in 38% of children and in only 3% of adults. Facial palsy in 26 of 40 childhood cases was bilateral in only 3, and was unassociated with pain, fever or neck stiffness. The diagnosis is based on inflammatory CSF changes and B. burgdorferi specific intrathecal antibody production (Hansen K, Lebech AM. The clinical and epidemiological profile of Lyme neuroborreliosis in Denmark 1985-1990. Brain April 1992;115:399-423). (Correspondence: Dr. Klaus Hansen, Borrelia Laboratory, Department of Infection-Immunology, Statens Seruminstitut, Artillerivej 5, DK-2300 Copenhagen S, Denmark.)

COMMENT. Neuroborreliosis in children is often less dramatic than in adults and may be insidious with fluctuating headache, loss of appetite, weight loss, slight meningeal signs but rare focal neurologic signs. Similar findings to the experience in Denmark are reported from the United States. (Belman AL. Neurologic complications of Lyme disease in children. Experience in an endemic area and review of the literature. Int Pediatr 1992;7:136-143.)-Editor. *Ped Neur Briefs* Aug 1992.

LYME DISEASE: PROGNOSIS WITH EARLY TREATMENT

The long-term outcome of 63 children with erythema migrans, treated early with antibiotics at the Wildwood Pediatrics Clinic, Essex, Connecticut, was determined by telephone interview 1 to 6 years after the initial episode of Lyme disease. Penicillin V (60% of patients), amoxicillin (25%), tetracycline (10%), or doxycycline (5%), had been given orally for 10 to 30 days. None of the patients had carditis, arthritis, or neurologic complications attributable to Lyme disease. A recurrence of erythema migrans was reported in 7 (11%). (Salazar JC et al. Long-term outcome of Lyme disease in children given early treatment. J Pediatr April 1993;122: 591-593). (Reprints: Michael A Gerber MD, Department of Pediatrics, University of Connecticut Health Center, 263 Farmington Ave, Farmington, CT 06030).

COMMENT. Treatment of Lyme disease at an early stage appears to protect from serious neurologic and other sequelae. A prospective study of the clinical and epidemiological features of 187 consecutive patients with neuroborreliosis recognized in Denmark over a 6-year period showed that 61% had Bannwarth's syndrome with paresis, a painful lymphocytic meningoradiculitis, during the second stage of the disease. CNS involvement in the early stages was rare; 4% had myelitis and 1 patient had acute encephalitis. The final morbidity after a 3 year median follow-up was low; disabling sequelae were reported in 9 (5%) patients. (Hansen K, Lebech A-M. Brain 1992;115:399-423). Measurement of intrathecal anti-*Borrelia burgdofferi* antibody is a reliable indicator of CNS infection. (Halperin JJ et al. Neurology 1991;41: 1571).-Editor. *Ped Neur Briefs* April 1993.

NEUROLOGIC COMPLICATIONS OF CAT-SCRATCH DISEASE

The neurologic complications of cat-scratch disease in 76 patients with an average age of 10 years are reported from the Jacksonville Health Education Program, University of Florida, and Department of Pediatrics, Uniformed Services, Bethesda, MD. The incidence of encephalopathy varied from 0.17%-2% in two groups of patients examined. Convulsions occurred in 28 (46%) of 61 patients, and combative behavior occurred in 39% of those who were semi-conscious during the recovery phase of a convulsive episode. Headache, lethargy and malaise were common and persistent. Less common findings were ataxia, bilateral VI nerve palsy, aphasia, transient hemiplegia, and profound hearing loss lasting eight months. Of 15 patients without encephalopathy, two had facial nerve paresis, ten neuroretinitis, and three peripheral neuritis. All 76 patients recovered within 12 months and 78% recovered within 1-12 weeks. There were no neurologic sequelae. Treatment with antibiotics and prednisone is usually ineffective. The authors recommend IV Gentamycin in severely ill patients. (Carithers HA, Margileth AM. Cat-scratch disease. Acute encephalopathy and other neurologic manifestations. AJDC Jan 1991;145:98-101).

COMMENT. Cat-scratch disease encephalopathy should be considered in a young patient presenting with sudden onset of coma and/or convulsions. The patient should be examined for lymphadenopathy and inoculation papule or conjunctival granuloma. The diagnosis can be confirmed by a cat-scratch skin test. The differential diagnosis includes Lyme encephalitis, drug intoxication, viral or bacterial infections, and Reye's syndrome.-Editor. *Ped Neur Briefs* Jan 1991.

NEUROLOGIC COMPLICATIONS OF CAT-SCRATCH DISEASE: STATUS EPILEPTICUS

An 8 year-old girl hospitalized with cat-scratch disease and recurrent generalized tonic-clonic seizures is reported from the Department of Pediatrics, Children's Hospital, The Ohio State University, Columbus, OH. The convulsant status and altered mental status lasted 4 hours and required ventilatory support. She received cefotaxime and gentamicin for 10 days and phenobarbital for 3 months. The lymph glands remained painful for several months but she ultimately made an uneventful recovery. (Tsao CY. Generalized tonic-clonic status epilepticus in a child with cat-scratch disease and encephalopathy. Clin Electroencephalogr April 1992;23:65-67). (Reprints: Chang Y. Tsao, M.D., Department of Pediatrics, Children's Hospital, 700 Children's Drive, Columbus, OH 43205).

COMMENT. Treatment with trimethoprim-sulfamethoxazole was superior to cephalosporins and other antibiotics in 71 children with cat-scratch disease. The nodes healed promptly and there was no suppuration or drainage. (Collipp PJ. AJDC April 1992;146:397-399.) A unique case of severe and lasting neurobehavioral changes after the acute episode of cat scratch encephalitis is reported from the Hopital Neurologique, Lyon, France. (Revol A et al. J Neur Neurosurg and Psychiat Feb 1992;55:133-135.) -Editor. *Ped Neur Briefs* May 1992.

BACTERIAL MENINGITIS

NEUROLOGIC SEQUELAE OF BACTERIAL MENINGITIS

The occurrence of chronic neurologic sequelae including late seizures or epilepsy was determined in a nine year follow-up study of 185 infants and children with bacterial meningitis at the Departments of Pediatrics and Neurology, Washington University School of Medicine, St. Louis, MD and the Department of Pediatrics, Baylor College of Medicine, Houston, TX. Seizures occurred in 58 patients (31%) during the acute phase of bacterial meningitis. Neurologic abnormalities developing during the acute illness had persisted at one month followup in 69 (37%) but many of these signs resolved within a one year period. Only 26 (14%) had persistent deficits; 18 (10%) had sensorineural hearing loss; 13 (7%) had one or more late seizures; and 8 (4%) had multiple neurologic deficits. Patients with serious neurologic abnormalities other than sensorineural hearing loss had a significantly increased risk of having at least one late seizure. Only two patients whose final neurologic examinations were normal had recurring seizures during follow-up. The occurrence of seizures during acute meningitis was strongly associated with the development of late seizures. Electroencephalographic abnornalities were also predictive of late seizures as was an initial CSF glucose concentration of less than 20 mg/dl. (Pomerov SL et al. Seizures and other neurologic sequelae of bacterial meningitis in children. N Engl J Med Dec 13, 1990;323:1651-7).

COMMENT. Children with persistent neurologic deficits from bacterial meningitis are at risk for epilepsy whereas those with a normal neurologic examination at time of discharge usually escape neurologic sequelae including epilepsy. Seizures during acute meningitis are highly predictive of late seizures and permanent neurologic deficits.

In a study of 97 school-aged children who had been treated for Haemophilus influenzae type b meningitis during infancy at the Children's Hospital of Toronto, Ottawa and Montreal, 14 (14%) had persisting neurologic sequelae, 11 had sensorineural hearing loss, and only 2% had a seizure disorder. The total sample of index children scored slightly below their siblings in reading ability but 56 children without acute phase neurologic complications (58%) were indistinguishable from their siblings on all neuropsychological tests. Neurologic sequelae were associated with lower socioeconomic status and a lower ratio of glucose in CSF to that in blood at the time of the meningitis. The prognosis was favorable for the majority of children treated for H. influenzae type b meningitis when followed for a mean of 9.6 years. (Taylor HG et al. The sequelae of Haemophilus influenzae meningitis in school-age children. N Engl J Med Dec 13, 1990;323:1657-63).-Editor. *Ped Neur Briefs* Jan 1991.

BRAIN ABSCESS: MANAGEMENT

A review of 130 children with brain abscesses treated over 21 years is reported from Hacettepe University School of Medicine, Sihhiye, Ankara,

Turkey. Four (3%) were infants, 45% were aged 3-8 years, and 30% were 68 years. The incidence decreased between ages 8 and 18 years. Chronic ear infection with mastoiditis occurred in 28 (21%) and congenital heart disease in 26 (20%). Infants had meningitis or ventriculitis. The abscess was supratentorial in 113. In children with congenital heart disease, the parietal lobes were commonly involved with a left-sided predilection (77%). Multiple abscesses occurred in 17 (13%). Primary or secondary excision was used in 74. The initial surgical procedure was aspiration in 71. Staphylococcus, Streptococcus and Proteus were the predominant microorganisms. Cephalosporins were used only recently and penicillin and chloramphenicol were the antibiotics used in earlier cases. Mortality was 15% overall, but 6% in the last 5 years and 0 in the last 3 years. Mortality in infants was 50% (Tekkok IH, Erbengi A. Management of brain abscess in children: review of 130 cases over a period of 21 years. Child's Nerv Sys Oct 1992;8:411-416). (Correspondence: I.H. Tekkok, M.D., Department of Neurosurgery, Hacettepe University School of Medicine, Sihhiye, Ankara 06100, Turkey.)

COMMENT. The medical cure of a brainstem abscess and serial brainstem auditory evoked potentials are reported from the Department of Pediatrics, Chang Gung Memorial Hospital, 199 Tung-Hua N. Road, Taipei, Taiwan, Republic of China (Wang HS et al. Dev Med Child Neurol Oct 1992;34:911-915). A 9 year-old girl with tetralogy of Fallot was cured after 6 weeks of parenteral antibiotic therapy, without surgical intervention. The initial brainstem auditory evoked potential showed poor demonstration of right waves IV and V, and delay of right wave III and left wave V. Serial follow-up showed improving latencies and wave forms but persistent abnormalities on the right side. The patient presented with a right-sided ptosis, abducens palsy and peripheral facial palsy and left hemiparesis. CT showed a hypodense lesion in the brain stem. Vancomycin and chloramphenicol were the antibiotics used in treatment.-Editor. *Ped Neur Briefs* Dec 1992.

LUMBAR PUNCTURE IN THE NEONATE

The diagnostic utility of lumbar punctures in neonates was evaluated in the Division of Neonatology, Department of Pediatrics, University of Miami, FL. Of 712 neonates with lumbar punctures during the first week of life, 8 had positive spinal fluid cultures but only 1 had a positive blood culture and a clinical course consistent with meningitis. In contrast, of 114 patients who underwent lumbar punctures after the first week of life, 7% had a positive culture approximating 5 times that observed during the first week of life. (Schwersenski J et al. Lumbar puncture frequency and cerebrospinal fluid analysis in the neonate. AJDC Jan 1991;145:54-58).

COMMENT. The authors conclude that the routine use of lumbar puncture as a part of the work-up for infection during the first week of life in an asymptomatic neonate should be reassessed. The results of the study suggest that lumbar puncture may not be justified in an asymptomatic at-risk neonate during the first week of life. After the first week, lumbar puncture may be indicated in the at-risk infant.-Editor. *Ped Neur Briefs* Jan 1991.

CT IN ACUTE MENINGITIS

The role of CT in the acute management of bacterial meningitis in 30 children was evaluated at the Department of Pediatrics, St. Mary's Hospital Medical School, London, England. Cranial CT was normal in 10 patients, 5 with raised intracranial pressure, 1 with focal neurological signs and 1 with generalized convulsions. Significant CT abnormalities were detected in 10 patients, 4 with subdural effusion, 4 with cerebral infarct, 1 hydrocephalus, and 1 empyema. CT identified a surgical abnormality in 2 patients with progressive focal neurological signs (Heyderman RS, Robb SA, Kendall BE, Levin M. Does computed tomography have a role in the evaluation of complicated acute bacterial meningitis in childhood? Dev Med and Child Neurol Oct 1992;34:870-875). (Correspondence: Dr. R.S. Heyderman, Department of Pediatrics, Queen Elizabeth the Queen Mother Wing, St. Mary's Hospital Medical School, South Wharf Road,

London W2 1NY.)

COMMENT. This study shows that the role of CT in the management of acute bacterial meningitis is limited, but CT may be valuable in those with progressive neurological signs for whom neurosurgical intervention may be necessary.

The long-term follow-up of acute bacterial meningitis in 74 children is reported from Taiyuan City, China (Yi LY, Qiong YS. Pediatr Neurol Sept/Oct 1992;8:404 (abstract). Neurologic sequelae occurred in 33.8% of survivors: 54% had mental retardation, 50% epilepsy, 33% paralysis, 16% sensorineural hearing loss and 4% blindness. Other abnormalities included growth retardation, hyperactivity and irritability. Dexamethasone reduced the incidence of hearing loss.

Cranial CT conducted in 199 children with tuberculous meningitis in Cape Town, Republic of South Africa, showed basal ganglia infarcts in 30%, which corresponded with hemiplegia (Schoeman JF et al. Pediatr Neurol Sept/Oct 1992;8:355 (abstract).-Editor. *Ped Neur Briefs* Dec 1992.

CNS COMPLICATIONS OF ASEPTIC MENINGITIS IN INFANTS

The incidence and outcome of neurological complications occurring during the acute stage of aseptic meningitis in 277 infants under 2 years of age are reported from Johns Hopkins University, Baltimore, and Dartmouth Medical School, Lebanon, NH. The dominant clinical findings were fever (88%) and irritability (78%). Meningeal irritation occurred in only 8.7%, and 8 (2.9%) infants had a single generalized seizure. Among 52 with neurologic abnormalities, 17 had a full fontanelle, 6 had complex seizures, 2 a large head circumference, and 2 diminished consciousness. Infants older than 3 months had more complications than younger infants. The type of enterovirus (Coxsackie or echo) and CSF indices were not correlated with risk of complications. Infants with CNS complications showed no sequelae on follow-up neurodevelopmental tests. (Rorabaugh ML et al. Aseptic meningitis in infants younger than 2 years of age: Acute illness and neurologic complications. Pediatrics Aug 1993;92:206-211). (Reprints: John F Modlin MD, Dept of Pediatrics, Dartmouth-Hitchcock Medical Center, Lebanon, NH 03754).

COMMENT. Acute "encephalitic" complications occurring in approximately 10% of young infants with aseptic meningitis are not associated with long-term neurologic or cognitive deficits.

Straussberg R and associates, at the Hasharon Hospital, Petach Tikvah, Israel, report two young children with posterior fossa tumors who presented with aseptic meningoencephalitis (Clin Pediatr Sept 1993; 552-4). Somnolence, stupor, and extreme nuchal rigidity were the major manifestations on admission. CSF showed pleocytosis and cultures were sterile. Surgical removal of the tumors revealed a fourth ventricle choroid plexus papilloma and a medulloblastoma. Head CT might avoid the dangers attending lumbar puncture in children with clinical manifestations that are common to both meningitis and posterior fossa tumor.-Editor. *Ped Neur Briefs* Oct 1993.

CORTICOSTEROIDS IN PNEUMOCOCCAL MENINGITIS

The records of 97 infants and children with pneumococcal meningitis, 41 receiving corticosteroid therapy, were examined at the Department of Pediatrics, University of Texas Southwestern Medical Center, Dallas, Texas. When steroid-therapy was given before or concurrently with antibiotic therapy, none of 30 steroid-treated versus 16 of 52 non-steroid-treated patients developed neurologic or cardiovascular instability after the first parenteral antibiotic dose was given. Bilateral moderate or greater hearing loss occurred in 9% of steroid-treated group compared to 21% of non-steroid group. The incidence of hearing loss was significantly lower in those survivors of overwhelming meningeal infection who had been treated with steroids (Kennedy WA et al. The role of corticosteroid therapy in children with pneumococcal meningitis. AJDC Dec 1991;145:1374-1378).

COMMENT. The data from this study were obtained retrospectively and a placebo-controlled double-blind study of dexamethasone in pneumococcal meningitis is indicated. The beneficial effect of corticosteroid adjunctive therapy has been demonstrated previously only in patients with Haemophilus meningitis. Since the incidence of H. influenzae meningitis will be reduced by immunization in the future, S. pneumoniae or N. meningitidis will be the causal agent in a larger percentage of children (Schuster V, Kreth HW, N Engl J Med Dec 5, 1991;325:1654). Dexamethasone in childhood meningitis is discussed in the correspondence section of this issue of the N Engl J Med.

A retrospective evaluation of 12 years experience in the treatment of neonatal meningitis is reported from The Departments of Paediatrics and Bacteriology, Goteborg and Molndal, University of Goteborg, Sweden (Tessin I et al. Acta Paediatr Scand Oct 1991;80:911-916). Initial treatment with ampicillin-aminoglycoside combination failed in 6 of 34 patients, despite organism sensitivity to the antibiotics.-Editor. *Ped Neur Briefs* Dec 1991.

INTRACRANIAL PRESSURE IN BACTERIAL MENINGITIS

The role of increased intracranial pressure and its effect on cerebral blood flow in the prognosis of children with bacterial meningitis is reviewed from the Division of Child Neurology, Loma Linda U Sch of Med, Loma Linda, CA. One-third have reduced cerebral flood flow (CBF) associated with cerebral edema and a poor prognosis. In patients with cerebral edema on CT or MRI and increased intracranial pressure (ICP), hyperventilation may reduce the ICP. The early use of diuretics, corticosteroids and mannitol is recommended. Ventriculostomy or ventricular tap may be necessary to decrease CSF volume in patients with increased ICP and signs of mass effect. The majority of subdural effusions require no specific treatment since spontaneous resolution will occur over time. In children with infarction, hyperventilation and diuretics may worsen the tissue injury whereas barbiturates or hypothermia may be of benefit. The authors recommend that interventional strategies must be started early and have a rapid onset of action if they are to be effective (Ashwal S et al. Bacterial meningitis in children: pathophysiology and treatment. Neurology April 1992;42:739-748).

COMMENT. This is an excellent review of the pathophysiology of bacterial meningitis and explains the continuing high morbidity despite the marked reduction in mortality resulting from newer antibiotics. Careful monitoring of intracranial pressure and use of neuroimaging in the early stages of meningitis should help in the selection of patients requiring early interventional treatments for the reduction of pressure and improvement in cerebral blood flow.-Editor. *Ped Neur Briefs* May 1992.

HEMOLYTIC-UREMIC ENCEPHALOPATHY

Twenty-seven children, ages 6 months - 13 years, with encephalopathy complicating hemolytic-uremic syndrome are reported from The University of British Columbia, Vancouver, Canada. Seventeen had seizures and 2 died. An increased risk for developing a neurological manifestation was correlated with the female sex, the prolonged use of an antimotility agent (e.g. codeine, anticholinergic drugs) and an increased hemoglobin (Cimolai N et al. Risk factors for the central nervous system manifestations of gastroenteritis-associated hemolytic-uremic syndrome. Pediatrics Oct 1992;90:616-621. (Reprints: N. Cimolai, M.D., Department of Pathology, British Columbia's Children's Hospital, 4480 Oak St., Vancouver, British Columbia, Canada V6H 3V4.)

COMMENT. These authors have previously found an association between the prolonged use of antimotility drugs and the likelihood for progression of E coli enteritis to hemolytic-uremic syndrome. Systemically absorbed verotoxins are thought to be responsible for the multiple organ involvement. A food reservoir and improper handling are the most likely vehicles for transmission of the E coli.-Editor. *Ped Neur Briefs* Nov 1992.

E COLI HEMORRHAGIC COLITIS AND NEUROLOGIC SYMPTOMS

The neurological manifestations of hemorrhagic colitis in seven kindergarten children with *Escherichia coli* 0157:H7 infection are reported from the Saitama Children's Medical Center, Saitama, Japan. Generalized convulsions, occurring in 5 comatose patients, were intractable in 3 and required toxic doses of anticonvulsants for their control. Two patients died after 5 and 7 days of illness. Transient symptoms, delayed in onset for 2 to 6 weeks and after consciousness improved, included phrenic nerve paralysis in 1 patient, neurogenic urinary incontinence in 3, gaze nystagmus in 3, action tremor and oral dyskinesia in 1, and vertigo in 1 patient. Pyrexia and hemolytic uremic syndrome were seen only in patients with neurologic complications. Diarrhea, bloody diarrhea, and abdominal pain were more frequent and severe in this group compared to 7 patients with no neurologic symptoms who were admitted to hospital. Contaminated well water was the source of infection, and verotoxin-I (Shiga-like toxin I) was the likely cause of neurological symptoms. (Hamano S et al. Neurological manifestations of hemorrhagic colitis in the outbreak of *Escherichia coli* 0157:H7 infection in Japan. Acta Paediatr May 1993;82:454-458). (Respond: S Hamano MD, Division of Neurology, S Children's Medical Center, 2100 Magome, Iwatsuki, Saitama 339, Japan).

COMMENT. Fever, high white blood cell count, young or old age, and prolonged antimotility drug use are risk factors for complications of this strain of E. *coli* infection. For a comprehensive review of neurologic and other complications of foodborne and waterborne infections, pollutants, and additives, see Millichap JG, Environmental Poisons in Our Food, Chicago, PNB Publishers, 1993.-Editor. *Ped Neur Briefs* June 1993.

CHAPTER 14

TOXIC DISORDERS

INTRODUCTION

Fourteen million children less than seven years of age are exposed to lead in the environment in the United States. Seventeen percent have blood lead levels sufficient to cause serious deficits in intelligence and disorders of behavior. Lead is just one of many poisons that contaminate our food and water and pose potential risks to the health of both children and adult populations. Despite government regulations designed to control hazardous wastes and the use of poisonous pesticides and insecticides in agriculture, dangerous levels of mercury, PCB, DDT, dioxin and other toxic residues contaminate inland lakes and waterways.

The pediatric neurologist needs to be aware of the symptoms and signs of these neurotoxic environmental pollutants and their long term effects on psychomotor development. In addition to articles concerning lead, manganese, and prenatal PCB exposure and toxicity, the effects of alcohol, cocaine, and tremorogenic aflatoxins are included in the following literature reviews and commentaries.- *Editor.*

LEAD POISONING

PRENATAL HEAVY METAL EXPOSURE AND COGNITION

The effects of prenatal exposure to heavy metals on childhood cognitive skills and health status are reported from the Robert Wood Johnson Medical School, New Brunswick, NJ. Cadmium, chromium, cobalt, lead, mercury, nickel and silver were determined in amniotic fluid taken from 92 pregnant women at 16 - 18 weeks gestation. A prenatal toxic risk score was based on the presence of a detectable level for the various metals. A correlation analysis indicated a negative relation between the toxic risk score and cognitive performance and a significant positive correlation between the toxic risk score and both the total number of atopic illnesses and infections assessed at 3 years of age. These findings indicate that health status as well as cognitive ability may show deficits as a consequence of prenatal heavy metal exposure. (Lewis M et al. Prenatal exposure to heavy metals: effect on childhood cognitive skills and health status. Pediatrics June 1992; 89:1010-1015.) (Reprints: Dr. Michael Lewis, Institute for the Study of Child Development, Dept. of Pediatrics, UMDNJ-Robert Wood Johnson Medical School, RWJ Professional Bldg. New Brunswick, NJ 08903-0019.)

COMMENT. Lead intoxication in infants is common and is of different origin from that in toddlers (Shannon MW, Graef JW. Lead intoxication in infancy. Pediatrics Jan 1992; 89:87-90). Formula preparation with lead contaminated water accounted for 9 of 50 infantile cases whereas paint chip ingestion was the most common cause among 47 children (86%) aged 18 through 30 months. These data support recent recommendations to initiate lead screening in children at 6 months of age.

A maintained average blood level of 25 mcg/dL or more during the second and third year of life was found to be detrimental to the child's attained stature at

33 months of age in a study from the University of Cincinnati (Shukla R et al. Lead exposure and growth in the early preschool child: A follow-up report from the Cincinnati lead study . Pediatrics 1991; 88: 886-892).- Editor. *Ped Neur Briefs* Aug 1992.

LOW LEVEL LEAD EXPOSURES AND IQ

The Port Pirie cohort study which began in 1979 at the Department of Community Medicine, University of Adelaide, Australia, has been followed into the primary school age range and examines intelligence at the age of 7 years in relation to lifetime exposure to lead. In 494 children from a lead smelting community, the IQ was inversely related to both antenatal and postnatal blood level concentrations. An increase in blood lead concentration from 10 to 30 mcg/dL was associated with a deficit in verbal IQ that varied according to age from 5.5 to 6.4 points. In full scale IQ, the estimated deficit was 4.4 - 5.3 points. (Baghurst PA et al. Environmental exposure to lead and children's intelligence at the age of seven years. N Engl J Med Oct 29, 1992; 327:1279-84.) (Reprints: Dr. Baghurst, CSIRO Division of Human Nutrition, P.O. Box 10041, Gouger St., Adelaide, SA 5000, Australia.)

COMMENT. Mahaffey KR from the National Institute of Environmental Health Sciences, North Carolina, comments in an editorial that the results of 3 longitudinal studies (Australia, Boston and Cincinnati) demonstrate that the lead associated decrements in intelligence are persistent across cultures, racial and ethnic groups, and social and economic classes. They are not limited to socially and economically disadvantaged children (N Engl J Med 1992; 327:1308). Meta-analysis of 7 studies showed an average decrease of 0.25 IQ points for each 1 mcg/dL increase in blood lead levels (BPb). This inverse relationship between IQ and BPb continued well below 10 mcg/dL (Rosen JF AJDC Nov 1992; 146:1278).

Lead encephalopathy was diagnosed in 10 Saudi Arabian children, ages 8-48 months, during 1984-1988. The mean BPb was 6.1 umol/L (range, 2.5-13 umol/L).

(Yaish HM et al. AJDC Nov 1992; 146:1257). In Washington, DC, 590 (20.8%) of children aged 9 months to 3 years examined showed blood lead concentrations of 0.5 umol/L or more, which exceeded the acceptable CDC limits. At levels between 0.5 and 1.2 umol/L, the free erythrocyte protoporphyrin (FEP) screening test was a very poor predictor of toxic blood lead values (Rifai N et al. AJDC Nov 1992; 146:1259).-Editor. *Ped Neur Briefs* Nov 1992.

LEAD EXPOSURE AND MOTOR DEVELOPMENT

The neuromotor assessment of 245 six-year-old urban inner-city children enrolled in the Cincinnati Lead Study is reported from the Departments of Environmental Health and Pediatrics, University of Cincinnati College of Medicine, and the Children's Hospital Medical Center, Cincinnati, OH. Quarterly measures of blood lead and development since birth showed that neonatal, but not prenatal blood lead levels were associated with impaired coordination, hand speed and dexterity. Postnatal blood lead levels were associated with similar impairments of coordination, and poorer scores on visual-motor control. Low to moderate lead exposure is associated with moderate deficits in gross and especially fine-motor development. Blood lead levels peaked at 2 years of age and then slowly declined; 87 children (35%) had levels of 25 mcg/dL or greater during the first 5 years of life, while 195 (80%) had at least one level at or above 15 mcg/dL during this period. Only 5% were chelated therapeutically. (Dietrich KN, Berger OG, Succop PA. Lead exposure and the motor developmental status of urban six-year-old children in the Cincinnati prospective study. Pediatrics Feb 1993; 91: 301-307). (Reprints: Dr Dietrich, University of Cincinnati College of Medicine, Dept of Environmental Health, Cincinnati, OH 45267.)

COMMENT. The cerebellum is particularly sensitive to lead intoxication in neonatal rats, and glial cell development and brain histogenesis are affected. In children of low socioeconomic status, motor development and coordination may be more sensitive indicators of the adverse effects of lead on the central nervous system than tests of intelligence and academic achievement. Lead poisoning is now defined as a blood lead level greater than or equal to 10 mcg/dL Children aged 6 months to 6 years and those living in older housing are the highest priority for screening, mandatory in many States.-Editor. *Ped Neur Briefs* March 1993.

COGNITIVE IMPROVEMENT FOLLOWING LEAD CHELATION

The short (7 weeks) and long (6 months) term effects of lowered blood lead levels on cognitive performance were measured in 154 previously untreated lead-poisoned children, aged 13 to 87 months, examined at the Department of Pediatrics, Albert Einstein College of Medicine, Montefiore Medical Center, Bronx, NY. Pre-treatment blood lead levels were 25-55 mcg/dL, and erythrocyte protoporphyrin levels were >0.65 mcmol/L, in children enrolled. Housing inspections and abatement procedures were performed as necessary, and an iron supplement (6 mg/kg day) was prescribed for children (39% of group) with ferritin levels <16 mcg/L. Those with positive lead mobilization tests (40% of group) were administered a 5 day course of EDTA. Cognitive development was measured by the Bayley and Stanford-Binet: 1) before treatment, 2) at 7 weeks, and 3) 6 months after enrollment. The Stanford cognitive index (CI) increased 1 point for every decrease of 3 mcg/dL in blood lead level after 6 months but not at 7 weeks after treatment. A moderate correlation of test performance with ferritin levels was the only significant change at short term: every increase of 3 mcg/L in serum ferritin was associated with an increase of 1 point on the CI. (Ruff HA et al. Declining blood lead levels and cognitive changes in moderately lead-poisoned children. JAMA April 7 1993; 269:1641-1646). (Reprints: Holly A Ruff PhD, Department of Pediatrics, Room 222, Kennedy Center, Albert Einstein College of Medicine, Bronx, NY 10461).

COMMENT. The results suggest an association between decreases in blood lead level and cognitive improvements in lead-poisoned children. The authors remain cautious in making causal correlations, and they admit a possible contribution of iron supplements or other factors in the cognitive improvements observed.

A study of lead-contaminated soil abatement in Boston and blood lead levels of 152 urban children less than 4 years of age showed that soil abatement around homes results in only a modest decline in blood lead levels (2.44 mcg/dL after an 11 month interval). The median surface soil lead levels were 2075 ppm before abatement and 105 ppm after abatement. Urban children with low-level lead exposure are not appreciably benefited by soil abatement programs. (Weitzman M et al. JAMA April 7 1993; 269: 1647-1654). An estimated 3 million children in the United States and 69% of children, 6 months to 5 years of age, in Boston have blood lead levels >10 mcg/dL, sufficient to impair intelligence and development. (Also see Editorial, Binder S, Matte T, JAMA 1993; 269: 1679).-Editor. *Ped Neur Briefs* April 1993.

MANGANESE POISONING IN ALAGILLE'S SYNDROME

An 8 year old girl with Alagille's syndrome who developed dystonia secondary to manganese toxicity is reported from the Pediatric Department, Hershey Medical Center, Hershey, PA. She had developed a mild sensory neuropathy secondary to vitamin E deficiency which was corrected. MRI revealed hyperintense lesions in the globus pallidus bilaterally on T1 weighted images. A CT scan was normal. The serum manganese was 27 mcg/L (normal: less than 3). Treatment with ursodeoxycholic acid resulted in a normal serum manganese level. The dystonia cleared within 2 months of therapy. (Barron TF et al. Manganese neurotoxicity in Alagille's syndrome: a case report. Ann Neurol Sept 1992; 32:453 (abstr).)

COMMENT. Long exposure to inhalation of manganese has been known to be associated with neurological syndromes. The present case is unusual because the manganese toxicity was dietary in origin and caused by an impairment of the normal excretion of manganese through the biliary tree. Also, the symptoms were reversible. Wilson's disease was considered and excluded.

Alagille D. and colleagues described a syndrome of hepatic duct hypoplasia associated with characteristic facies, vertebral malformations, retarded physical, mental and sexual development and cardiac murmur (J Pediatr 1975:86-63). He also published on the clinical aspects of neonatal hepatitis (AMJ Dis Child 1972; 123:287). The above case of Alagille's syndrome was characterized by paucity of intrahepatic bile ducts with chronic cholestasis and pulmonic stenosis. Toxicity from dietary sources of manganese appears to require a prolonged period of exposure before neurological symptoms develop.-Editor. *Ped Neur Briefs* Nov 1992.

COCAINE ADDICTION AND EEG IN INFANTS

Thirty-five consecutive infants of cocaine-addicted mothers hospitalized for a comprehensive health assessment and 51 healthy, age-matched infants were studied with electroencephalography at the Children's Hospital of Philadelphia, PA. No definite EEG seizures were recorded in any of the patients. In infants of cocaine-addicted mothers there was a tendency for electroclinical sleep discordance, and the frequency of early acquisition of a mature pattern of quiet sleep (continuous, slow-wave sleep) was significantly higher than in the comparison group below conceptional age 45 weeks. The significance of precocious maturity of quiet sleep was unclear, but may indicate accelerated biological development. (Legido A et al. Electroencephalographic and behavioral-state studies in infants of cocaine-addicted mothers. AJDC June 1992; 146:748-752.) (Reprints: Dr. Legido, St. Christopher's Hospital for Children, Section of Neurology, Erie Avenue at Front Street, Philadelphia, PA 19134-1095.)

COMMENT. The authors suggest that the longitudinal assessment of sleep disturbance and its relation to later development might permit tracking of the long-term effects of prenatal exposure to cocaine. Other complications of cocaine exposure in utero are small head circumference, abnormal behavior, cerebral infarction or hemorrhage, seizures and SIDS.- Editor. *Ped Neur Briefs* July 1992.

COCAINE AND THE DEVELOPING BRAIN

The effects of cocaine on corticogenesis in the developing murine brain were examined at the University of Louvain Medical School, Brussels, Belgium, and the Massachusetts General Hospital, Boston, MA. Two groups of 5 pregnant mice were injected with 20-40 mg/kg/day of cocaine hydrochloride from the 8th day of gestation until term. Examination of brains of embryos from embryonic day 15-18, post-natal pups from birth to 10 days, and adults showed disturbances of corticogenesis and brain growth and reductions in the number of live pups per litter. Neocortical architecture was disrupted and various steps of gliogenesis were altered. Interference with neurogenesis in the germinative zone could be attributed to cocaine-induced recurrent ischemia and inhibition of DNA synthesis (Gressens P, Kosofsky BE, Evrard P. Cocaine-induced disturbances of corticogenesis in the developing murine brain. Neuroscience Letters 1992; 140:113-116). (Correspondence: Professor P. Evrard, Laboratoire de Neurologie du Developpement, Av. Hippocrate 10/1303, B-1200 Brussels, Belgium.)

COMMENT. An estimated 10-15 % of pregnant mothers deliver infants who have been exposed to cocaine in utero. Some develop behavioral impairments and structural brain abnormalities at birth (Kosofsky BE. NIDA research monograph 1991). In a separate series of experiments the same authors injected rat pups ages 8, 15 and 28 days and adult rats with cocaine 30 mg/kg. As early as 8 days, a 5-6 fold induction of striatal mRNA was evident before cortical-immediate early gene-induction was demonstrable. Cocaine induced alterations in gene transcription during critical developmental periods may alter CNS form and function and may relate to the gestational timing of the cocaine exposure (Kosofsky BE et al. Neuroanatomical consequences of exposing developing brain to cocaine: a rodent model. Ann Neurol Sept 1992; 32:426 (abstract)).-Editor. *Ped Neur Briefs* Nov 1992.

ALCOHOL AND MENTAL DEVELOPMENT

In a prospective follow-up study at the University of Helsinki, Finland, 60 children exposed to alcohol in utero were assessed by a psychologist (Bayley Mental scale) and a speech therapist (Reynell Verbal Comprehension scale) at a mean age of 27 months. Forty-eight non-exposed children were also examined to set the -2 SD limit for subnormal performance. In children exposed to heavy drinking during the first trimester only, no definite effect on mental or language development was demonstrated. Children exposed throughout pregnancy scored significantly lower than those subjected to alcohol during the first trimester only. The diagnosis of fetal alcohol syndrome was made in 7 children, 1 exposed during the first and second trimesters, and 6 exposed throughout pregnancy. The lower limit for heavy drinking was more than 10 drinks a week, or more than 45 drinks per month. The drinking patterns of these mothers varied from 1 to 20 drinks per day. (Autti-Ramo I et al. Mental development of 2-year-old children exposed to alcohol in utero. J Pediatr May 1992; 120:740-746.) (Reprints: Dr. Ilona Autti-Ramo, Peuramaentie 1 H 18, 02700 Kauniainen, Finland.)

COMMENT. Fetal alcohol exposure causes a continuum of developmental defects ranging from mental retardation to slight developmental difficulties. The identification of mothers who are heavy drinkers in early pregnancy and effective counseling should help to preserve the developmental potential of the fetus.-Editor. *Ped Neur Briefs* June 1992.

PRENATAL MARIHUANA, CIGARETTES, ALCOHOL AND ATTENTIONAL BEHAVIOR

A follow-up study of intentional behavior in 6 year old children exposed prenatally to marihuana, cigarettes and alcohol is reported from the Department of Psychology, Carleton University, Ottawa, Ontario, Canada. Discriminant function analysis in 126 children revealed a dose response association between prenatal cigarette exposure and impulsive behavior. Performance on memory tasks requiring verbal recall was negatively associated with maternal cigarette use. Prenatal marihuana was associated with omission errors in vigilance tasks reflecting a deficit in sustained attention. The mother's rating of impulsive hyperactive behavior was also higher. Low levels of maternal alcohol consumption were related to decreased impulsive responding, assessed by mothers' reports. (Fried PA et al. A follow-up study of attentional behavior in 6-year-old children exposed prenatally to marihuana, cigarettes, and alcohol. Neurotoxicol Teratol Sept/Oct 1992; 14:299-311). (Reprints: Dr. Peter A. Fried, Department of Psychology, Carlton University, Ottawa, Ontario, Canada KlS 5B6.)

COMMENT. There was no negative relationship between prenatal alcohol exposure and attention related variables noted in this study. The only differences related to maternal alcohol consumption were in decreased impulsivity: fewer responses were made in the delay tasks and a decreased degree of impulsivity/hyperactivity in the child was reported by the mother. Others have reported an increased reaction time associated with maternal alcohol consumption in 4 and 7 year old children on vigilance tasks. The timing of the exposure to the alcohol was not determined in this present study, and relatively low levels of alcohol were consumed by the mothers. This could account for the absence of negative association between attentional behavior and maternal alcohol use.-Editor. *Ped Neur Briefs* Dec 1992.

PRENATAL PCB EXPOSURE AND COGNITIVE DEVELOPMENT

IQ scores of 118 Taiwanese children who had been exposed prenatally to high levels of heat-degraded polychlorinated phenyls (PCBs) in contaminated rice oil and compared with controls are reported from the National Cheng Kung University Medical College,

Tainan, Taiwan, and the National Institute of Environmental Health Sciences, Research Triangle Park, North Carolina. Exposed children scored 5 points lower on the Chinese versions of the Stanford-Binet and WISC-R at ages 4 - 5 and 6 - 7 years, respectively. Children born up to 6 years after maternal exposure and tested at 6 and 7 years of age were as affected as those born within a year after exposure. (Chen Y-CJ, Rogan WJ et al. Cognitive development of Yu-Cheng ("oil disease") children prenatally exposed to heat-degraded PCBs. JAMA Dec 9 1992; 268: 3213-3218). (Reprints: Dr Chen, Department of Psychiatry, National Cheng Kung University Medical College, 138 Sheng Li Rd, Tainan 70428, Taiwan, Republic of China).

COMMENT. In the US children born to women who routinely consumed Lake Michigan sportfish had poorer short-term memory function on both verbal and quantitative tests in a dose-dependent fashion (Jacobson JL et al. Effects of in utero exposure to polychlorinated biphenyls and related contaminants on cognitive functioning in young children J Pediatr 1990; 116: 38). Rogan WJ, an author of the Taiwan report, has written several articles on the in utero effects of PCBs on child development, a hazard that requires effective governmental disposal. (Also see Environmental Poisons in our Food. Millichap JG, Chicago, PNB Publ, 1993, 271 pp).-Editor. *Ped Neur Briefs* March 1993.

ORGANOPHOSPHATE AND POLYNEUROPATHY

A 3-year-old boy was admitted to the North Shore University Hospital, Manhasset, NY, with acute organophosphate (Dursban) roach poisoning. He was comatose, his pupils were pinpoint, and he had tachycardia, frothy oral secretions, and fasciculations of the eyelids and extremities. Following treatment with atropine and phenytoin, he recovered consciousness and the fasciculations ceased. On the 11th day, he developed severe stridor, bilateral vocal cord paralysis, and areflexia with proximal neuropathy. By day 27, deep tendon reflexes had returned, and EMG and NCS were normal. (Aiuto LA et al. Life-threatening organophosphate-induced delayed polyneuropathy in a child after accidental chlorpyrifos ingestion. J Pediatr April 1993; 122: 658-660). (Reprints: Leslie A Aiuto MD, Div of Pediatric Critical Care Medicine, Dept of Pediatrics, North Shore University Hospital, 300 Community Dr, Manhasset, NY 11030).

COMMENT. Organophosphate-induced delayed polyneuropathy has been described previously only in adults. Clinical manifestations begin 1 to 3 weeks after the acute cholinergic crisis. Signs of a distal, symmetric, motor polyneuropathy may be complicated by pyramidal tract and CNS involvement. Residual deficits are common.-Editor. *Ped Neur Briefs* April 1993.

IPECAC-INDUCED NEUROMUSCULAR WEAKNESS

A 15-month-old girl was admitted to the University of Maryland, Department of Pediatrics, with recurrent vomiting after two previous hospitalizations for vomiting, proximal weakness, and ataxia. Weakness and hypotonia progressed, she could not sit, and deep tendon reflexes were depressed. She was hypotensive, the heart was enlarged, and the pulse rapid. Liver enzymes were markedly elevated. Muscle biopsy was consistent with a myopathy of undetermined cause. By day 12, the endotracheal tube was removed, and by day 14 she could walk. The mother had discovered an empty bottle of ipecac in the infant's toy box some 2 weeks before the initial hospitalization and 4 weeks before the onset of weakness. (Carraccio C et al. Sudden onset of profound weakness in a toddler. J Pediatr April 1993; 122: 663-667). (Reprints: Carol Carraccio MD, Dept of Pediatrics, Room N5W56, University of Maryland, 22 S Greene St, Baltimore, MD 21201).

COMMENT. The ipecac poisoning in this case was accidental but is sometimes intentional and a chemical method of child abuse. Emetine produces a neuromuscular weakness of moderate to severe degree by a direct toxic effect on muscle. Cardiomyopathy is an additional side effect of emetine overdose.-Editor. *Ped Neur Briefs* April 1993.

TREMOROGENIC TOXIC ENCEPHALOPATHY

A 16 year old boy who developed tremorogenic toxic encephalopathy as a result of inhalation and/or ingestion of mouldy silage containing aspergillus fumigatus, flavus and clavitus is reported from Halifax, Nova Scotia and Kingston, Ontario, Canada. Malaise, fatigue and headache were followed by fever, chills and vomiting. On recovery from these symptoms the boy had progressive dullness of mentation, an incapacitating tremor and rigidity. He was disorientated, his fund of knowledge was reduced and he could not add 2 digit numbers. The trembling and encephalopathy resolved after 7 days and his recovery has appeared to be complete. (Gordon K, Masotti R, Waddell W. Tremorogenic toxic encephalopathy: a role of mycotoxins in the production of CNS disease in humans? Ann Neurol Sept 1992; 32:453 (abstr)).

COMMENT. Reye's syndrome has been attributed to the ingestion of aflatoxins, a form of naturally occurring mycotoxin found on corn (Dvorackova I et al. Aflatoxin and encephalopathy with fatty degeneration of viscera (Reye). Ann Nutr Aliment 1977; 31:977-989.) Other foods sometimes contaminated by the aspergillus flavus and aflatoxins include peanuts, rice, cereals, soybeans and peas. Corn produced in southeastern United States has contained more than 20-100 ppb aflatoxin in 30% of samples tested. The tremorogenic mycotoxins induce rye grass staggers and bermuda grass tremors in sheep and cattle, but more commonly the aflatoxins are known for their effects on the liver and kidneys of animals and humans.-Editor. *Ped Neur Briefs* Nov 1992.

ASPARTAME AND ABSENCE SEIZURES

The effect of aspartame on epilepsy was studied in 10 children with previously untreated generalized absence seizures using a double blind challenge of 40 mg/kg aspartame as a single dose at the Children's Hospital, Halifax, Canada. Ambulatory cassette recording of the EEG and quantification of numbers and length of spike wave discharges on 2 consecutive days showed that the number of seconds spent in spike wave discharge per hour of recording was significantly increased following aspartame compared with the control day when the children received sucrose. (Camfield PR et al. Aspartame exacerbates EEG spike-wave discharge in children with generalized absence epilepsy: a double-blind controlled study. Neurology May 1992; 42:1000-1003.) (Reprints: Dr. Peter Camfield, IWK Children's Hospital, Box 3070, Halifax, Nova Scotia, Canada B3J 3G9).

COMMENT. Anecdotal claims that aspartame may exacerbate epilepsy appear to have scientific validity based on this EEG double blind controlled study in 10 children with absence seizures.

In support of the FDA decision to clear aspartame for general consumption, excepting phenylketonuric children, a study of 126 apparently healthy children and adolescents showed that there were no clinically significant differences documented between the children taking aspartame and those taking sucrose for a 13 week period, regardless of age between 2 and 21 years. Aspartame appeared to be a safe sweetening agent for use by healthy children aged 2 or older. (Frey GH. J Toxicology Environmental Health 1976; 2 401). However, studies of aspartame in children with neuropsychiatric problems are limited, and adequate data are not available to establish its safety and freedom from adverse effects. Until more specific investigations are completed to determine the effects of aspartame on seizure control it might be advisable to limit or avoid the ingestion of aspartame products in children with seizures and particularly poorly controlled absence seizures (Camfield et al. 1992). See Millichap JG. Nutrition. Diet and Child's Behavior. Charles C. Thomas, Springfield, 1986 for a review of the effects of aspartame on diseases of the nervous system in children.-Editor. *Ped Neur Briefs* June 1992.

Addendum: Aspartame exacerbation of seizures and epileptiform discharges was not observed in 10 epileptic children tested for a period of 2 weeks at Yale University School of Medicine, New Haven, CT

(Shaywitz BA et al. Ann Neurol Jan 1994; 35:98-103). Neither sucrose nor aspartame had statistically significant adverse effects on behavior or cognitive performance of 23 school-age children described by their parents as sensitive to sugar in a study at Vanderbilt University, Nashville, TN, and the University of Iowa College of Medicine, Iowa City. (Wolraich ML et al. N Engl J Med Feb 3, 1994; 330:301-7).

REYE SYNDROME AND ANTI-EMETICS

A drug-induced encephalopathy mainly by anti-emetics in two children with a diagnosis of Reye syndrome is reported from the Department of Paediatrics, University Hospital, Gasthuisberg, Leuven, Belgium. A 6 year-old girl presented with fixed stare, stupor alternating with agitation, confusion and wild delirium and signs of liver disease. The illness was preceded by headache, muscular aching, abdominal pain and anorexia. Vomiting had been treated with domperidone and metoclopramide. Dystonic reactions and oculogyric crises occurred one day before referral. When medication was omitted the neurological examination became normal 24 hours later. The preceding viral syndrome was due to influenza-A. The patient recovered completely after 10 days. Case 2 consisted of an 11 month-old baby who later proved to have cytomegalovirus infection. Anti-emetic domperidone had been prescribed for severe vomiting and 60 hours later bizarre arm movements and eye movements developed. A diagnosis of Reye syndrome prompted admission to hospital. The infant had impaired consciousness, stupor and upwards fixed gaze. The liver was enlarged and hypoglycemia and raised transaminases were noted. The encephalopathy and dystonic reactions were considered secondary to the anti-emetic drug in combination with liver disease most probably due to viral infection. Neurological examination was normal after 36 hours and the patient recovered completely after 10 days. The author stresses the need to consider drugs other than salicylates in the etiology of Reye syndrome and particularly the use anti-emetics (Casteels-VanDaele M. Reye syndrome or side effects of anti-emetics? Eur J Pediatr May 1991;

150:456-459).

COMMENT. In the 1960's several cases of toxic encephalopathy resembling Reye syndrome were reported in patients who had received the anti-emetic Tigan. Dr. John Pepper, the Director of Toxicological Studies at Hoffman Laroche Company investigated these reports with customary thoroughness and with the aid of many consultants. No specific correlation between the use of Tigan and the toxic encephalopathy was determined. The lack of association of Reye syndrome with aspirin use has been reported from Australia (Orlowski J P et al. A catch in the Reye Pediatrics 1987; 80:638. See Ped Neur Briefs Nov 1987).-Editor. *Ped Neur Briefs* July 1991.

MITOCHONDRIAL ENZYMES IN REYE'S SYNDROME

A nonuniform decrease in several mitochondrial residual enzyme activities in the liver and brain of a 42 year old woman who died with Reye's syndrome is reported from the Departments of Neurology and Pediatrics, Columbia Presbyterian Medical Center, New York, NY. Pyruvate carboxylase activity was negligible whereas subunits II and IV of cytochrome c oxidase were in normal quantities. There was no evidence for a specific insult to mitochondrial DNA or intramitochondrial protein synthesis. The trigger that precipitates the initial disturbance in the chemical micro environment of the mitochondrial matrix remains unknown. Restoration of mitochondrial ATP concentration repairs the disturbance of intramitrochondrial enzyme processing and is followed by recovery of organ function (Van Coster RN, De Vivo DC et al. Adult Reye's syndrome: a review with new evidence for a generalized defect in intramitochondrial enzyme processing. Neurology Nov 1991; 41:1815-1821).

COMMENT. In a review of the literature the authors found 26 additional cases of adult onset Reye's syndrome. Viral studies showed influenza A or B in 11, varicella in 1, dengue in 1, and not reported in 14. 12 recovered. The incidence of Reye's syndrome has decreased since 1981 and in 1988 there were only 20 cases reported. The relationship between Reye's syndrome and aspirin is debated (Casteels-Van Daele M. Lancet Nov 30, 1991; 338:1408) and the choice of alternative antipyretic management of fever is discussed in an editorial (Lancet Oct 26, 1991; 338:1049). Chronic paracetamol poisoning is reported in Australia and ibuprofen is suggested as an alternative.-Editor. *Ped Neur Briefs* Dec 1991.

CHAPTER 15

METABOLIC DISORDERS

INTRODUCTION

John H. Menkes, M.D.
Professor Emeritus of Neurology and Pediatrics
University of California, Los Angeles

Those of us who attended scientific meetings some two to three decades ago will remember the ongoing debates between "lumpers" and "splitters." Lumpers believed that the same genetic disease could have many different clinical presentations. Splitters, on the other hand, insisted that an identical clinical picture could result from a variety of different genetic mutations. In the intervening years the votes have come in, and the splitters have won, hands down. This should not come as a surprise to anyone who has reflected on the relatively restricted repertoire with which the immature nervous system can respond to disease. It is now evident that the same clinical picture can result from different mutations either at the same gene locus or at different loci. There are numerous examples to support this statement.

At this point in time, at least 37 mutations at the genetic locus that codes for phenylanaline hydroxylase have been recognized. All of these result in the clinical picture of phenylketonuria. Whereas in some mutations a small amount of functional phenylalanine hydoxylase has been preserved, in other mutations the enzyme is totally absent or non-functional, and consequently there is no tolerance for phenylalanine. A similarly diverse, but even more complex picture has emerged for GM2 gangliosidosis (Tay-Sachs disease). From these data we can now conclude that when the same clinical disease manfests itself in different ethnic groups, it probably results from different genetic mutations.

With a relatively limited clinical picture, how does the physician distinguish the child with a metabolic disorder from one in whom neurologic symptoms result from other causes? The triad of drowsiness, tachypnea and seizures represents a typical presentation of an organic aciduria. (Propionic acidemia. Ped Neur Briefs 1992;6:85-86). Atypical presentations are not unusual however. These include motor deterioration and the appearance of a movement disorder. (Methylglutaconic aciduria. Ped Neur Briefs 1992;6:55).

The clinical manifestations of mitochondrial disorders are particularly diverse, and almost any neurologic deficit has resulted from deletions or point mutations in the mitochondrial genome. (Alternating hemiplegia: mitochondrial dysfunction. Ped Neur Briefs 1993;7:48. Mitochondrial myopathy with DNA deletions. Ped Neur Briefs 1993;6:11. Leigh's syndrome with two mitochondrial defects. Ped Neur Briefs 1992;6:11-12).

The best advice is to consider a metabolic disorder whenever other causes for the neurologic disease are not readily apparent. Neuroimaging studies have been of little diagnostic help in these disorders, and a complete metabolic evaluation is much less expensive,

Treatment of metabolic disorders remains problematical. Dietary control, the mainstay for most entities, is not totally successful; in fact, for some conditions it is of little help. (Propionic acidemia: Prognosis. Ped Neur Briefs 1992;6:85-86). Gene therapy with direct insertion of the defective genetic material, or treatment with the missing gene product has been attempted for some entities, notably Gaucher disease and metachromatic leukodystrophy, with varying success. The costs and ethical problems inherent in these procedures have yet to be fully addressed.

Have we reached an end to the number of diagnosable metabolic disorders, and are we to content ourselves with delineating deletions and point mutations? This complaint which echoes that of young Alexander, who thought that his father, Philip of Macedonia, would not leave him any lands to conquer, is probably premature. Witness the molybdenum cofactor deficiency (Ped Neur Briefs 1993;7:93: and Ped Neur Briefs 1993;7:52), and the newly discovered defect in cholesterol biosynthesis responsible for Smith-Lemli-Opitz syndrome (Ped Neur Briefs 1994;8:11). Doubtlessly, there are many other metabolic disorders left to be described; it only requires a high index of suspicion, and a little bit of luck. - *John H, Menkes, M.D., Professor Emeritus of Neurology and Pediatrics, University of California, Los Angeles, CA.*

MITOCHONDRIAL DISEASES

DYSTONIA AND CYTOCHROME B DEFICIENCY:

An 18 year old female with idiopathic torsion dystonia associated with mitochondrial encephalomyopathy is reported from the Departments of Neurology, Pediatrics and Biochemistry, Wayne State University School of Medicine, Detroit, Michigan. At the age of 2 1/2 years she developed weakness and disuse of the right leg with a febrile illness. Within one week the weakness extended to the right upper limb. During the next six months she developed progressive dysarthria and dystonia of the right leg and trunk. The dystonia progressively involved all extremities over the next four years. At the age of 7 years CT revealed bilateral putaminal hypodensities. Mitochondrial encephalomyopathy was suspected because of persistent lactic acidemia and myopathy. Studies of oxidative metabolism on skeletal muscle mitochondria revealed partial cytochrome b deficiency indicating a defect in cytochrome b-Cl complex (Nigro MA et al. Partial cytochrome b deficiency in generalized dystonia. Pediatr Neurol Nov/Dec 1990; 6:407-410).

COMMENT. Children with Leigh encephalopathy may develop dystonia and putaminal degeneration. H magnetic resonance spectroscopy was used to demonstrate regional variation in brain lactate in an 11 month old infant with Leigh syndrome at the University of Pennsylvania, Philadelphia. (Detre JA et al. Regional variation in brain lactate in Leigh syndrome by localized H magnetic resonance spectroscopy. Ann of Neurol Feb 1991; 29:218-221). Elevations in brain lactate were observed throughout the brain, but were most pronounced in the basal ganglia and brain stem regions with an abnormal MRI appearance. The increase in lactate was consistent with a deficiency in oxidative substrate utilization. The measurement of brain lactate is significant in patients where blood lactate levels may not always be elevated.

Symptomatic dystonias secondary to birth asphyxia, birth trauma, Wilson's disease, other degenerative disorders, encephalitis, neuroleptic drugs and mitochondrial disorders are distinguished from idiopathic or primary torsion dystonias. A genetic study of *idiopathic* focal dystonias has shown that 25% of index patients had relatives with dystonia. The results of segregation anslysis suggested an autosomal dominant gene or genes with reduced penetrance as a common cause for focal dystonia and a single autosomal dominant gene mutation responsible for inherited dystonia in the majority of patients, irrespective of distribution or severity. Severity is largely determined by age of onset, with generalized idiopathic dystonia developing before the age of 20 and focal dystonias developing in adult life. (Waddy HM et al. Ann Neurol March 1991; 29:320-324).-Editor. *Ped Neur Briefs* April 1991.

MITOCHONDRIAL MYOPATHY WITH DNA DEPLETION

Five children with mitochondrial myopathy associated with depletion of muscle mtDNA are reported from the Departments of Neurology and Genetics and Development, Columbia University College of Physicians and Surgeons, New York, NY and other centers in Germany, Belgium and the U.S.A. Symptoms manifested within or soon after the first year of life and muscle biopsies showed ragged red fibers and decreased respiratory chain activity. There was good correlation between clinical severity and degree of mtDNA depletion in muscle. An infant who died at 2 months had lactic acidosis and less than 2% of the normal level of mtDNA, while 4 children with relatively milder myopathy had no lactic acidosis and 8-34% residual mtDNA (Tritschler H-J et al. Mitochondrial myopathy of childhood associated with depletion of mitochondrial DNA. Neurology Jan 1992; 42:209-217). (Reprints: Dr. Eric A. Schon, Department of Neurology, Rm. BB324, Columbia University, 630 West 168th St., New York, NY 10032.)

COMMENT. Depletion of mtDNA is considered a distinct entity distinguished from other known mitochondrial disorders with COX deficiency or with multiple respiratory chain defects (fatal and benign infantile myopathies, Leigh's syndrome, Kearns-Sayre syndrome). The principal clinical features of patients with mtDNA depletion and mitochondrial myopathy are weakness, hypotonia and respiratory distress.-Editor. *Ped Neur Briefs* Feb 1992.

MITOCHONDRIAL MYOPATHY WITH DNA DELETIONS

Deletions of mitochondrial DNA (mtDNA) are reported in 19 of 56 patients with mitochondrial myopathy examined in the Department of Neurology and Neuromuscular Research Laboratory, Mayo Clinic, Rochester, MN. All 19 patients had progressive external ophthalmoplegia and 12 had complete or partial Kearns-Sayre syndrome. The age at onset varied from 4 to 48 years, 10 presenting in childhood. Patients with more than 50% deleted mtDNA had an earlier onset of symptoms and a higher proportion of ragged red fibers and cytochrome c oxidase negative fibers than patients with less than 50% deleted mtDNA (Yamamoto M et al. Mitochondrial DNA deletions in mitochondrial cytopathies: observations in 19 patients. Neurology Nov 1991; 41:1822-1828). (Reprints: Dr. Andrew G. Engel, Department of Neurology, Mayo Clinic, Rochester MN 55905.)

COMMENT. This paper confirms that large scale mtDNA deletions are present in a high proportion of patients with mitochondrial myopathy associated with progressive external ophthalmoplegia and that these deletions are a hallmark of Kearns-Sayre syndrome. Kearns-Sayre syndrome consists of progressive external ophthalmoplegia, pigmentary retinopathy, cardiac conduction abnormalities, and mitochondrial myopathy involving facial, cervical and limb muscles and increased CSF protein.-Editor. *Ped Neur Briefs* Feb 1992.

LEIGH'S SYNDROME WITH TWO MITOCHONDRIAL DEFECTS

A female infant with a biochemical defect of the respiratory chain and of *B*-oxidation and neuropathological changes typical for Leigh's disease is reported from the Department of Neurology, University of Wurzburg, Departments of Pediatrics and Pathology, University of Hamburg, and Department of Pediatrics, University of Freiburg, Germany. The infant was seen at age 2 months because of hypotonia, delayed motor development and lactic acidosis. Decreased activities of both cytochrome c oxidase and long chain acyl coenzyme A dehydrogenase were found in a muscle specimen of 11 months and in a liver specimen obtained post mortem at 13 months. Myoclonic seizures accompanied by multifocal EEG epileptic discharges were treated with valproate. Seizures were controlled, but her general condition deteriorated within 2 months, respiratory insufficiency worsened and the acidosis became intractable. Post mortem examinations showed severe demyelination in the capsula interna, calcification in the brain stem ganglia, and gliosis in the pons and medulla. The liver was enlarged with centrolobular fatty infiltration. A rare occurrence of two independent mitochondrial enzyme defects is suggested (Reichmann H et al. Cytochrome c oxidase deficiency and long-chain acyl coenzyme A dehydrogenase deficiency with Leigh's subacute necrotizing encephalomyelopathy. Ann Neurol Jan 1992; 31:107-109). (Correspondence: Dr. Reichmann, Department of Neurology, University of Wurzburg, Josef-Schneider-Strasse 11, D-8700 Wurzburg, Germany.)

COMMENT. Valproate administration was not considered the cause but may have worsened the palmitoyl CoA dehydrogenase deficiency. Leigh's syndrome, first described in 1951, appears to be non-specific biochemically as well as clinically. Consistent early clinical features in the infantile cases are a quiet immobility with lack of crying and hypotonia. In addition to the COX deficiency and dehydrogenase deficiency described above, defects of the pyruvate dehydrogenase multi-enzyme complex and pyruvate carboxylase have been reported.-Editor. *Ped Neur Briefs* Feb 1992.

LEIGH ENCEPHALOPATHY

Histologic and biochemical analyses of muscle biopsies from 33 patients with Leigh encephalopathy were performed at the National Institute of Neuroscience, Tokyo and Tokushima University School of Medicine, Japan. Cytochrome c oxidase activity was decreased or absent in 7 patients (21%), 10 patients (30%) had biochemical defects including 2 with pyruvate dehydrogenase complex, 4 with cytochrome c oxidase, 1 with NADH-cytochrome c reductase and 3 with multiple complex deficiencies. None had DNA deletions in the muscle mitochondria. (Nagai T et al. Leigh encephalopathy: histologic and biochemical analyses of muscle biopsies. Pediatr Neurol Sept/Oct 1992; 8:328-332.) (Communications: Dr. Nagai, Division of Ultrastructural Research, National Institute of Neuroscience, NCNP, Kodaira, Tokyo 187, Japan.)

COMMENT. A mitochondrial DNA mutation in the ATPase 6 gene was reported in 7 of 40 patients with neuropathologically or MRI defined Leigh syndrome but no known biochemical defect (Santorelli FM et al. Ann Neurol Sept 1992; 32:467). A high abundance of the "NARP" mutation (neuropathy, ataxia, and retinitis pigmentosa) can cause Leigh syndrome and should be looked for in patients without biochemical defects. In another report, a 7 year old girl presented with a partial pyruvate carboxylase deficiency and basal ganglia lesions compatible with Leigh's disease (Schrank Wl et al. Ann Neurol Sept 1992; 32:468). The biochemical defects in Leigh encephalopathy are probably heterogeneous.-Editor. *Ped Neur Briefs* Nov 1992.

FAMILIAL SPASTIC PARAPARESIS AS A MITOCHONDRIAL DISORDER

A girl presenting at 6 years with familial spastic paraparesis and having deficiencies of respiratory chain enzyme complex I, III and IV is reported from the Departments of Pediatrics and Neurology, Loyola University Medical Center, Maywood, IL. Her gait was clumsy and her maternal grandmother had a spastic gait with onset at age 40. Deep tendon reflexes were brisk at the knees. Plantar responses were extensor bilaterally and ankle clonus was unsustained. The tone was increased in both lower extremities. The gait was wide based with hip circumduction. A 3 centimeter cyst in the left parietal region on MRI appeared to be coincidental. Efforts to treat the deficiencies of mitochondrial enzymes with various respiratory chain co-factors (coenzyme Q, vitamin K and C) and a mitochondrial substrate entry carrier (carnitine) were rewarded with no further progression of symptoms and some mild improvement clinically. The mitochondria were structurally normal by electron microscopy and ragged red fibers were absent on muscle biopsy (Beltran RS, Coker SB. Familial spastic paraparesis: a case of a mitochondrial disorder. Pediatr Neurosurg Oct 1991; 16:40-42). (Reprints: Dr. Beltran, Department of Pediatrics, Loyola University Medical Center, 2160 South First Ave., Maywood, IL 60153.)

COMMENT. Familial spastic paraparesis or *Stumpell's disease* is characterized by a progressive gait disturbance with lower extremity spasticity and weakness, without associated sensory, cerebellar or cranial nerve deficits. The age of onset ranges from 1-55 years and varies within specific kindreds. Heredity may be autosomal dominant, autosomal recessive or sex-linked. Involvement of the spinal cord is unique for a mitochondrial disorder.-Editor. *Ped Neur Briefs* Feb 1992.

EPILEPSY IN A MITOCHONDRIAL DISORDER

Epilepsy in 9 (22 %) of 37 members of a family with maternally inherited mitochondrial disease is reported from the Department of Neurology, University Hospital, Tromso, Norway. The epilepsy began in infancy or childhood in 3 patients and during adult life in the remainder. The different clinical expressions of epilepsy in the family were myoclonus, partial epilepsy and generalized tonic-clonic seizures. The neuropsychiatric disorders included intellectual deterioration, muscle weakness, pigmental retinal degeneration, progressive hearing loss, cerebellar ataxia and in 1 patient a hemiplegia and paranoid psychosis. The CT scan showed cerebral atrophy, cerebellar atrophy and calcification in the basal ganglia. The EEG abnormalities included slowing and spikes, sometimes focal, and a bilateral paroxysmal response to photic stimulation. A muscle biopsy from the proband revealed a mild defect in the NADH-ubiquinone oxidoreductase step (complex 1) in the respiratory chain (Torbergsen T et al. Epilepsy in a mitochondrial disorder. J Neur Neurosurg & Psych Dec 1991; 54:1073-1076). (Correspondence: Dr. Torbergsen, Department of Neurology, 9038 University Hospital, Tromso, Norway.)

COMMENT. The various clinical manifestations of epilepsy including partial motor and/or complex partial epilepsy in different branches of this family were remarkable and worthy of publication. The authors postulate that mitochondrial dysfunctions may be the cause of some epileptic syndromes of undetermined etiology.-Editor. *Ped Neur Briefs* Feb 1992.

MITOCHONDRIAL MYOPATHY AND CONGENITAL CATARACT

The autosomal recessive syndrome characterized by mitochondrial myopathy of cardiac and skeletal muscle, congenital cataract and lactic acidosis is described in two forms following a retrospective study of 16 patients at the University of Nijmegen, The Netherlands. Four patients with the fatal form died from hypertrophic obstructive cardiomyopathy in the neonatal period. In those with the relatively benign form, cardiomyopathy developed late, causing death in 7 patients at a median age of 23 years. The prognosis in patients without subvalvular aortic stenosis is dependent on the metabolic function of skeletal muscle. It varies between moderate exercise intolerance and wheelchair existence. In both forms, bilateral cataracts, lactacidemia and mitochondrial myopathy are present from birth. If a propositus has an affected sib, he will probably suffer from the same form, and genetic counselling is important. (van Ekeren GJ et al. A retrospective study of patients with the hereditary syndrome of congenital cataract, mitochondrial myopathy of heart and skeletal muscle and lactic acidosis. Eur J Pediatr 1993; 152(3): 255-259). (Respond: Dr RCA Sengers, Dept of Paediatrics, University of Nijmegen, PO Box 9101, NL-6500 HB Nijmegen, The Netherlands).

COMMENT. Cataracts present at birth are the first manifestation of the syndrome in most patients. Some present with muscular hypotonia, and others with cardiac symptoms. The metabolic cause is unknown. Skeletal muscle biopsy showed abnormal mitochondrial structure or number with matrix vesicles, and the sarcoplasm contained large quantities of lipid or glycogen. Morphometric analysis demonstrated an increased volume density of subsarcolemmal mitochondria, a possible compensatory mechanism for a deficit in energy production. The findings were similar in the fatal and benign forms. Mitochondrial function showed no abnormalities. Qualitative and quatitative defects in mitochondrial DNA in infants with fatal metabolic disorders are discussed by Moraes CT (Int Pediatr 1993; 8: 40).-Editor. *Ped Neur Briefs* May 1993.

ALTERNATING HEMIPLEGIA: A MITOCHONDRIAL DYSFUNCTION

Mitochondrial function in 4 patients with alternating hemiplegia (AH) was evaluated by magnetic resonance spectroscopy of resting muscle at the Montreal Neurological Institute, McGill University, Montreal, Canada. All patients had abnormally high resonance intensities from inorganic phosphate and an abnormally low calculated cytosolic phosphorylation potential. These changes were consistent with mitochondrial dysfunction. (Arnold DL et al. Evidence for mitochondrial dysfunction in patients with alternating hemiplegia of childhood. Ann Neurol June 1993; 33: 604-607). (Respond: Dr Arnold, Montreal Neurological Institute, 3801 University Street, Montreal, Quebec, H3A 2B4 Canada).

COMMENT. Alternating hemiplegia of childhood may represent a phenotype of mitochondrial disease. Mitochondrial diseases share with AH the occurrence of alternating hemiplegia, seizures, and neuro-developmental deterioration. The clinical characteristics and differential diagnosis of AH are reviewed in a report of 22 cases from the Hopital des Enfants Malades, Paris, France. (Bourgeois M et al. J Pediatr May 1993; 122: 673-9). SPECT images of two patients showed focal areas of decreased uptake of the radiotracer, representing impaired regional blood flow during and between hemiplegic episodes and a possible mechanism of the neurologic deficits.(Siemes H, Cordes M. Dev Med & Child Neur April 1993; 35: 346).-Editor. *Ped Neur Briefs* June 1993.

ORGANIC ACIDURIAS

METHYLGLUTACONIC ACIDURIA

Two siblings with 3-methylglutaconic aciduria with normal enzyme activity and neurological abnormalities are reported from the Department of Pediatrics, Beilinson Medical Center, Petah Tiqva, Sackler School of Medicine, Tel Aviv University, Israel. Patient 1, an 11 month old infant was referred for evaluation of deterioration of motor development beginning at 5 months of age. There was an arrest of weight gain and head circumference growth. He was restless and had choreoathetoid movements of hands, head and mouth, deep tendon reflexes were hyperactive, plantar responses were extensor and optic discs atrophied. At 2 years of age he sat with support, crawled and walked with help. MRI and CT showed prominent frontal lobe atrophy. Urinary organic acid analysis showed a prominent peak of 3-methylglutaconic and 3-methylglucrylic acid. Patient 2, the 14 year old sister of patient 1, developed ataxia of gait at age 2 years, and optic atrophy at 8 years of age. Examination showed variable muscle tone with brisk tendon reflexes and extensor plantar responses. Choreoathetoid movements were prominent in the upper limbs, head and mouth and funduscopic examination showed prominent optic atrophy. Her IQ on the WISC was 87. CT and MRI showed generalized brain atrophy. Urinary organic acid excretion showed a prominent peak of methylglutaconic and methylglutaric acids. The patients represent a new clinical variant of the methylglutaconic aciduria syndrome with a relatively favorable prognosis. (Zeharia A, Weitz R et al. 3-methylglutaconic aciduria: a new variant. Pediatrics June 1992; 89:1080-1082.) (Reprints: Avraham Zeharia, M.D., Department of Pediatrics B, Beilinson Medical Center, Petah Tiqva 49100, Israel.)

COMMENT. 3-Methylglutaconic aciduria is the hydrolysis product of 3-methylglutaconyl coenzyme and an intermediate in the degradation pathway of leucine. Two syndromes are described - one with deficient methylglutaconyl coenzyme A and the other with normal enzyme activity, but prominent neurological deterioration. The present case reports were unique in the relatively normal cognitive and intellectual development and the relatively mild neurological manifestations. The boy had demonstrated developmental improvement in his second year of life and his sister developed well with normal school performance.-Editor. *Ped Neur Briefs* July 1992.

SYNDROMES OF 3-METHYLGLUTACONIC ACIDURIA

The most common clinical syndromes associated with 3-methylglutaconic (MGC) aciduria are reviewed by researchers from various centers; Courtwright and Summers Metabolic Disease Center and Baylor Research Institute, Dallas, TX; Shaare Zedek Medical Center, Jerusalem; Free University of Amsterdam; Loewenstein Hospital, Tel-Aviv Univ, Raanana, Israel; and Kennedy Krieger Institute, Baltimore, MD. Three distinct syndromes are described: *Type I 3-MG-CoA Hydratase Deficiency.-* (autosomal recessive) 3 patients had delayed speech and macrocephaly, increased urinary excretion of 3-MGC acid, 3-M Glutaric(MGR) and 3-hydroxyisovaleric acids, elevated CPK and serum carnitine, and hypoglycemia. Urinary 3-MGC excretion is decreased by restriction of L-leucine intake. *Type II Barth Syndrome.- (* X-linked) dilated cardiomyopathy, recurrent infection, neutropenia, growth retardation. Improves with age. Increased urinary excretion of 3-MGC, 3-MGR, fumaric, and 2-ethylhydracrylic acids. *Type III Costeff Optic Atrophy Syndrome.*(autosomal recessive) A Behr-like syndrome described in 39 patients of Iraqi-Jewish origin living in Israel. Optic atrophy, choreoathetosis, spastic paraparesis, cerebellar ataxia. Nonprogressive. 3-MGC and 3-MGR aciduria. An *Unclassified 3-MGC aciduria* includes patients presenting in the first year of life with neurologic impairment, seizures, retinal pathology, and a fatal course. Cardiomyopathy, hepatic dysfunction, hypoglycemia, lactic acidosis, and dysmorphia are associated manifestations. Defects of the mitochondrial respiratory chain are suggested. (Gibson KM et al. Multiple syndromes of 3-methylglutaconic aciduria. Pediatr Neurol March/April 1993; 9: 120-123). (Respond:

Dr Gibson, Baylor Research Institute, 3812 Elm Street, Dallas, TX 75226).

COMMENT. This review will assist the neurologist in the differential diagnosis of patients with 3-MGC aciduria. Some cases are multisystemic and progressive, with onset from birth to several years, some are primarily neurologic and non-progressive, while others involve the heart muscle and may improve with age.-Editor. *Ped Neur Briefs* May 1993.

HYDROXYGLUTARIC ACIDEMIA

Increased urinary excretion of L-2-hydroxyglutaric acid, found in 8 mentally retarded patients from 5 unrelated families including 3 pairs of siblings seen in various centers in Europe, was reported from University Hospital Amsterdam, the Netherlands. The first symptoms occurred between 1 and 5 years of age and consisted of abnormal gait. Febrile seizures occurred in 7 of 8 patients. Cerebellar dysfunction was the principle neurological abnormality in later childhood and adulthood. MRI revealed subcortical leukoencephalopathy, cerebellar atrophy, and changes in the putamina and dentate nuclei. L-2-hydroxyglutaric acid was also increased in the CSF and plasma. Lysine was increased in CSF and plasma and glutaric acid was increased in the plasma of 2 patients. Loading and dietary studies failed to reveal the origin of the L-2-hydroxyglutaric acid. (Barth PG et al. L-2-Hydroxyglutaric acidemia: a novel inherited neurometabolic disease. Ann Neurol July 1992; 32:66-71.)

COMMENT. Glutaric acidemia, an autosomal recessively inherited disease caused by deficiency of glutaryl-Coenzyme A dehydrogenase, was manifested by acute dystonia in 3 infants reported from the Children's Hospital of Pittsburgh, PA (See Ped Neurol Briefs Jan 1989). Dystonia was also reported in 3 of the 8 patients with L-2-hydroxyglutaric acidemia.-Editor. *Ped Neur Briefs* Sept 1992.

PROPIONIC ACIDEMIA: PROGNOSIS

The neurologic outcome of 20 patients with propionic acidemia was evaluated at the Medical Unit, Institute of Child Health, London, England. In 11 patients who presented in the first week of life, the death rate was high and all were mentally retarded (IQ less than 60), and 3 had mild chorea or dystonia. Of 9 patients with onset after the neonatal period, 4 had a severe movement disorder that evolved following an episode of metabolic derangement. In the late onset group, CT disclosed transient basal ganglia lucencies after episodes of metabolic decompensation. CSF neurotransmitter metabolites were unchanged (Surtees RAH et al. Neurologic outcomes of propionic acidemia. Pediatr Neurol Sept/Oct 1992; 8:333-337). (Respond: Dr. Surtees, Medical Unit, Institute of Child Health, 30 Guilford Street, London WCIN 1EH, England.)

COMMENT. A biotin-responsive propionic acidemia in a newborn is reported from Buenos Aires, Argentina and Paris, France (Cayssials AE et al. Pediatr Neurol Sept/Oct 1992; 8:409 (abstract)). The infant presented at the 4th day of life with partial feeding rejection, drowsiness, tachypnea, hypothermia and hepatomegaly. He developed generalized tonic-clonic seizures and required mechanical respiratory support. Enzyme studies in fibroblasts showed a profound deficiency of propionyl-CoA carboxylase activity and normal values for pyruvate carboxylase. Lab results showed severe metabolic acidosis and ketonuria. Treatment with carnitine and biotin was followed by clinical improvement and normal urine organic acids. One patient in the early onset group of the London study was treated with biotin and lived to 6 years of age. The outcome for patients with propionic acidemia is generally poor, although there is a wide variation.

Propionic acidemia (ketotic hyperglycinemia) should be distinguished from non-ketotic hyperglycinemia which is characterized by hypotonia, lethargy and seizures beginning on the first day of life. Some infants succumb within a few weeks, whereas others develop mental retardation and extrapyramidal signs (Menkes JH. Textbook of Child Neurology 3rd Ed., Philadelphia, Lea & Febiger 1981).-Editor. *Ped Neur Briefs* Nov 1992.

BIOTINIDASE DEFICIENCY AND SEIZURES

The clinical features of 78 symptomatic children with biotinidase deficiency were reviewed and the response to antiepileptic drugs and biotin therapy in 43 (55%) with seizures are reported from the Medical College of Virginia, Richmond, VA. Seizures were the presenting symptom in 30 (38%) patients, with onset between 2 and 24 months (mean, 8 months). Seizure patterns were generalized tonic-clonic or clonic in 56%, infantile spasms or myoclonic in 16%, and partial in only 5%. EEGs were abnormal in 16 (76%) of 21 patients tested; spike or other epileptiform discharges were reported in 9. Antiepileptic drugs controlled seizures in 22 (51%) patients, but treatment was withdrawn without relapse after biotin therapy was initiated. Biotin orally, 5 to 10 mg daily, stopped seizures within 24 hours in 12 of 16 (75%) children whose seizures were uncontrolled by AEDs. Five infants died and 3 sustained permanent brain damage before the biotinidase deficiency was diagnosed. (Salbert BA, et al. Characterization of seizures associated with biotinidase deficiency. Neurology July 1993; 43: 1351-1355). (Reprints: Dr Barry Wolf, Dept of Human Genetics, Medical College of Virginia, Box 33, MCV Station, Richmond, VA 23298).

COMMENT. Early diagnosis by newborn screening is recommended by the authors. Biotinidase enzyme deficiency and a trial of biotin should be considered in infants or young children with poorly controlled seizures, especially in those with hypotonia, ataxia, skin rash, alopecia, metabolic ketoacidosis, or organic aciduria. Symptoms resolve rapidly after biotin therapy, but neurologic damage may be irreversible if diagnosis is delayed. (see Ped Neur Briefs, Jan 1990).-Editor. *Ped Neur Briefs* July 1993.

MAPLE SYRUP URINE DISEASE AND CEREBRAL EDEMA

Cerebral edema causing death in four children

with maple syrup urine disease (MSUD) is reported from St. Christopher's Hospital for Children, Temple University School of Medicine, Philadelphia, PA. An intercurrent infection that caused severe dehydration and acidosis precipitated the cerebral edema when the children were three to five years of age. All four had been adequately managed with few problems before the intercurrent illness. The diagnosis of cerebral edema was established by autopsy in one patient and demonstrated by CT in two, one also having a subarachnoid hemorrhage. The authors recommend early hospitalization and cautious rehydration in all children with MSUD in whom intercurrent infections develop in association with decreased nutrient intake or vomiting, or both. Early treatment of dehydration and acidosis may prevent the catastrophic consequences observed (Riviello JJ Jr et al. Cerebral edema causing death in children with maple syrup urine disease. J Pediatr July 1991; 119:42-45).

COMMENT. Acute metabolic decompensation in MSUD during otherwise minor illnesses has generally been presumed to result from massive release of leucine from protein catabolism. The dynamics of protein metabolism and implications for management are reported from the Murdoch Institute and the Department of Dietetics, Royal Children's Hospital, Melbourne, Australia, and the Nutrition Research Group, Clinical Research Centre, Harrow, UK (Thompson GN et al. J Pediatr July 1991; 119:35-41). Fasting appeared to be a more important cause of increased leucine levels than the catabolic effect of infection. Branched-chain amino acid restriction should be commenced at the start of minor illness in children with MSUD and the intake of other nutrients should be increased. Dietary supplementation reduces the risk of metabolic decompensation during acute illnesses. Early and meticulous treatment of MSUD results in intellectually normal children, according to a study from the Division of Biochemical Development and Molecular Diseases, Children's Hospital of Philadelphia, University School of Medicine, Philadelphia (Kaplan P et al. J Pediatr July 1991; 119:46-

50). Affected children treated pre-symptomatically had higher IQ scores than their siblings treated when their disease was symptomatic.-Editor. *Ped Neur Briefs* Sept 1991.

MENKES MAPLE SYRUP URINE DISEASE: TREATMENT

Five patients with maple syrup urine disease were treated intravenouslv with branched-chain amino acid-free solution of amino acids during nine episodes of acute illness and are reported from the Children's Hospital of Philadelphia, PA. In a regimen of total parenteral nutrition a 9% branched-chain amino acid-free solution of amino acids reduced plasma leucine levels in acutely ill infants and young children with maple syrup urine disease. The steps in treatment included rapid correction of dehydration or acidosis; recommended dietary allowance of calories; age dependent minimal requirement of amino acids; supplements of isoleucine or valine to prevent deficiency; and treatment of hyperglycemia with insulin. The use of the modified parenteral nutrition was associated with relief from vomiting, improvement in consciousness, and return to the maple syrup urine disease formula. The authors stress the value of this therapy in all acutely ill patients with plasma leucine levels hetween 1 and 2 mmol per liter who cannot tolerate enteral nutritional therapy. (Berry GT et al. Branched-chain amino acid-free parenteral nutrition in the treatment of acute metabolic decompensation in patients with maple syrup urine disease. N Engl J Med Jan 17, 1991; 324:175-179).

COMMENT. Peritoneal dialysis and hemodialysis have proved effective in the treatment of acute metabolic decompensation in these patients but in those who are not comatose, this form of modified nutritional therapy may be more appropriate. The treatment was thought to lower the plasma leucine levels by favoring the flux of branched-chain amino acids into body protein.-Editor. *Ped Neur Briefs* Feb 1991.

NON-MENKES TYPE COPPER DEFICIENCY

A two year old girl with copper deficiency, progressive neuronal disorder and granulocytopenia is reported from the Department of Pediatrics, Kyoto University, Japan. A familial granulocytopenia was noted at one month of age and she developed truncal ataxia and progressive neurologic regression at age two years, shortly after a ten day fever. She was admitted with a diagnosis of acute cerebellar ataxia and later developed dysarthria, mild dysphagia and was then unable to speak two word sentences. She was referred to the Utano National Hospital, Kyoto, three months after the onset. She was well nourished, her hair was normal, and she had no hepatosplenomegaly. Truncal and limb ataxia, horizontal nystagmus, increased reflexes and extensor plantar reflexes were noted. CT showed cerebellar atrophy and symmetric low-density areas in the bilateral periventricular white matter. Sural nerve biopsy revealed axonal degeneration. Blood lactate levels were high (25.8 mg/dl) and serum levels of copper and ceruloplasmin and urinary excretion of copper were low. Cultured skin fibroblasts showed normal copper uptake. Copper given orally 0.1 mg/kg daily for three days resulted in increased serum copper and ceruloplasmin levels, normal granulocyte count, hemoglobin level, blood lactate and pyruvate levels, but neither clinical improvement nor normalization of copper, lactate and pyruvate levels in the CSF were noted. The patient deteriorated slowly, the MRI showed extension of high signal T2-weighted images and newly appearing lesions in the basal ganglia. At age three years (11 months after onset) she had spastic tetraplegia with respiratory difficulty and was placed on a respirator. (Fujii T et al. Non-menkes-type copper deficiency with regression, lactic acidosis, and granulocytopenia. <u>Neurology</u> August 1991; <u>41</u>:1263-1266).

COMMENT. The clinical and MRI features of this patient ruled out the diagnosis of Wilson's disease. Menkes' disease was unlikely in the absence of pili torti and with a normal copper uptake in cultured fibroblasts. The authors speculated that copper transport across the intestinal wall and across the blood brain barrier was impaired in their patient, and that long-term copper deficiency in the brain might have caused irreversible damage to cytochrome c oxidase production.-Editor. *Ped Neur Briefs* Sept 1991.

MENKES DISEASE: COPPER-HISTIDINE THERAPY

The response to subcutaneous copper-histidine treatment (50 - 150 mcg Cu/kgm/daily) in seven children with Menkes disease (Kinky-Hair disease) is reported from the Hospital for Sick Children and University of Toronto, Canada. Two patients, ages 16 and 6 years, whose therapy began within 1 month of birth, did well neurologically but have skeletal deformities and muscle weakness. Both have normal IQs and no seizures. The other 5 patients whose treatment was initiated at 2 to 7 months of age failed to thrive and had progressive neurological deterioration. Treatment with copper-histidine is recommended and should be started before 1 month of age. (Sarkar B, Lingertat-Walsh K, Clarke JTR. Copper-histidine therapy for Menkes disease. J Pediatr Nov 1993;123:828-830). (Reprints: B Sarkar PhD, Head, Department of Biochemistry Research, Hospital for Sick Children, Toronto, Ontario M5G IX8, Canada).

COMMENT. In a 13-week-old boy with Menkes disease treated with copper-histidine by daily intramuscular injections, Cu and ceruloplasmin in serum and Cu in CSF became normal after 6 weeks, epileptic discharges and infantile spasms were reduced, muscle tone was improved, motor activities increased, and developmental regression stopped. A marked improvement in osseous changes at 6 months was also noted. (Kreuder J et al. Clinical and biochemical consequences of copper-histidine therapy in Menkes disease. Eur J Pediatr Oct 1993; 152:828-832). This report from Children's Hospital, Justus Liebig University, Giessen, Germany, is the first to demonstrate normalization of dopamine and dopamine /norepinephrine ratio in CSF after copper-histidine therapy.

The recent reports from three independent

laboratories of the isolation of a Menkes' gene candidate have narrowed the search for the defective or missing factor in this sex-linked, recessive neurodegenerative disorder. A copper-transporting ATPase may be the important factor in normal copper metabolism. (Harris ED. Menkes' disease: Perspective and update on a fatal copper disorder. Nutrition Reviews Aug 1993;51:235-245).-Editor. *Ped Neur Briefs* Nov 1993.

BIOCHEMICAL MARKER FOR MENKES DISEASE

Plasma and CSF levels of catechols in 10 patients with Menkes disease, ranging in age from 9 days to 27 months, were compared with control groups and patients with congenital absence of dopamine-B-hydroxylase (DBH) at the National Institutes of Health, Bethesda, MD. The neurochemical pattern in Menkes disease patients was characterized by high dihydroxyphenylalanine (DOPA), dopamine (DA), and dihydroxyphenylacetic acid (DOPAC) levels, reduced dihydoxyphenylglycol(DHPG) levels, and high ratios of DOPA:DHPG and DOPAC:DHPG. In contrast to patients with absent DBH, norepinephrine (NE) levels were normal in 4 Menkes patients and in the CSF of all 10 patients. The pattern was consistent with partial deficiency of DBH activity and compensatory increases in catecholamine biosynthesis in sympathetic nerves and brain. The changes may provide a biochemical marker for Menkes disease. (Kaler SG et al. Plasma and cerebrospinal fluid neurochemical pattern in Menkes disease. Ann Neurol Feb 1993; 33: 171-175). (Correspondence: Dr Kaler, National Inst of Health, Bldg 10, Rm 9S 242, 9000 Rockville Pike, Bethesda, MD 20892).

COMMENT. Menkes disease (Kinky-Hair disease) is a sex-linked recessive, neurodegenerative disorder of gray matter involving copper metabolism. Clinically, it is characterized by failure to thrive, cherubic facies, twisted and fractured hair, seizures, hypotonia, and progressive psychomotor deterioration. Biochemically, serum copper and ceruloplasmin levels are reduced or low-normal, and copper uptake by cultured fibroblasts is abnormally increased, permitting intrauterine diagnosis of the disease. Copper levels in liver and brain are low, but are high in the intestine and kidney. The incorporation of copper into enzymes such as DBH requiring this cofactor is impaired. DBH activity was assessed in the present study by measuring levels of DA, NE, and metabolites to provide a picture of catecholamine synthesis and turnover in infants with Menkes disease.-Editor. *Ped Neur Briefs* Feb 1993.

CEREBELLAR SYMPTOMS IN CRIGLER-NAJJAR TYPE I DISEASE

Three children with Crigler-Najjar (CN) type I disease who had cerebellar symptoms as the initial manifestation of kernicterus are reported from the Hopital Antoine Beclere, Clamart Cedex, France. Patient 1, a 3600 gram boy, was admitted with jaundice and a serum total bilirubin of 507 umol/L unconjugated on day 2. After two exchange transfusions and continuous phototherapy the jaundice persisted and a therapeutic trial with phenobarbital was of no benefit. The bilirubin UDPG-T hepatic activity assayed at 3 months was absent. At age 6 years during an episode of fever and headache with respiratory viral infection the jaundice increased and ataxia and dysmetria developed. Liver transplantation was performed with apparent success. In all 3 children the cerebellar symptoms began after an infectious episode or an interruption of phototherapy. The neurotoxicity was associated with an elevated saturation of albumin by bilirubin of 61% to 75%. In 8 patients without neurotoxicity this parameter remained below 58%. (Labrune PH et al. Cerebellar symptoms as the presenting manifestations of bilirubin encephalopathy in children with Crigler-Najjar type I disease. Pediatrics April 1992; 89:768-770.) (Reprints: P.H. Labrune,M.D.,Service de Pediatrie, Hopital antoine Beclere, 157 rue de la Porte de trivaux, 92141 Clamart Cedex, France.)

COMMENT. Cerebellar symptoms are rare features of kernicterus despite the known occurrence of bilirubin staining of the dentate nuclei in pathological studies. The absence of reports of cerebellar involvement in the neonate may be explained by the difficulty in detection of cerebellar signs. Since neurological impairment may be permanent and is potentially preventable, patients with CN-1 disease are candidates for liver transplantation performed when phototherapy is ineffective and prior to the development of kernicterus. Therapy of jaudice in the newborn is reviewed by Newman TB and Maisels MJ in Pediatrics May 1992; 89:809-818.-Editor. *Ped Neur Briefs* July 1992.

FOLATE DEFICIENCY, PORPHYRIA, AND SEIZURES

A 12 year old, learning-disabled boy with epilepsy was admitted to the University of Connecticut Health Center, Farmington, CT because of symptomatic folate deficiency and newly diagnosed acute intermittent porphyria. Seizures and global developmental delays were noted by 12 months of age. Seizures required multiple drug combinations, and optimal control was obtained with carbamazepine, valproate, and methsuximide. The patient was hospitalized because of abdominal pain, vomiting, anorexia, and behavioral changes. He developed hypertension, hyponatremia, and anemia. The urine became brown in color, positive for urobilinogen, and showed elevated coproporphyrins, uroporphyrins, aminolevulinic acid, and porphobilinogen (PBG). Erythrocyte and maternal PBG deaminase measurements were decreased. RBC folate levels were deficient. Oral folate, 0.5 mg/d, resulted in correction of the anemia and no recurrence of porphyric crises. (DiMario FJ Jr et al. Folate deficiency and acute intermittent porphyria in a 12-year-old boy. Neurology July 1993; 43: 1438-1439). (Reprints: Dr Francis J DiMario Jr, Pediatric Neurology, Bldg 12, UCONN Health Center, Farmington, CT 06030).

COMMENT. Serum folate should be determined in patients with acute intermittent porphyria requiring chronic anticonvulsant therapy. A folate deficiency induced by the AEDs may further reduce red blood cell production and precipitate a porphyric crisis. Folate supplements are beneficial as an adjunct to the carbohydrate loading in therapy for a porphyric crisis or its prevention.-Editor. *Ped Neur Briefs* July 1993.

MOLYBDENUM-COFACTOR DEFICIENCY AND SEIZURES

The clinical, biochemical, and neuropathological findings in two neonates with molybdenum-cofactor deficiency presenting with convulsions are reported from the Academic Medical Center, Amsterdam, The Netherlands. Patient 1 was admitted at day two with feeding problems, jitteriness, an abnormal cry, apneic spells, and partial and generalized seizures. Head circumference, weight and length were above the 97th percentile. EEGs showed a burst suppression pattern. CT revealed diffuse hypodense ischemic changes. Plasma and urinary cysteine were decreased, and urine sulphite, S-sulphocysteine, taurine, and thiosulphate were increased. Purine analysis showed elevated xanthine and hypoxanthine in the urine, while uric acid was very low. Seizures were refractory, and the infant died on the 10th day. Cultured fibroblasts from a skin biopsy showed absent sulfite oxidase activity. Autopsy findings were meningeal fibrosis, loss of cortical neurons, gliosis and cystic lysis of white matter. Patient 2 was admitted at age 4 days with feeding difficulties, hypertonia, jitteriness, opisthotonus, and high-pitched cry. Generalized and partial tonic-clonic seizures were resistant to treatment. EEG was a multifocal epileptic pattern. An initial diagnosis of postanoxic encephalopathy was changed to molybdenum-cofactor deficiency at 3 years, on reexamination prompted by the revelation of parental consanguinity. Clinically deteriorated, he had spastic tetraplegia, intractable epilepsy, and characteristic metabolic changes. He died 8 months later. Diagnosis was confirmed by liver biopsy and sulfite oxidase and xanthine oxidase analyses. Lens dislocation, a frequent feature of the syndrome, was absent. (Slot HMJ et al. Molybdenum-cofactor deficiency: an easily missed cause of neonatal convulsions. Neuropediatrics June 1993; 24: 139-142). (Respond: Mrs HMJ Slot MD, Dept of Neonatology, Academic Medical Center, Meibergdreef 9, 1105 AZ Amsterdam, The Netherlands).

COMMENT. Molybdenum-cofactor deficiency is an inborn error of metabolism that results in characteristic biochemical and clinical symptoms of sulphite oxidase and xanthine dehydrogenase deficiences. Diagnosis can be made simply with a sulphite strip test in fresh urine and by measuring uric acid excretion. Antenatal diagnosis is possible by chorionic villus sampling and sulphite oxidase assay.- Editor. *Ped Neur Briefs* July 1993.

MOLYBDENUM COFACTOR DEFICIENCY: DIETARY THERAPY

Moderate short-term clinical improvement was obtained with dietary methionine restriction and cysteine supplementation in a 5-month-old-girl with molybdenum cofactor deficiency (MoCD) treated at Yale University School of Medicine, New Haven, CT. Born to first-cousin parents, the infant's head circumference fell from the 25th percentile at birth to <5th at age 2 months. Developmental delay, spastic quadriplegia, opisthotonus, and irritability were remarkable at 3 months, and a CT showed multiple infarcts. Focal seizures began at 4 months. Laboratory abnormalities included an elevated plasma lactate level, low plasma cysteine, low serum uric acid, and urine positive for sulfites and S-sulfocysteine, consistent with sulfite oxidase deficiency. The diagnosis of MoCD was confirmed by absent urinary urothione. Within one month of dietary restriction of methionine to 30 mg/kg/d and supplementation of cysteine to 70 mg/kg/d the infant was more active and alert, irritability resolved, head growth resumed, and seizures were controlled. Urinary sulfites were undetectable. Dietary parental noncompliance resulted in recurrence of irritability, spasticity, opisthotonus, frequent infantile spasms and hypsarrythmia, lack of head growth, regression to a vegetative state by 16 months of age, and elevated sulfites in the urine, >400 mg/L. (Boles RG et al. Short-term response to dietary therapy in molybdenum cofactor deficiency. Ann Neurol Nov 1993;34:742-744). (Respond: Dr Boles, Dep of Genetics, Yale Univ School of Medicine, WWW 305, 333 Cedar street, New Haven, CT 06510).

COMMENT. MoCD is an autosomal recessive inborn error of metabolism involving 3 molybdenum-requiring enzymes: sulfite oxidase, xanthine dehydrogenase, and aldehyde oxidase. An infant with delayed development, microcephaly, refractory seizures, and lactic acidosis, should be tested for urinary sulfites and serum hypouricemia. Dietary therapy appears promising. The appearance of ectopia lentis, a characteristic finding, is often delayed. For MoCD as an overlooked cause of neonatal seizures, see Ped Neur Briefs July 1993;7:52.-Editor. *Ped Neur Briefs* Dec 1993.

MUCOPOLYSACCHARIDOSIS: MRI STUDY

Characteristic changes in the MRI of 2 brothers with mucopolysaccharidosis type I are reported from the Departments of Paediatrics, Neuroradiology and Neurology, University of Ancona, Italy. One patient was mentally retarded and the other had a normal IQ. The MRI showed a honeycomb-like appearance of the thalami, hypoplasia of the cerebellum and an enlarged ventricular system, with changes in the white matter behind the occipital horns. These changes were not correlated with the mental retardation. (Gabrielli O et al. Cerebral MRI in two brothers with mucopolysaccharidosis type I and different clinical phenotypes. Neuroradiology Aug 1992; 34:313-315.) (Correspondence: Dr. O. Gabrielli, Department of Pediatrics, University of Ancona, Via F. Corridoni 11, I-60123 Ancona, Italy.)

COMMENT. Glycosaminoglycans and glycolipids accumulate in the cells of the central nervous system in mucopolysaccharidosis type I. It is suggested that the mental retardation could be tied to neuronal damage caused by lysosomal storage of these substances. The cell biology of glycosaminoglycans in regulating normal cerebrospinal fluid absorption is reviewed by Knepper PA and McLone DG, Children's Memorial Hospital and Northwestern University Medical School, Chicago (Pediat Neurol Sci 1986; 12:240-251).-Editor. *Ped Neur Briefs* Sept 1992.

HARP SYNDROME

The clinical and laboratory studies of an 11 year old girl with hypoprebetalipoproteinemia, acanthocytosis, retinitis pigmentosa and pallidal degeneration are reported from the Developmental and Metabolic Neurology Branch, National Institute of Neurological Disorders and Stroke and Clinical Pathology Department, National Institutes of Health, Bethesda, MD. Development was normal until age 3 years, when spasticity began in the lower extremities and this was followed by language deterioration, generalized dystonia, orofacial dyskinesia, progressive dementia, and deterioration of visual acuity. At age 11 the fundi showed atypical retinitis pigmentosa. The MRI showed a marked signal decrease in the pallidal nuclei on T2 weighted images and the "eye-of-the-tiger" sign. Thirty to 40% acanthocytes were present in the peripheral blood, and high resolution lipoprotein electrophoresis revealed an absence of the pre-beta fraction. Phase-contrast microscopy of whole blood showed 80-90% acanthocytes, confirmed by electron microscopy. Previous reports in 6 patients linking Hallervorden-Spatz disease with acanthocytosis have not included the orofacial dyskinesia and abnormal lipoproteins seen in this patient (Higgins Jl et al. Hypoprebetalipoproteinemia, acanthocytosis, retinitis pigmentosa, and pallidal degeneration (HARP syndrome). Neurology Jan 1992; 42:194-198). (Reprints: Dr. Joseph J Higgins, Developmental and Metabolic Neurology Branch, NIND&S, National Institutes of Health, Bldg. 10, Rm. 3D03, Bethesda, MD 20892.)

COMMENT. This group of signs described by the acronym HARP syndrome has features in common with the rare association of Hallervorden-Spatz disease and acanthocytosis (Swisher CN, Menkes IH, Cancilla PA, Dodge PR. Trans Am Neurol Assoc 1972; 97:212) and with the syndrome of choreoacanthocytosis (Feinberg TE et al. Neurology 1991; 41:1000). A defect of vertical gaze noted in the present case report was also recorded in 3 sisters reported by Swisher and associates. -Editor. *Ped Neur Briefs* Feb 1992.

METABOLIC PIGMENTARY RETINOPATHIES

The diagnosis and management of inborn errors of metabolism associated with retinal degeneration are reviewed from the Clinique et Unite de Recherche de Genetique Medicale, the Hopital des Enfants Malades and the Opthalmologic Department et Formation Associee de Recherches Claude Bernard, Hopital Necker-Enfants-Malades-Laennec, Paris, France. Pigmented retinopathies are divided into two groups: (1) primary RP confined to the eyes; and (2) secondary RP associated with single or multiple organ system disease. Secondary RP is most often associated with nervous system involvement, morphological abnormalities, deafness, myopathy, nephropathy, and skin abnormalities. Some are well defined non-metabolic genetic syndromes and others are related to inherited metabolic disorders. In a patient presenting with retinal abnormalities the search for a metabolic disorder will concentrate on (1) errors of lipid metabolism; (2) errors of peroxisomal functions; and (3) errors of mitochondrial functions including the respiratory chain. Biochemical investigation should be considered in patients with ocular deficits that are associated with the following abnormalities: (1) neurological involvement including muscle hypotonia, seizures, peripheral neuropathies, cerebellar signs, sensorineural hearing deficit, cerebral abnormalities, mental retardation; (2) craniofacial abnormalities; (3) hepatological abnormalities; (4) renal abnormalities; (5) cardiomegaly; (6) skeletal abnormalities; (7) skin abnormalities; (8) failure to thrive; (9) hormonal disturbances; and (10) progression of symptoms. The screening procedure for metabolic disorders includes (1) peripheral blood for acanthocytes; (2) lipid pattern including lipoproteins; (3) redox status including lactic acid, pyruvate and ketones; (4) amino acid pattern; (5) organic acid pattern in the urine; (6) very long chain fatty acids and phytanic acid; and (7) enzymatic studies (Poll-The BT et al. Metabolic pigmentary retinopathies: diagnosis and therapeutic attempts. Euro J Pediatr Jan 1992;151:2-11).

COMMENT. This excellent review of the metabolic retinal degenerations includes case reports of the major errors of metabolism associated with retinal degeneration including abetalipoproteinemia, neuronal ceroid lipofuscinosis, classical and infantile Refsum diseases, hydroxydicarboxylic aciduria, Sjogren-Larsson syndrome, Kearns-Sayre syndrome and peroxisomal disorders (see Progress in Pediatric Neurology, Millichap JG ed. 1991 pp. 470-474).-Editor. *Ped Neur Briefs* Feb 1992.

SEIZURES AND PARTIAL HYPOPARATHYROIDISM

Neonatal hypocalcemia and seizures in three infants who developed recurrence of hypocalcemia later in childhood are reported from the Department of Paediatrics, The Hospital for Sick Children, Toronto, Ontario, Canada. Hypocalcemia resolved in 1 week, 3 months, and 14 months and recurrences were noted at 4, 7 and 12 years of age. Plasma parathyroid hormone concentrations were low but detectable. One patient born full term with normal birth weight became irritable and developed tonic-clonic convulsions on the first day of life. The plasma calcium was 1.43 mmol/L; magnesium, 0.86 mmol/L; and phosphate 1.95 mmol/L. She was hospitalized again at 4 weeks of age for asymptomatic hypocalcemia. Except for generalized development delay first noted at 7 months of age, she had no clinically important illness until 12-1/2 years of age when she experienced difficulty bending her fingers and numbness of her hands and feet. Several months later, following a minor viral illness, she lost consciousness while watching television and developed convulsions. The plasma calcium was 1.35 mmol/L and ionized calcium 0.69 mmol/L. She has received therapy with calcitriol for the last 3 years and has maintained a normal plasma calcium concentration. In patients 2 and 3 the childhood hypocalcemia developed gradually over several years. The authors caution that congenital hypoparathydroidism is not always transient, neonatal hypocalcemia may signal permanent partial hypoparathyroidism, and hypocalcemia in an otherwise normal neonate should be followed up with blood calcium measurements during childhood and adolescence. (Kooh SW, Binet A. Partial hypoparathyroidism. A variant of transient congenital hypoparathyroidism. A J D C August 1991; 145:877-880).

COMMENT: The authors note that DiGeorge syndrome most closely resembles congenital partial hypoparathyroidism and includes immunologic and cardiac abnormalities. Patients with MEDAC (multiple endocrine deficiency, Addison's disease, and candidiasis) may also have partial parathyroid hormone deficiency.-Editor. *Ped Neur Briefs* Aug 1991.

ADRENAL, ALACRIMAL, ACHALASIA SYNDROME

The results of a British and European Paediatric Endocrinology Society, multicenter collaborative, questionnnaire study of the neurological complications of familial glucocorticoid deficiency syndrome are reported from the Hospital for Sick Children, Great Ormond Street, London. Of 20 patients identified, ages 2 to 29 years, all had impaired cortisol secretion, 19 absent tear secretion, 15 achalasia of the cardia, and 17 had neurologic abnormalities including hyperreflexia, hypertonia, Babinski signs, muscle weakness and/or wasting, ataxia, dysarthria, and sensory impairment. Impaired autonomic function in 11 patients was manifested by postural hypotension and anisocoria. Eleven were intellectually impaired. Ten had hyperkeratosis and fissures of their palms. Siblings were affected in 3 families, and 7 siblings had died in childhood. (Grant DB et al. Neurological and adrenal dysfunction in the adrenal insufficiency /alacrima/achalasia (3A) syndrome. Arch Dis Child 1993; 68: 779-782). (Respond: Dr DB Grant, Hospital for Sick Children, Great Ormond Street, London WClN 3JH).

COMMENT. The most frequent presenting symptom was hypoglycemia, often associated with addisonian skin pigmentation. In 4 cases the diagnosis of achalasia preceeded the recognition of cortisol deficiency. The authors recommend a test of cortisol secretion in children with achalasia, if associated with alacrima or with any of the above neurologic abnormalities.-Editor. *Ped Neur Briefs* July 1993.

CHAPTER 16

HEREDO-DEGENERATIVE AND DEMYELINATING DISORDERS

INTRODUCTION

Paul Richard Dyken, M.D.
Department of Neurology
University of South Alabama, Mobile, AL

Progressive neurological symptomatology and ongoing neuropathological sequences characterize the heredo-degenerative and demyelinating diseases. These disorders also are called the neurodegenerative diseases or, less often, the progressive encephalomyelopathies. Often the diseases are of unknown etiology; however, the majority are abnormalities of inheritance, immunopathology, or the result of slow virus infections, such as subacute sclerosing panencephalitis (SSPE). SSPE represents a hallmark demyelinating process that is degenerative. Some of these degenerative diseases reflect drug refractory epilepsies and are due to epileptogenic or kindling mechanisms. There are also a host of toxic, nutritional, vascular and even neoplastic diseases that could represent the etiological basis for some diseases previously considered of unknown etiology (Dyken, Krawiecki, 1983).

In classifying neurodegenerative diseases, all diseases characterized by neurological deterioration beyond that seen in the normal aging process should be included, regardless of etiology. This expanded definition includes disorders ranging in scope from those of long duration and mild form to those fulminating processes which end in death within weeks. Almost 28% of patients admitted to an inpatient service of academic pediatric neurology were neurodegenerative diseases. Classifications have used an etiological basis, or pathoanatomical and pathophysiological criteria, but each has its limitations. The most complete and satisfactory classification is based on clinical dynamics. which separates neurodegenerative diseases by age of onset, clinical course, clinical characteristics and duration of disease.(Table I).

Table I. Classification of Neurodegenerative Diseases of Childhood Based On Clinical Dynamics.

I. Infantile Neurodegenerations (Onset 0-2 years)
- A. Acute Monophasic: Tay-Sachs disease
- B. Chronic Monophasic: Pelizaeus-Merzbacher
- C. Chronic Heterophasic: Menkes disease

II. Childhood Neurodegenerations (Onset 2-5 years)
- A. Acute Monophasic: Bielschowsky disease
- B. Chronic Monophasic: Rett disease
- C. Chronic Heterophasic: Rubella encephalitis

III. Juvenile Neurodegenerations
- A. Acute Monophasic:Adrenoleukodystrophy
- B. Chronic Monophasic: Batten disease
- C. Chronic Heterophasic: SSPE

The clinical characterization of infantile, childhood, and juvenile neurodegenerations in the developing organism is dependent upon interplay of growth or developmental factors and death or degenerative factors. Each of these disorders represents an imbalance of neurodevelopmental and neurodegenerative factors, as illustrated by Fig. 1. They are the hallmarks of the so-called abiotrophies suggested by Sir William Gowers.

Figure 1.

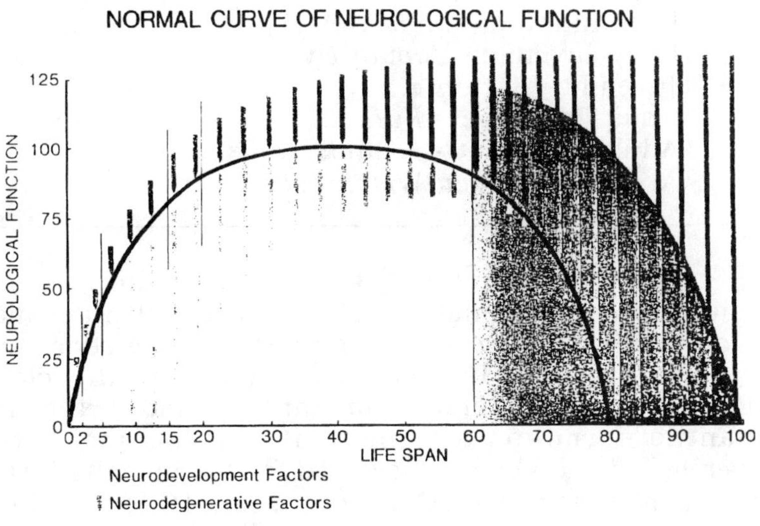

Probably the most satisfying outcome of efforts to classify the neurodegenerative diseases concern the neuronal ceroid-lipofuscinoses. These are neuro-degenerative disorders in which autofluorescent lipopigments accumulate within neurons and other cells, both in the nervous system and systemically. The disorders were originally separated from other neurodegenerative diseases by their clinical onset, dynamics, and characteristics. It is now recognized that the disorders are not amaurotic familial idiocies, as originally suggested, for they have a different genetic, pathoanatomical, pathophysiological and pathobiochemical basis. These differences allowed further subclassification. It is now universally accepted that the neuronal ceroid-lipofuscinoses are not the same disease, but a series of separate genetic diseases (Dyken, Wisniewski, in press). The universally accepted classification of these diseases is shown in Table II.

Table II. Forms of Neuronal Ceroid-Lipofuscinoses.

Infantile - *Santavuori*
Late Infantile - *Bielschowsky*
Early Juvenile - *Zeman-Dyken*
Juvenile - *Batten*
Adult-Recessive - *Kufs*
Adult-Dominant - *Boehme*
Atypical - *Dyken-Wisniewski*

Since 15 atypical forms have now been identified, approximately 21 subtypes of neuronal ceroid-lipofuscinoses now exist. Most of these represent separate diseases. This is substantiated by the clear identification of defects on chromosome 1 for the infantile form, on chromosome 13 for the early juvenile form, on chromosome 16 for the juvenile form, and on neither chromosome 1, 13, nor 16 for the late infantile form of neuronal ceroid-lipofuscinosis. The diseases in question are uniquely separated on clinical and pathological grounds. Because a real classification exists, we recognize their genetic differences and now have a near total mastery of our understanding of them. - *Paul Richard Dyken, M.D., Department of Neurology, University of South Alabama, Mobile, Alabama.*

BIBLIOGRAPHY

Dyken P, Krawiecki N. Neurodegenerative disease of infancy and childhood. Ann Neurol 1983;13:351-364.

Dyken P, Maertens P, Moser H, Swaiman K. Pediatric

neurodegenerative diseases. In Manual for Course No. 342, American Academy of Neurology, Dyken P, (ed), Washington, DC, May 8, 1994.

Dyken P, Wisniewski K. Reclassification and atypical forms of neuronal ceroid-lipofuscinoses. Fifth International Conference on Neuronal Ceroid-Lipofuscinoses. May 19-21, 1994, Newark, NJ (in press).

Maertens P, Dyken P: Inborn errors of metabolism I. Neurologic degenerative diseases, In Pediatric Neurology for the Clinician. RB David ed. Chap 13. Norwalk, Appleton and Lange, 1992.

CHILDHOOD DEGENERATIVE DISORDERS AND ADULT DEMENTIA

An approach to the evaluation of dementia in adults related to pediatric metabolic and degenerative diseases is reviewed from the Department of Neurology, University Medical Center, Maywood, IL. A list of 17 neurodegenerative disorders that ordinarily occur in childhood but may be present in adults includes adrenoleukodystrophy, metachromatic leukodystrophy, Krabbe's disease, Alexander's disease, Lafora's disease, Kufs' disease, mucopolysaccharidosis, Gaucher's type 1, Niemann-Pick disease, and gangliosidosis 1 and 2. Diagnosis is important for genetic counseling and some are treatable. A history of myoclonus suggests Kufs' disease, Lafora's disease, and mitrochondrial disorders. Easy tanning on sun exposure suggests adrenoleukodystrophy. Bone pain occurs with Gaucher's disease. Extrapyramidal symptoms suggest gangliosidosis. Muscle weakness is seen with gangliosidosis and mitochondrial disorders. Depressed deep tendon reflexes may occur with metachromatic leukodystrophy, adrenoleukodystrophy and gangliosidosis. Organomegaly is present in Gaucher's disease, Niemann-Pick disease and mucopolysaccharidosis. Macrocephaly can occur with Alexander's disease and metachromatic leukodystrophy. Special studies to be considered in young adults with idiopathic dementia include: 1) very long-chain fatty acids (adrenoleukodystrophy); 2) mucopolysaccharide screen; 3) arylsulfatase A (metachromatic leukodystrophy); 4) bone marrow for foam cells (Niemann-Pick disease); 5) copper and ceruloplasmin (Wilson's disease). (Coker S.B. Diagnosis of childhood neurogenerative disorders presenting as dementia in adults. Neurology June 1991; 41:794-798).

COMMENT. This review should be of value to the adult neurologist specializing in Alzheimer's disease and other causes of dementia. A knowledge of childhood neurodegenerative disorders would be important in the differential diagnosis of adult dementia.-Editor. *Ped Neur Briefs* July 1991.

MOLECULAR BASIS OF METACHROMATIC LEUKODYSTROPHIES

Arylsulfatase A alleles were analyzed in 68 patients with metachromatic leukodystrophy in the Department of Biochemistrv II, Georg-August-Universitat Gottingen, Gosslerstr, Gottingen, Germany. Of the 68 patients 50 carried at least one of the two metachromatic leukodystrophy alleles (I or A). Twenty-three patients were homozygous for either allele I or allele A or heterozygous for both alleles. In 18 patients neither allele I nor allele A was found. These two alleles accounted for about half of all arylsulfatase A alleles in this selection of patients. Patients were classified clinically as late infantile, juvenile, or adult forms. All six patients with MCL homozygous for allele I had the late infantile form. Five who were homozygous for allele A had the adult form and three had the juvenile form. Seven with both allele I and allele A had the juvenile onset MCL. The authors conclude that like many lysosomal storage disorders MCL shows clinical heterogeneity that reflects genetic heterogeneity. Allele I is associated with late infantile and more severe disease and allele A occurs with the adult form and juvenile forms of MCL. (Polten A, Gieselmann V et al. Molecular basis of different forms of metachromatic leukodvstrophy. N Engl J Med Jan 3, 1991; 324:18-22).

COMMENT. Three forms of metachromatic leukodystrophy are distinguished according to the age of onset: late infantile (1-2 years), juvenile (3-16), and adult (older than 16 years). The incidence is estimated at 1:40,000. These authors describe four genotypes as combinations of two arylsulfatase A alleles that cause MCL and a pseudo deficiency allele. These genotypes are associated with levels of residual arylsulfatase A activity from 0 to 10% and represent the infants and children affected most severely to adults who may be asymptomatic or suffer from a slowly progressive form of MCL. The authors had identified two persons with compound heterozygosity for the pseudo deficiency allele and the MCL allele I. This conbination reduces arylsulfatase A to about 10% of normal activity. Both persons were in their third decade of life and were asymptomatic. The most severe type of MCL is associated with homozygosity for allele I. One copy of allele A lessens the severity and produces the juvenile form, and two copies of a1lele A results in the mildest or adult form of MCL. One copy of arylsulfatase A pseudo deficiency allele permits a normal phenotype. Patients with the juvenile or adult form of MCL were thought to be better candidates for bone marrow transplantation than those with the late infantile form since less enzyme needed to be replaced.-Editor. *Ped Neur Briefs* Feb 1991.

ADRENOLEUKODYSTROPHY: CHILDHOOD AND ADULT FORMS COMPARED

Saturated, very long-chain fatty acids in erythrocyte membranes, blood plasma, and mononuclear cells were studied in 4 patients with childhood-adolescent adrenoleukodystrophy, 4 patients with adult adrenoleukodystrophy and 19 normal control subjects in the Department of Neurology, National Chikugo Hospital and the Neurological Institute, Kyusu University, Fukuoka, Japan. The ratios of C26:0 to C22:0 in patients were significantly higher than those of normal control subjects. Ratios of C26:0 to C22:0 in mononuclear cells were significantly higher in patients with childhood-adolescent adrenoleukodystrophy than in patients with adult adrenoleukodystrophy, whereas no significant difference in the ratios in erythrocyte membranes and blood plasma were noted. The results suggest that there is a correlation between phenotype and ratio of C26:0 to C22:0 within mononuclear cells in patients with adrenoleukodystrophy. (Antoku Y et al. Adrenoleukodystrophy: a correlation between saturated very long-chain fatty acids in mononuclear cells and phenotype (Ann Neurol July 1991;30: 101 -103).

COMMENT. Adrenoleukodystrophy is an X-linked recessive disorder characterized by adrenal insufficiency and demyelination of the CNS along with accumulation of saturated very long-chain fatty acids in tissues. Adrenoleukodystrophy has a wide phenotypical variation including childhood-adolescent forms, adrenomyeloneuropathy with adult onset and adult rare forms. Variable phenotypes in a family kindred have been described. Marsh W.W. and Hurst D.L. reported a 20 month-old male who presented with a sudden onset of status epilepticus and cortical blindness; the patient died before his affected 5 year-old brother exhibited any features of ALD (Pediatr Neurol Jan-Feb 1991; 7:50-52).-Editor. *Ped Neur Briefs* July 1991.

ADRENOLEUKODYSTROPHY: LORENZO OIL THERAPY

Dietary therapy with glycerol trioleate and glycerol trierucate (Lorenzo oil) was tested in 108 adult patients with adrenomyeloneuropathy phenotype of adrenoleukodystrophy (ALD) at Johns Hopkins Hospital and the Kennedy Krieger Institute, Baltimore, MD. Pattern-reversal visual evoked potentials were used to evaluate visual pathways before and after treatment for 1 year. Very-long-chain fatty acid (VLCFA) levels were markedly reduced, but visual evoked potentials remained abnormal or became abnormal. No patients improved, and there was no evidence that reduction in VLCFA levels benefited or retarded demyelination of visual pathways. (Kaplan PW, Moser HW et al. Visual evoked potentials in adrenoleukodystrophy: a trial with glycerol trioleate and Lorenzo oil. Ann Neurol Aug 1993;34:169-174). (Respond: Dr Kaplan, Department of Neurology, Francis Scott Key Medical Center, 4940 Eastern Avenue, Baltimore, MD 21224).

COMMENT. Moser, in an editorial (Ann Neurol Aug 1993;34:121-122), reviews the development of therapies for adrenoleukodystrophy and describes Lorenzo oil as "a prematurely amplified hope." Trials of the oil in Europe and the USA have failed to demonstrate a significant effect on the rate of progression of the childhood cerebral form of ALD. A possible preventive effect of Lorenzo oil in patients who have not yet developed the neurological disability is under investigation. Of 61 asymptomatic patients treated for a few months up to 4 years at the Kennedy Krieger Institute, one has developed childhood cerebral ALD and 7 have shown progressive demyelination on the MRI. Longer follow-up is required to determine the outcome in the 53 who remain asymptomatic. A depression in platelets was an unexpected side effect of Lorenzo oil therapy.-Editor. *Ped Neur Briefs* Aug 1993.

METACHROMATIC LEUKODYSTROPHY VARIANTS

Clinical, pathological, imaging, and genetic findings in a family with multiple allelic mutations of metachromatic leukodystrophy (MLD) are reported from McGill University, Montreal, and McMaster University, Hamilton, Canada. The propositus, a 23-year-old man, presented at age 18 with a 3-year history of clumsiness and stiffness of gait. Two maternal uncles, ages 48 and 56, were also neurologically impaired. Two siblings, a brother aged 30 and sister aged 25, the mother, and father were clinically normal and had normal electrical studies and MRIs, but their arylsulfatase activity was reduced. Allele-specific amplification confirmed the pseudodeficiency (PD) allele, with no clinical dysfunction, in the mother and her 2 unaffected children. The mother was a PD/MLD compound heterozygote since she was an obligate MLD carrier. The father was a normal (N/MLD) heterozygote. The family was unique in the unusual occurrence of MLD in consecutive generations in the absence of consanguinity. (Francis GS et al. Metachromatic leukodystrophy: multiple nonfunctional and pseudodeficiency alleles in a pedigree: problems with diagnosis and counseling. Ann Neurol Aug

1993;34:212-218). (Respond: Dr Francis, Department of Neurology, Montreal Neurologic Institute, McGill University, 3801 University Street, Montreal, Quebec, Canada H3A 2B4).

COMMENT. Three phenotypes of MLD are recognized based on age of onset: late infantile (0-2 years), juvenile (3-16 years), and adult. The time of onset is determined by the amount of residual arylsulfatase A activity, those retaining some activity having a delayed onset of the disease. A variety of allelic mutations has been identified, including a pseudodeficiency allele with no clinical dysfunction. Cloning of the enzyme gene and genotype identification at the molecular level for the PD and MLD mutations allow appropriate genetic counselling for the families. With these advances in diagnosis, the authors conclude that unnecessary testing of spouses and prenatal screening of pregnancies can be avoided.- Editor. *Ped Neur Briefs* Aug 1993.

CANAVAN'S DISEASE: MAGNETIC RESONANCE SPECTROSCOPY

The neuroradiological evaluation of Canavan's disease in a 38 month-old girl is reported from the Alfred I. duPont Institute, Wilmington, DE and Children's Hospital, Philadelphia, PA. A female child of Ashkenazic Jewish heritage presented at age 5 months with psychomotor retardation and macrocephaly. At age 7 months cerebral brain biopsy confirmed a suspected diagnosis of Canavan's disease. Over the last 30 months she developed severe spastic quadriparesis, optic atrophy and dysphagia which was treated by gastrostomy at age 27 months. CT showed diffuse symmetrical low attenuation values of the subcortical and deep cerebral white matter. MRI demonstrated symmetrical diffuse low signal density on T1-weighted images and high signal intensity on T2-weighted images. Magnetic resonance spectroscopy showed elevated levels of N-acetylaspartic acid in the occipital lobe. The in vivo measurement of N-acetylaspartic acid in the brain by magnetic resonance spectroscopy offered an additional non-invasive diagnostic test for Canavan's disease (Marks H G et al. Use of computer tomography, magnetic resonance imaging, and localized 1H magnetic resonance spectroscopy in Canavan's disease: a case report. Ann Neurol July 1991; 30: 106-110).

COMMENT. Canavan's disease or spongy degeneration of the brain in infancy is a rare autosomal recessive leukodystrophy most prevalent among Ashkenazi Jews and Saudi Arabians. Matalon and co-workers have demonstrated an excessive amount of acetylaspartic acid in urine, blood, CSF and a deficiency of aspartoacylase in cultured skin fibroblasts and brain tissue in children with Canavan's disease (Matalon R et al. Am J Med Genet 1988; 29 :463). The diagnosis may now be confirmed by magnetic resonance imaging followed by localized 1H magnetic resonance spectroscopy.-Editor. *Ped Neur Briefs* July 1991.

WOLFRAM SYNDROME

Two unrelated patients with Wolfram syndrome (diabetes insipidus, diabetes mellitus, optic atrophy, and deafness) in whom MRIs of the brain provide evidence of a diffuse neurodegenerative process are reported from the Departments of Neurology and Ophthalmology, University of California at San Francisco, CA. Patient 1 was mildly mentally retarded and had a 5-year history of ataxia. Diabetes mellitus and diabetes insipidus had developed at age 3, and bilateral optic atrophy was diagnosed at age 13. Deep tendon reflexes were diminished and plantar responses were extensor. An audiogram showed bilateral high frequency hearing loss. Her parents were first cousins. Patient 2 was admitted for treatment of diabetic ketoacidosis at age 21. She had severe bilateral optic atrophy and horizontal nystagmus. Her gait was ataxic. Deep tendon reflexes were diminished and the plantar responses were flexor. MRI showed atrophy of brain stem and cerebellum and ventricles were dilated. (Rando TA, et al. Wolfram syndrome: evidence of a diffuse neurodegenerative disease by magnetic resonance imaging. Neurology June 1992; 42:1220-1224.) (Reprints: Dr. Thomas A. Rando, Department of Pharmacology, Stanford University Medical Center, Stanford, CA 94305-5332.)

COMMENT. Wolfram syndrome is inherited as an autosomal recessive disorder or it may be sporadic. Reported neurologic features include ataxia, nystagmus, vertigo, dysarthria, dysphagia, mental retardation, seizures, psychiatric disorders, pigmentary retinopathy, tremor, dystonia, hyporeflexia and neurogenic bladder. Endocrine abnormalities include delayed sexual maturation, growth retardation, hypothyroidism, and testicular atrophy. Recurrent urinary tract infections are associated with bilateral hydronephrosis. The differential diagnoses include olivopontocerebellar atrophy, Friedreich's ataxia, Refsum's syndrome, Laurence-Moon-Biedl syndrome, and Alstrom syndrome. The childhood presentation of diabetes mellitus, diabetes insipidus, and optic atrophy together with gait ataxia should suggest the diagnosis of Wolfram syndrome and indicate the need for an MRI, audiogram and renal sonogram.-Editor. *Ped Neur Briefs* July 1992.

NEURODEGENERATION WITH TRICHORRHEXIS INVAGINATA

Two siblings are reported from the Medical College of Ohio with an autosomal recessive syndrome characterized by hair and skin abnormalities, hypoplastic nails, hypotonia, areflexia, and progressive neurological deterioration. Mutiple abnormalities were observed at birth, and apneic episodes secondary to laryngomalacia occurred in the neonatal period. At 10 months, CT showed early cortical atrophy, and EEG revealed seizure activity and encephalopathy. At 12 months, neuromotor deterioration had progressed and the child was no longer able to suck, did not smile, and did not move her legs. Apneic episodes and respiratory difficulties worsened and she died at 16 months. The sibling with a similar syndrome was alive at 27 months. (Gyure KA et al. Autosomal recessive neurodegenerative disorder with trichorrhexis invaginata and ectoderma dysplasia. Pediatr Neurol Nov/Dec 1992; 8: 469-72). (Correspondence: Dr TW Kurczynski, Dept of Pediatrics, Medical College of Ohio, PO Box 10008, Toledo, OH 43699).

COMMENT. Trichorrhexis invaginata, or bamboo hair, is an hair-shaft defect usually found with ichthyosiform dermatoses and Nethertons syndrome. Its significance in relation to the present neuro-degenerative disorder is unknown. Hair-shaft abnormalities occur as a feature of various neurological diseases, including Menkes disease, biotin deficiency, and Pollitt syndrome. Electron micrographs of hair samples may be of diagnostic importance in children with neurologic disorders.-Editor. *Ped Neur Briefs* Jan 1993.

MRI IN INFANTILE NEUROAXONAL DYSTROPHY

The MRI findings in four children aged 3 to 10 years with infantile neuroaxonal dystrophy are reported from the Chiba Children's Hospital, Japan. T_2-weighted images showed bilateral diffuse hyperintensity of the cerebellar cortex and cerebellar atrophy. Autopsy changes in one patient included cerebellar atrophy, ventricular dilatation, spheroids in the gray matter, loss of neurons, axonal swellings, and extensive astrogliosis. (Tanabe Y et al. The use of magnetic resonance imaging in diagnosing infantile neuroaxonal dystrophy. Neurology Jan 1993; 43: 110-113). (Reprints: Dr Y Tanabe, Division of Neurology, Chiba Children's Hospital, 579-1 Heta-cho, Midori-ku, Chiba 266, Japan).

COMMENT. The authors comment that these MRI findings may be specific to infantile neuoaxonal dystrophy and permit early diagnosis. The clinical picture includes upper and lower motor neuron deficits, including progressive weakness, difficulty in walking, hypotonia, muscle atrophy, hyperactive reflexes, Babinski signs, and optic atrophy. Diagnosis is confirmed by peripheral nerve biopsy, which shows globular swellings on the axons. Axonal swelling may also occur in Hallervorden-Spatz disease, Friedreich's ataxia, and other neurodegenerative diseases, however.-Editor. *Ped Neur Briefs* Feb 1993.

MRI IN INFANTILE KRABBE DISEASE

Serial MRI findings paralleling the clinical deterioration of a year-old child with Krabbe disease are reported from the University of Rochester Medical Center, New York. At 13 months, an abnormal high signal on T_2-weighted images in the frontoparietal white matter and cerebellar white matter was correlated with severe developmental delay, increased tone, and hyperextension (stage 2). At 32 months, MRI changes had progressed to include central and cortical atrophy, decreased white matter volume, thalamic and caudate atrophy, and abnormal high signal in all motor tracts except the anterior limb of the internal capsule. Clinically, the child was in stage 3, with spasticity of the upper extremities, peripheral neuropathy, and no response to auditory or visual stimuli. (Farley TJ et al. Serial MRI and CT findings in infantile Krabbe disease. Pediatr Neurol Nov/Dec 1992; 8: 455-458). (Respond: Dr Ketonen, Dept Radiology, University of Rochester Medical Center, Box 648, 601 Elmwood Ave, Rochester, NY 14642).

COMMENT. The 3-stages of Krabbe disease described by Hagberg begin with hyperirritability, restlessness, and frequent crying. Convulsions may develop, induced by sensory stimuli. Development becomes delayed, tone is increased, and later, reflexes are difficult to elicit and are absent in the lower limbs. Terminally, the infant is flaccid and blind. CSF protein is elevated and nerve conduction is delayed. The absence of the enzyme galactosyl ceramide B-galactosidase in leukocytes and skin fibroblasts is diagnostic, a test result common to all variants and stages of Krabbe disease, including antenatal forms.- Editor. *Ped Neur Briefs* Feb 1993.

NYSTAGMUS OF PELIZAEUS-MERZBACHER DISEASE

Magnetic search-coil oculography of three brothers, aged 20, 22, and 25, with Pelizaeus-Merzbacher disease (PMD) was used to demonstrate nystagmus not obvious on inspection at the W. K Kellogg Eye Center, University of Michigan, Ann Arbor, MI. The method uncovered binocular elliptical pendular nystagmus in two patients and upbeat nystagmus in all three patients. This combination of elliptical pendular and upheat nystagmus is not described in any other childhood neurodegenerative disease. In conjunction with MRI findings and supportive clinical signs a diagnosis of PMD is strongly indicated. (Trobe JD et al. Nystagmus of Pelizaeus-Merzbacher disease. A magnetic search-coil study. Arch Neurol Jan 1991; 48:87-91).

COMMENT. PMD may be classified by age of onset into a classical infantile type, congenital type, and adult onset type. The classical and congenital forms have X-linked recessive inheritance whereas the adult onset type is autosomal dominant in inheritance. Nystagmus and head tremor are the first signs followed by spasticity, ataxia, choreoathetosis, optic atrophy, and dementia. PMD must be differentiated from congenital nystagmus or spasmus nutans, metachromatic leukodystrophy, adrenoleukodystrophy, Krabbe's disease, and Cockayne's syndrome. The MRI in PMD shows brain atrophy, increased T_2 signal in white matter, and decreased signal in basal ganglia and thalami. Pathological correlations of upbeat nystagmus have shown dysmyelination of the pontomedullary tegmentum.-Editor. *Ped Neur Briefs* Feb 1991.

ACETAZOLAMIDE IN VESTIBULOCEREBELLAR SYNDROME

Five patients withh long-standing episodic vertigo and ocular motor signs are reported from the Department of Neurology, UCLA School of Medicine, Los Angeles, CA. Because of the clinical similarity to the familial periodic ataxia syndromes, these patients and affected family members were treated with acetazolamide. The episodic vertigo was either abolished or markedly decreased in frequency and severity. The age of onset of the vertigo varied from age two to 32. The episodes lasted from several hours to several days and were complicated by nausea and vomiting and later, a mildly progressive ataxia. Associated symptoms included horizontal or vertical diplopia, slurred speech, and positional downbeat and rebound nystagmus between attacks. The findings suggested a lesion of the vestibulocerebellum. In seven patients examined the MRI was normal. (Baloh RW, Winder A. Acetazolamide-responsive vestibulocerebellar syndrome: Clinical and oculographic features. Neurology March 1991; 41:429-433).

COMMENT. The familial periodic ataxia syndromes have been divided into two types, 1) a vestibulocerebellar syndrome and 2) diffuse cerebellar ataxia, as described by Parker, in which vertigo is infrequent and ataxia is more pronounced. Both syndromes appear to respond to acetazolamide.-Editor. *Ped Neur Briefs* May 1991.

X-LINKED ATAXIC SYNDROME

An X-linked recessive disease with a fatal course in early childhood is reported in a five-generation Dutch family from the Netherlands. Twelve boys were affected and 13 female carriers were identified, some with hearing impairment. Neurological deterioration coincided with recurrent respiratory infections at 1 year of age or earlier and was characterized by hypotonia, ataxia, weakness, absent deep tendon reflexes, nystagmus, and visual and hearing loss. Autopsy in one patient revealed absence of myelin in posterior columns of the spinal cord, and axonal degeneration in the peripheral nerves. The brain was normal in appearance. No biochemical or immunological defects were detected. (Arts WFM et al. X-linked ataxia, weakness, deafness, and loss of vision in early childhood with a fatal course. Ann Neurol May 1993; 33:535-539). (Respond: Dr Arts, Dept of Neurology, Westeinde Hospital, PO Box 432, 2501 CK The Hague, The Netherlands).

COMMENT. Mitochondrial encephalomyelopathy and other known metabolic or degenerative diseases were excluded. The autopsy findings in one patient resembled those of Friedreich's ataxia, but the age of onset and early death were atypical.-Editor. *Ped Neur Briefs* May 1993.

LATE-ONSET FRIEDREICH'S ATAXIA

Three adult patients from one family with late-onset Friedreich's ataxia (LOFA) presenting after 25 years (mean age, 30 yrs) were compared with 13 children with classical FA presenting before 20 years (mean age, 13 yrs) and reported from the University of Tubingen, Germany, and St Mary's Hospital, London, England. Clinical presentation of LOFA and FA were similar, except that muscle wasting, foot deformity, and cardiomyopathy were absent in LOFA patients. Genetic linkage analysis using markers tightly linked to the FA locus on chromosome 9 showed that all affected members of the LOFA family, but not their unaffected siblings, had inherited identical paternal and maternal genotypes. LOFA may result from mutation within the FA locus, giving rise to a more benign and slowly progressive disorder. (Klockgether T, Chamberlain S et al. Late-onset Friedreich's ataxia. Molecular genetics, clinical neurophysiology, and magnetic resonance imaging. Arch Neurol Aug 1993;50:803-806). (Reprints: Dr Klockgether, Department of Neurology, University of Tubingen, Hoppe-Seyler-Str 3, W-7400 Tubingen, Germany).

COMMENT. With the exception of age of onset, all patients with LOFA satisfied the basic diagnostic criteria for classical Friedreich's ataxia: 1) progressive ataxia; 2) family history with autosomal-recessive inheritance; 3) loss of tendon reflexes in lower limbs; 4) dysarthria; and 5) posterior column signs. The more benign 'Acadian' subtype (Barbeau et al, 1984) has previously been differentiated from the classical, French and French Canadian, type of FA and has been attributed to a mutation at the same locus (Keats BJ, Chamberlain S et al. Am T Med Genet 1989;33:266).-Editor. *Ped Neur Briefs* Aug 1993.

VITAMIN E DEFICIENCY FAMILIAL ATAXIC SYNDROME

A total of 8 members of two consanguineous Tunisian families affected with Friedreich's ataxia (FA) phenotype not linked to chromosome 9 were found to have very low levels of serum vitamin E (0.5 mcg/ml cf 8 mcg/ml in controls) in a study at the Institut National de Neurologie, Tunis, and at Centers in Cyprus and France. All patients had typical signs of FA: severe ataxia, bilateral Babinski signs, pes cavus, scoliosis, and absent tendon reflexes and proprioception. The mean age at onset was 11 years, and 6 patients were wheelchair-bound at examination at 20 - 30 years of age. Cardiomyopathy was found in 5. Parents and healthy sibs had normal serum vitamin E levels, pointing to an autosomal recessive trait in affected members. Cystic fibrosis, abetalipoproteinemia, and fat malabsorption syndromes were excluded as possible causes of vitamin E deficiency. This FA with selective vitamin E deficiency was mapped to chromosome 8q, confirming its specificity. (Hamida MB et al. Friedreich's ataxia phenotype not linked to chromosome 9 and associated with selective autosomal recessive vitamin E deficiency in two inbred Tunisian families. Neurology Nov 1993;43:2179-2183). (Reprints: Prof Mongi Ben Hamida, Institut National de Neurologie, La Rabta 1007 Tunis, Tunisia).

COMMENT. The neurological syndrome of vitamin E deficiency is reviewed in an editorial by Dr HJ Kayden, Dept of Medicine, New York University Medical Center, New York (Neurology Nov 1993;43:2167-2169). Abetalipoproteinemia and cholestatic liver disease are characterized by fat malabsorption, resulting in steatorrhea and vitamin E deficiency. In familial isolated vitamin E deficiency, lipid and vitamin E absorption and plasma lipoproteins are normal but conservation of plasma a-tocopherol is poor due to impaired secretion in very low-density lipoproteins. Patients must maintain continuous supplementation with vitamin E (600 IU twice daily, 5 - 10 mg/kg).

The observation that some patients with typical signs of Friedreich's ataxia have a familial vitamin E deficiency syndrome emphasizes the recommendation that all patients with ataxia and neuropathy should have plasma vitamin E determinations. Early supplementation with vitamin E should halt progression of ataxia, and genetic linkage analysis may establish the diagnosis. Asymptomatic sibs should be tested in early childhood, since vitamin E may prevent the onset of ataxia in those affected.-Editor. *Ped Neur Briefs* Dec 1993.

CEREBRAL METABOLISM IN MULTIPLE SCLEROSIS

Alterations in regional cerebral metabolism have been demonstrated by in vivo proton magnetic resonance spectroscopy of 8 children (7 - 16 years) with established multiple sclerosis at the Max-Planck-Institut fur biophysikalische Chemie, Postfach, and Abt. Kinderheilkunde, Schwerpunkr Neuropadiatrie, Georg-August-Universitat, Gottingen, Federal Republic of Germany. MS plaques showed a decrease in N-acetylaspartate and creatines, and an increase in cholines and myo-inositol. Cortical gray matter related to MS lesions showed a reduction of N-acetylaspartate. Functional impairment in MS was linked to gross metabolic disturbances of neuronal cell chemistry. (Bruhn H et al. Multiple sclerosis in children: cerebral metabolic alterations monitored by localized proton magnetic resonance spectroscopy in vivo. Ann Neurol Aug 1992; 32:140-150.) (Correspondence: Dr. Bruhn, Max-Planck-Institut fur biophysikalische Chemie, Postfach 2841, D-3400 Gottingen, Federal Republic of Germany.)

COMMENT. Proton magnetic resonance spectroscopy has revealed metabolic alterations associated with multiple sclerosis in focal lesions and in the adjacent cortex. The method could aid in the differentiation of MS plaques from other disorders and in monitoring response to therapy. For additional articles on MS in children see Progress in Pediatric Neurology, Millichap JG, Chicago, PNB Publ, 1991, 507-510.-Editor. *Ped Neur Briefs* Sept 1992.

FOCAL TUMOR-LIKE DEMYELINATING LESIONS

Thirty-one patients with large, focal cerebral demyelinating lesions are reported from the University of Kansas School of Medicine, Kansas City. The lesions presented clinically and radiologically as brain tumors or as multiple cysts. The demyelinating pathology was established through biopsy and a significant improvement with corticosteroid therapy. Four patients were children, ages 8 - 12 years, and one was an adolescent, aged 18. One young adult had received an influenza vaccine 10 days before the onset of symptoms. The clinical course favored postinfectious/postvaccination encephalitis, but the tumor-sized masses of demyelination were atypical. (Kepes JJ. Large focal tumor-like demyelinating lesions of the brain: intermediate entity between multiple sclerosis and acute disseminated encephalomyelitis? A study of 31 patients. Ann Neurol Jan 1993; 33: 18-27). (Correspondence: Dr Kepes, Department of Pathology and Oncology, University of Kansas College of Health Sciences and Hospital, 39th and Rainbow Blvd, Kansas City, KS 66103).

COMMENT. The author rules out Schilder's disease, a progressive childhood diffuse sclerosis, which often presents with asymmetrical, large focal hemispheric lesions and smaller lesions, sometimes difficult to differentiate from multiple sclerosis. (See Greenfield's Neuropathology, Baltimore, Williams and Wilkins, 1963). Many reported cases of Schilder's disease are now thought to represent either adrenoleukodystrophy or acute forms of multiple sclerosis (Menkes JH. Textbook of Child Neurology. 3rd ed. Philadelphia, Lea & Febiger, 1985).-Editor. *Ped Neur Briefs* Feb 1993.

HEPATOCEREBRAL DEGENERATION OR VALPROATE TOXICITY

Six children with refractory seizures and focal neuronal damage who died of liver failure are reported from the Washington University School of Medicine, St Louis, MO. Four were treated with valproic acid (VPA) and developed liver failure within 30 - 68 days. Two of these children each had one sibling who was not exposed to VPA and developed the same clinical picture, but liver failure was delayed. Siblings receiving VPA survived only 3 and 5 months after onset of seizures, whereas those not treated with VPA lived for 7 to 16 months. (Bicknese AR et al. Early childhood hepatocerebral degeneration misdiagnosed as valproate hepatotoxicity. Ann Neurol Dec 1992; 32: 767-775). (Correspondence: Dr WE Dodson, St Louis Children's Hospital,

400 S Kingshighway Blvd, St Louis, MO 63110).

COMMENT. The authors propose that many of the reported patients with VPA-associated hepatotoxicity represent undiagnosed hepatocerebral degeneration, the Huttenlocher variant of Alpers' syndrome. Their experience suggests that liver failure is accelerated by exposure to VPA, and an alternative antiepileptic treatment should be employed in young children with resistant seizures and mental and motor regression, indicative of cerebral degeneration. Recurrence of this syndrome in family members suggests an autosomal recessive inheritance, but the biochemical basis remains undetermined. Of 13 similar cases reported from the Hospital for Sick Children, London (Egger J et al. Clin Pediatrics 1987; 26: 167), only 4 had received VPA and 2 may have died from VPA-hepatotoxicity.(See Ped Neur Briefs July 1987).-Editor. *Ped Neur Briefs* Jan 1993.

ALPERS SYNDROME WITH HEPATIC CIRRHOSIS

Four children, from two families, with fatal degeneration of the cerebral grey matter and terminal hepatic dysfunction are reported from the Royal Belfast Hospital for Sick Children, Northern Ireland. The disease presented with intractable generalized or partial seizures during infancy in 3 and at 5 years of age in one patient. Epilepsia partialis continua was associated with ataxia and progressive neurologic deterioration. The EEG showed high amplitude slow waves with smaller poyspikes. Visual evoked responses were delayed, and CTs showed cerebral atrophy. Post mortem findings in one patient included neuronal loss and gliosis and hepatic cirrhosis. (Wilson DC et al. Progressive neuronal degeneration of childhood (Alpers syndrome) with hepatic cirrhosis. Eur J Pediatr 1993; 152(3): 260-262). (Respond: Dr DC Wilson, Neonatal Unit, Royal Maternity Hospital, Grosvenor Road, Belfast BT126BJ, N Ireland).

COMMENT. Valproic acid, sometimes implicated in deaths of young infants with this syndrome, was apparently not a factor in these cases. Early diagnosis allows appropriate genetic counselling.-Editor. *Ped Neur Briefs* May 1993.

ATYPICAL LEBER'S OPTIC NEUROPATHY

The diagnosis of Leber's hereditary optic neuropathy (LHON) in 6 female atypical cases seen at Harvard, Emory, and Johns Hopkins Medical Centers required molecular analysis and demonstration of the 11778 mitochondrial DNA mutation for accurate confirmation. Features atypical for LHON included a negative family history, a normal fundus, bitemporal hemianopia, optic disc cupping, and premonitory episodes of transient monocular visual loss. Molecular analysis allows accurate identification of most cases. The 11778 point mutation accounts for 50%. (Weiner NC et al. Atypical Leber's hereditary optic neuropathy with molecular confirmation. Arch Neurol May 1993; 50: 470 473). (Reprints: Nancy J Newman MD, Neuro-ophthalmology Unit, Emory Eye Center, 1327 Clifton Rd NE, Atlanta, GA 30322).

COMMENT. In typical cases of LHON, males predominate and the fundus is characterized by circumpapillary telangiectatic microangiopathy and pseudoedema. The diagnosis should also be considered in females with an unexplained optic neuropathy, a negative family history and a normal fundus. Genetic analysis has allowed for a broader view of what constitutes the clinical phenotype of LHON. (Newman NJ. Leber's hereditary optic neuropathy. New genetic considerations. Arch Neurol May 1993; 50: 540-548).-Editor. *Ped Neur Briefs* May 1993.

ANGELMAN'S SYNDROME: PATHOLOGICAL STUDY

The first pathological descriptions of Angelman's happy puppet syndrome based on an autopsy study of a 21 year old woman are reported from the Division of Neuropathology, The Hospital for Sick Children, University of Toronto, Canada. The diagnosis was first made at age 12 on the basis of severe mental retardation, absent speech, seizures, ataxia, hyperactive reflexes, extensor plantars, inappropriate laughter, microcephaly, brachycephaly, prognathism, and widely spaced teeth. She had been treated with multiple anticonvulsants and she died of recurrent pneumonia, pulmonary abscess, and hemoptysis. Autopsy findings showed a small brain with marked cerebellar atrophy, loss of Purkinje and granule cells, and Bergmann's gliosis. Dendrite morphology was abnormal with decreases in arborization and numbers of dendritic spines. Neurochemical studies showed reduced gamma-aminobutyric acid in the cerebellar cortex and elevated glutamate content in frontal and occipital cortices. (Jay V et al. Puppet-like syndrome of Angelman: A pathologic and neurochemical study. Neurology March 1991; 41:416-422).

COMMENT. The cause of the cerebellar pathology was unknown. Since seizures began at ten months of age and the patient had received multiple anticonvulsants, the possibility of a secondary cerebellar degeneration could not be excluded. The dendritic pathology was similar to that found in Down syndrome and could be developmental or a consequence of dendritic atrophy. In familial cases of Angelman's syndrome there is evidence for a dominant inheritance at the chromosome 15q11-13 locus.(Clayton-Smith J et al. Am J Med Genet 1992;44:256-260). -Editor. *Ped Neur Briefs* May 1991.

CHAPTER 17

RETT SYNDROME

INTRODUCTION

John Wilson, PhD, FRCP.
Great Ormond Street
Children's Hospital Trust, London, UK

In the 1991 edition of **"Progress in Pediatric Neurology,"** most of the section on Rett syndrome explored clinical features and some biochemical aspects. As yet a distinctive biochemical marker has not been identified. It has been suggested that the Rett syndrome is primarily a mitochondrial disorder but there is no confirmatory laboratory evidence.

There is understandably, a pervasive sense of therapeutic impotence, and palliative measures such as physiotherapy, music therapy, aroma therapy and spinal bracing dominate therapeutic endeavour viz. Hanks SB (Brain Dev 1990;12:157-61).

The most favoured genetic explanation of the condition is that there is a sex-linked dominant mutation lethal to the male fetus which is aborted, whilst the rare occurrence of second-affected children is explained as an example of gonadal mosaicism. Attention has focussed on the X-chromosome and a panoply of the latest techniques of molecular genetics have been applied. These have been more successful in excluding rather than identifying candidate loci.

Anvret et al (Am J Med Genet 1990;37:31-35) reported a girl with classical Rett syndrome with a mildly affected aunt, but no chromosomal abnormality was identified. Zoghbi et al (Am J Med Genet 1990;35:148-51) identified a de novo X;3 translocation in one patient out of 28 studied, and concluded that a candidate gene might be distal to Xp21 and proximal to Xp22. Further study (Ellison KA et al. Am J Med Genet 1993;47:1124-34) has identified a 179-kb YAC clone at the breakpoint which maps to Xp21.3 between the DMD gene and the DXS28 (C7) locus. The same group has also reported an increased frequency of non-random X-inactivation in patients, and in the mother of two affected half-sisters (Zoghbi et al. Brain Dev 1990;12:131-5).

Journel et al (Am J Med Genet 1990;35:142-7) identified a translocation t(X;22) (211.22; p11) in a patient, her mother, and in her mildly affected sister. Wahlstrom et al (Brain Dev 1990;12:128-30) demonstrated a statistically significant increase of fragile X (p.22) in a small series. By contrast, Gordon et al (Am J Med Genet 1993;46:142-4) desbribed the classical feratures of Rett syndrome in a patient with 18q-mosaicism. Alternative hypotheses proposing autosomal inheritance are less persuasive. The first example of affected mother and daughter has been reported from Sweden (Hagberg B, personal communication). *John Wilson PhD, FRCP, Consultant Neurologist, Great Ormond Street Childrens Hospital Trust, London, UK.*

RETT SYNDROME SYMPTOMS IN ADULT MALES

A survey of 297 institutionalized adults with mental retardation to determine the prevalence of symptoms of Rett syndrome is reported from the Medical Center Rehabilitation Hospital, Grand Forks, ND and University of North Dakota School of Medicine. The survey suggests that a) male and female adults as a group express the individual symptoms of Rett syndrome with equal frequency, b) as individuals, only females appear to exhibit the full criteria for Rett syndrome, c) males do exhibit particular symptoms of the syndrome, and d) no individual symptom or two symptoms separate males and females. The prevalence rate for Rett syndrome in the institutionalized population of persons with mental retardation was 1:46 for females and 1:116 for both sexes. Midline hand stereotypies, hyperventilation, impaired ambulation, seizures, and absence of prenatal complications all occurred with equal frequency in both sexes. (Burd L et al. Rett syndrome symptomatology of institutionalized adults with mental retardation: Comparison of males and females. AJMR March 1991; 95:596-601).

COMMENT. The oldest of the four females who met the strict and necessary criteria for the diagnosis of Rett syndrome was 40 years of age. The female sex is no longer considered a necessary diagnostic criterion and a less restrictive symptom complex is proposed by some authorities.-Editor. *Ped Neur Briefs* May 1991.

RETT SYNDROME AND MITOCHONDRIAL ENZYME DEFICIENCIES

Three children with Rett syndrome and normal muscle mitochondrial structure but abnormalities in mitochondrial respiratory chain enzymes are reported from the Departments of Neurology and Pediatrics, Loyola University, Stritch School of Medicine, Maywood, IL. The children, all girls, were three, four, and 13 years of age. The 13 year old had normal development until 15 months of age when she stopped talking and developed an abnormal gait and loss of hand use. At six years of age, self-injurious behavior and head hitting developed and at age nine years, she had atonic and clonic seizures. Her behavior was autistic and hyperactive. Hand wringing and mouthing were constant while awake. The head circumference was 49 cm (below the 2nd percentile). There were low levels of cytochrome c-oxidase and succinate cytochrome c-reductase in all cases. Muscle morphology by light and electron microscopy was normal. (Coker SB, Melnyk AR. Rett syndrome and mitochondrial enzyme deficiencies. J Child Neurol April 1991; 6:164-166).

COMMENT. Mitochondrial alterations in muscle, including distention, vacuolation, and membranous changes, have been described in children with Rett syndrome. (See Ped Neur Briefs Sept 1989).-Editor. *Ped Neur Briefs* May 1991.

CEREBRAL LIPIDS IN RETT SYNDROME

The lipid membrane composition of cerebral tissue from five patients, age 12-30 years, and from 14 age-matched controls was studied at the Departments of Psychiatry and Neurochemistry and Pediatrics, University of Goteborg, Goteborg, Sweden. A selective loss of myelin-associated lipids and an enrichment of gangliosides was demonstrated in the temporal white matter. The ganglioside pattern showed an increase of astroglial cell-associated gangliosides and reduced proportions of gangliosides GDla and GTlb. The fatty acid compositions of ethanolamine phosphoglyceride, choline phosphoglyceride, and galactosylceramide were normal. (Lekman AY, Hagberg BA, Svennerholm LT. Membrane cerebral lipids in Rett syndrome. Pediatr Neurol May/June 1991; 7:186-190).

COMMENT: There is as yet no specific biochemical marker for Rett syndrome. These changes in lipid membranes are thought to be secondary, confirming the neuropathologic finding of slight demyelination in Rett syndrome. PET studies performed on six patients with Rett syndrome at the Division of Child Neurology, National Center Hospital for Mental Disorders, Kodaira, Tokyo, Japan showed that cerebral blood flow and oxygen metabolism were abnormal and the cerebral metabolic rate of oxygen and oxygen extraction fraction were low. Impaired oxidated metabolism in Rett syndrome is suggested by this study. (Yoshikawa H et al. J Child Neurol July 1991; 6:237-242).

A significant increase in B-endorphin in the cerebrospinal fluid, an elevation of the CSF/Plasma B-endorphin ratio and a decrease in CSF cortisol are reported in a study of 15 girls with Rett syndrome at the Unite de Neuropediatrie, Centre Gui de Chauliac, Montpellier, France. The plasma cortisol and B-endorphin levels were similar in the patient and control groups (Echenne B et al. J Child Neurol July 1991; 6:257-262). The authors comment that the inconsistent nature of the CSF endorphin increase exclude its use as a biologic marker of Rett syndrome.- Editor. *Ped Neur Briefs* Sept 1991.

NEUROCHEMICAL MARKERS IN RETT'S SYNDROME

The levels of endogenous biogenic amines and neurotransmitter receptors in the brains of 5 patients with Rett's syndrome and 6 normal controls were examined at The Johns Hopkins University, Kennedy Institute for Handicapped Children, The Department of Neurology and Pediatrics, The Johns Hopkins Hospital, Baltimore, MD and The National Institute of Mental Health, Washington, D.C. The patients with Rett's syndrome were all female and they had died at ages 4, 10, 12, 15, 21 years. The cause of death was unknown in 2, asphyxiation in 1, drowning in 1 and pneumonia, 1. The level of choline acetyltransferase activity was lower in many cortical and subcortical regions in the Rett syndrome brains as compared with the mean level in the controls. Endogenous dopamine levels in the superior frontal and superior temporal gyri, occipital cortex, and putamen were reduced. The authors note that these results suggest neurochemical features in Rett's syndrome similar to those found in Parkinson's and Alzheimer's diseases (Wenk GL, Moser H et al. Altered neurochemical markers in Rett's syndrome. Neurology Nov 1991; 41:1753-1756).

COMMENT. The dopamine agonist, bromocriptine,

used to treat girls with Rett's syndrome, has made them more relaxed, sociable, affectionate and attentive, the stereotyped hand-washing movements diminished and some patients spoke for the first time (Zappella M, Genazzani A. Wien Med Wochenschr 1986; 122:98). The hypothesis that a disturbance in the function of central dopaminergic systems in Rett's syndrome is related to a defect in maturation may also be extended to include the cholinergic neural system. The search for a biochemical marker for Rett's syndrome continues.- Editor. *Ped Neur Briefs* Dec 1991.

STAGES OF RETT SYNDROME

The late infantile regression period (stages I and II) was analyzed retrospectively in 91 girls and women at the Department of Pediatrics, University of Goteborg and Pediatric Clinic, Ostersund Hospital, Sweden. The median age at onset of developmental stagnation (stage I) was 11 months, and loss of acquired skills (stage II) began at 19 months and lasted for 19 months. The onset of regression was distinct in 43%, dramatic in 16%, and insidious in 41%. The first observed signs of disease were delay in reaching expected gross motor milestones, dissociation of motor development, and disequilibrium. A triad of manifestations characterized the deterioration or loss of acquired skills: contact/communication, hand use/skill, babble/words. End of regression occurred at mean age 2.5 years. The girls gradually became more alert and showed an interest to act and interact. Handedness showed a preference for the left hand compared to the right, and was associated with spike activity in the left central leads in the EEG in 13 of 20 girls. (Engerstrom IW. Rett syndrome: the late infantile regression period - a retrospective analysis of 91 cases. Acta Paediatr Feb 1992; 81:167-172.) (Correspondence: Dr. Ingegerd Witt Engerstrom, Pediatric Habilitation Center, Tallasvagen 4, S-83142 Ostersund, Sweden.)

COMMENT. This further delineation of the stages of Rett syndrome may help in the diagnosis and pathophysiology of the disorder. In a study involving the analysis of beta-endorphin, as well as lactate, pyruvate and metabolites of norepinephrine, dopamine and serotonin in CSF from 12 girls with Rett's syndrome, the most consistent and significant difference from a control group was the elevation of beta-endorphin immunoreactivity in the CSF. Myer EC et al. from the Department of Child Neurology, Medical College of Virginia, Richmond, VA found increased levels of beta-endorphin immunoreactivity in lumbar CSF in 90% of 158 Rett syndrome patients. (Neurology Feb 1992; 42:357-360.) The authors note that the symptoms of Rett syndrome are similar to the effects of centrally administered beta-endorphin or other opioids in experimental animals.-Editor. *Ped Neur Briefs* July 1992.

RETT SYNDROME: GROWTH AND NUTRITION

Feeding problems, dietary intake and the growth and nutrition of 10 girls with Rett syndrome were reported from the University of Oslo, Norway. All patients had birth weight and length within the normal range until 6 to 24 months of age. A fall off in linear growth occurred in the first 2 years of life, and at follow-up between 3 and 16 years of age, all but 1 had height and/or weight below the 2.5 percentile of healthy children. Oral-motor dysfunctions were common. The mean energy intake was 70% of the U.S. recommendations according to age and 108% according to body weight. The intakes of thiamin, vitamin D, calcium and iron were low. None was anemic (Thommessen M et al. Growth and nutrition in 10 girls with Rett syndrome. Acta Paediatr Sept 1992; 81:686-690). (Correspondence: Dr. M. Thommessen, Oslo City Department of Environmental Health, Saint Olavs plass 5, 0165 Oslo 1, Norway.)

COMMENT. The authors conclude that feeding problems and inadequate intake of nutrients contribute to the poor weight and growth of girls with Rett syndrome. Consultation with a dietician is important in children with Rett syndrome.

Rett syndrome in a pair of full sisters is reported from Sao Paulo, Brazil (Kok F et al. Pediatr Neurol

Sept/Oct 1992; 8:381 (abstract)). The occurrence of familial cases is very rare and up to now, 3 pairs of full sisters, 2 pairs of half sisters, and 1 aunt/niece pair had been reported. All 2 pairs of female dizygotic twins have been discordant and all 8 pairs of monozygotic twins have been concordant for the disease. The parents of the reported sisters with Rett syndrome were unrelated.-Editor. *Ped Neur Briefs* Dec 1992.

RETT SYNDROME:MITOCHONDRIAL DYSFUNCTION?

Ultrastructural and biochemical alterations of muscle mitochondria are reported in two girls, aged 4 years, with Rett syndrome examined at the Institute of Neurological Sciences, University of Siena, Italy. Mitochondria were abnormally swollen and dumb-bell-shaped, and cytochrome c oxidase and NADH cytochrome c reductase were decreased in activity. The primary or secondary role of this mitochondrial pathology in the pathogenesis of the syndrome is undetermined. (Dotti MT et al. Mitochondrial dysfunction in Rett syndrome. Brain & Development March/April 1993; 15: 103-106). (Respond: Prof A Federico, Instituto di Scienze Neurologiche, Policlinico Le Scotte, 53100 Siena, Italy).

COMMENT. In contrast to the above, phosphorus magnetic resonance spectroscopy, proton MRS, muscle biopsies, and determination of pyruvate and lactate in plasma of 5 girls with Rett syndrome, examined at the John F Kennedy Institute, Glostrup, Denmark, failed to detect evidence for a mitochondrial disorder. (Nielsen JB, Lou HC et al. Brain & Development March/April 1993; 15: 107-112).-Editor. *Ped Neur Briefs* June 1993.

MRI NEUROANATOMY OF RETT SYNDROME

The neuroanatomy of 11 females with Rett syndrome (RS) and 15 control subjects investigated in vivo with quantitative MRI is reported from Johns Hopkins University, Baltimore, MD. Compared to age- and gender-matched controls, RS patients had 1) significantly reduced cerebral volume; 2) reduction in brain tissue volumes, especially affecting gray matter; 3) regional variation in cortical gray matter, frontal regions showing the largest decrease; 4) volume reduction of caudate nucleus and midbrain; and 5) increased CSF volume. There was no evidence of an ongoing degenerative process in these patients. (Reiss AL et al. Neuroanatomy of Rett syndrome: a volumetric imaging study. Ann Neurol Aug 1993;34:227-234). (Respond: Dr Reiss, Behavioral Genetics and Neuroimaging, Kennedy Kreiger Institute, 707 North Broadway, Baltimore, MD 21205).

COMMENT. These findings are consistent with one previous neuropathological report, whereas cerebellar pathology was emphasized in another autopsy report of 5 patients (Oldfors A et al. Pediatr Neurol 1990;6:310). See Progress in Pediatric Neurology, Chicago, PNB Publ, 1991.-Editor. *Ped Neur Briefs* Aug 1993.

CHAPTER 18

NUTRITION, DIET AND NERVOUS SYSTEM DISORDERS

INTRODUCTION

The role of nutrition and diet in the cause and management of nervous system diseases is often discounted in the practice and teaching of child neurology. This compilation of articles points to the importance of nutritional and dietary factors as the basis for certain neurobehavioral and cognitive disorders, neural tube and other fetal malformations, familial ataxias and degenerative diseases, seizures, and foodborne toxic encephalopathies. -*Editor.*

CHLORIDE-DEFICIENT DIET AND COGNITIVE DEFICITS

Distinctive cognitive impairments and a specific neurobehavioral syndrome are reported in 11 of 13 children who had failed to thrive on chloride-deficient formula during infancy. They were examined four to nine years later at the Division of Pediatric Neurology, UCLA School of Medicine, Los Angeles, CA and the Department of Neurology, Boston University School of Medicine, Boston, MA. All patients during infancy had developed symptoms of hypokalemic, hypochloremic metabolic alkalosis and/or growth deceleration, concurrently with their exposure to chloride-deficient Neo-Mull-Soy formula. Head circumference at follow-up was within normal limits, three children had hypotonia, two diffuse hyperreflexia, one had choreiform movements and one bilateral intention tremor. The EEG was abnormal in six, with paroxysmal discharges seen in five children. CT and MRI studies were normal. Intelligence was within the average range for 11 of the 13 children tested. All had a neurobehavioral syndrome consisting of a language disorder primarily involving articulation, word finding and naming; visual-motor and fine motor difficulties; and attention deficit disorder often featuring repetitive behaviors, withdrawal and "over-focus". (Kaleita TA, Kinsbourne M, Menkes JH. A neurobehavioral syndrome after failure to thrive on chloride-deficient formula. Dev Med Child Neurol July 1991; 33:626-635).

COMMENT. A syndrome characterized by loss of appetite, failure to gain weight, muscular weakness, lethargy, vomiting and severe hypochloremic, hypokalemic, metabolic alkalosis has been described in infants fed chloride-deficient soy-based infant formulas. Clinical features resemble Bartter Syndrome, but the renal biopsy is normal and infants recover when dietary chloride supplements are provided. Previous follow-up reports have drawn attention to developmental delay (Chutorian et al. Pediatr Neurol 1985;1:334-341) and the present study demonstrates specific cognitive, language and attentional deficits in later childhood.-Editor. *Ped Neur Briefs* Sept 1991.

SUGAR AND AGGRESSIVE AND INATTENTIVE BEHAVIOR

The effect of a sucrose challenge on aggressive behavior and sustained attention in a sample of young hyperactive boys and age-matched control subjects was studied at the Schneider Children's Hospital, Long Island Jewish Medical Center, New York, and Albert Einstein College of Medicine, Bronx, New York. The index group met DSM-III criteria for ADD-H and oppositional disorder as determined by interviews using the diagnostic interview for children and adolescents. They also scored at least 14 or above on the hyperkinesis index of parent and teacher revised questionnaires. Baseline testing was followed by a breakfast containing 8 oz of an orange colored and flavored drink containing either 35 g of sucrose or adjusted to equal sweetness with either saccharine (175 mg) or aspartame (175 mg). The sugar and placebo challenges were given with a breakfast high in carbohydrate. There were no significant effects of sugar or placebo on the aggressive behavior of either group. Inattention measured by a continuous performance task increased in the ADD-H group following sugar, but not with saccharine or aspartame control. (Wender EH, Solanto MV. Effects of sugar on aggressive and inattentive behavior in children with attention deficit disorder with hyperactivity and normal children. Pediatrics Nov 1991; 88:960-966.) (Reprint- Dr Wender, Scbneider Children's Hospital, New Hyde Park, NY 11042)

COMMENT. A deterioration in attention following sugar ingestion has been reported in one other study by Connors et al. in which sugar was administered with a high carbohydrate breakfast. When a negative effect was observed in 3 other studies the sugar was given either in a fasting state or with a protein breakfast. Further studies are indicated.-Editor. *Ped Neur Briefs* Jan 1992.

Addendum. Wolraich ML and associates, at Vanderbilt University, Nashville, TN, and Iowa College of Medicine, Iowa City, testing 25 normal preschool children (3 to 5 years of age), and 23 school-age children (6 to 10 years) described by their parents as sensitive to sugar, found no significant differences in behavior and cognitive performance during three-week diet periods high in sucrose or aspartame. (N Engl J Med Feb 3, 1994;330:301-7). Despite these negative results in a well controlled study, parents and some physicians cite cane sugar as a frequent trigger of hyperactive behavior in children. It may be argued that certain children are sensitive to sugar and aspartame but adverse effects are difficult to document by limited trial periods in the children selected for specific studies.

FOOD-INDUCED HYPERKINESIS

The results of a controlled trial of hyposensitization with intradermal EPD (beta-glucuronidase and food antigens) in 40 children with the hyperkinetic syndrome are reported from the Universitatskinderklinik, Lindwurmstrasse, Munchen, Germany and The Allergy Unit, London, UK. The study was in 3 phases: the first consisted of the oligoantigenic diet; children who responded to the diet entered the reintroduction of foods, phase II; and those with food-induced hyperkinetic syndrome entered phase III, a double-blind, placebo-controlled trial of EPD, 3 intradermal doses at 2 monthly intervals. Of 20 patients who received the hyposensitization active treatment, 16 became tolerant toward provoking foods, compared with 4 of 20 who received placebo ($p<0.001$). The authors conclude that EPD permits children with food-induced hyperkinetic syndrome to eat foods that had previously been identified as responsible for their symptoms (especially chocolate, colorings, cow milk, egg, citrus, wheat, nuts and cheese). Food allergy is considered a possible mechanism of the hyperkinetic syndrome. (Egger J et al. Controlled trial of hyposensitization in children with food-induced hyperkinetic syndrome. Lancet May 9, 1992; 339:1150-1153.) (Correspondence: Dr. J. Egger, Universitatskinderlclinik, Lindwurmstrasse 4, 8000 Munchen 2, Germany .)

COMMENT: Dr. Egger also reports a beneficial effect of the hypoallergenic diet in 12 children who suffered from enuresis in association with migraine and the hyperkinetic syndrome (Egger J et al. Clin Pediatr May 1992; 31:302-307). In an editorial Fitzwater D and Macknin ML (Clin Pediatr 1992; 31:308-310) recommend additional studies before dietary therapy can be introduced as a standard therapy for enuresis. Given the hazards of pharmacological therapy and the practical disadvantages of the alarm system, Dr. Egger's dietary and hyposensitization methods deserve attention. For reviews of previous articles on the hypoallergenic diet, see Progress in Pediatric Neurology, Ed Millichap JG, Chicago, PNB Publ, 1991, p. 88-89.-Editor. *Ped Neur Briefs* Aug 1992.

FOLIC ACID AND NEURAL TUBE DEFECTS

The results of a randomized double-blind prevention trial conducted at 33 centers in seven countries to determine the effects of folic acid supplements around the time of conception in the prevention of neural tube defects are reported by the MRC Vitamin Study Research Group, Department of Environmental and Preventive Medicine, Medical College of St. Bartholomew's Hospital, London EC1, UK. A total of 1,817 women at high risk of having a pregnancy with a neural tube defect were allocated at random to one of four groups - folic acid, other vitamins, both, or neither. Of 27 mothers giving birth to a child with a neural tube defect, six were in the folic acid groups and 21 in the two other groups, a 72% protective effect. Other vitamins showed no significant protective effect. Capsules for those in the folic acid group contained 4 mg of folic acid, one a day until 12 weeks of pregnancy (Wald N et al. Prevention of neural tube defects: results of the Medical Research Council vitamin study. Lancet July 20, 1991; 338:1311 37) .

COMMENT. This study establishes the specific role of folic acid in the prevention of neural tube defects. Folic acid supplementation in a dose of 4/mg/day is now recommended for all women who have had a previously affected pregnancy, and the diet of all women who may bear children should contain an adequate amount of folic acid. An editorial in this issue of The Lancet comments that this supplement did not prevent all neural tube defects and six unsuccessful cases were not accounted for by unusually low serum folic acid concentrations. A heterogeneous etiology for this group of disorders is suggested. The dosage of folic acid necessary to prevent neural tube defects is not entirely established, and the optimal duration of treatment before conception is uncertain. Can culturally appropriate dietary guidelines be prepared as a matter of urgency for all ethnic groups? Can the requisite folic acid be eaten in food instead of given as a supplement? Providing specific dietary advice about the prevention of malformations to women before pregnancy is a challenging public health problem.-Editor. *Ped Neur Briefs* Sept 1991.

Addendum. In July 1993, the US Center for Disease Control and Prevention in Atlanta, and later, the FDA proposed that all flour and other grains should be fortified with folic acid to prevent spinal and brain defects in newborns. This general supplementation of diets could lead to complications in some individuals, particularly in patients with pernicious anemia.-Editor.

VITAMIN E DEFICIENCY FAMILIAL ATAXIC SYNDROME

A total of 8 members of two consanguineous Tunisian families affected with Friedreich's ataxia (FA) phenotype not linked to chromosome 9 were found to have very low levels of serum vitamin E (0.5 mcg/ml cf 8 mcg/ml in controls) in a study at the Institut National de Neurologie, Tunis, and at Centers in Cyprus and France. All patients had typical signs of FA: severe ataxia, bilateral Babinski signs, pes cavus, scoliosis, and absent tendon reflexes and proprioception. The mean age at onset was 11 years, and 6 patients were wheelchair-bound at examination at 20 - 30 years of age. Cardiomyopathy was found in 5. Parents and healthy sibs had normal serum vitamin E levels, pointing to an autosomal recessive trait in affected members. Cystic fibrosis, abetalipoproteinemia, and fat malabsorption syndromes were excluded as possible causes of vitamin E deficiency. This FA with selective vitamin E deficiency was mapped to chromosome 8q, confirming its specificity. (Hamida MB et al. Friedreich's ataxia phenotype not linked to chromosome 9 and associated with selective autosomal recessive vitamin E deficiency in two inbred Tunisian families. Neurology Nov 1993;43:2179-2183). (Reprints: Prof Mongi Ben Hamida, Institut National de Neurologie, La Rabta 1007 Tunis, Tunisia).

COMMENT. The neurological syndrome of vitamin E deficiency is reviewed in an editorial by Dr HJ Kayden, Dept of Medicine, New York University Medical Center, New York (Neurology Nov 1993;43:2167-2169). Abetalipoproteinemia and cholestatic liver disease are characterized by fat malabsorption, resulting in steatorrhea and vitamin E deficiency. In familial isolated vitamin E deficiency, lipid and vitamin E absorption and plasma lipoproteins are normal but conservation of plasma a-tocopherol is poor due to impaired secretion in very low-density lipoproteins. Patients must maintain continuous supplementation with vitamin E (600 IU twice daily, 5 - 10 mg/kg). The observation that some patients with typical signs of Friedreich's ataxia have a familial vitamin E deficiency syndrome emphasizes the recommendation that all patients with ataxia and neuropathy should have plasma vitamin E determinations. Early supplementation with vitamin E should halt progression of ataxia, and genetic linkage analysis may establish the diagnosis. Asymptomatic sibs should be tested in early childhood, since vitamin E may prevent the onset of ataxia in those affected.-Editor. *Ped Neur Briefs* Dec 1993.

PYRIDOXINE DEPENDENT EPILEPSY

Four children with pyridoxine dependent seizures beginning at 2 to 19 months are reported from the Loyola University Medical Center, Maywood, IL. Patients were identified out of 51 treated routinely with pyridoxine for refractory seizures and seen over a 6 year period. The dose of pyridoxine was 50 mg orally twice daily. The seizure types were atypical absence, myoclonic, generalized clonic and simple partial and complex partial. The authors suggest that pyridoxine should be tried in all children with seizure disorders with onset at any age who are poorly responsive to anticonvulsant drugs. (Coker SB, Postneonatal vitamin

B_6 - dependent epilepsy. Pediatrics Aug 1992; 90:221-223.) (Reprints: S.B. Coker, M.D., Loyola University Medical Center, 2160 S. First Ave., Maywood, IL 60153.)

COMMENT. Pyridoxine dependent epilepsy may present after the neonatal period and may be manifested by many seizure types. Many of us have been discouraged by failure to uncover pyridoxine dependency in drug resistant epilepsies in children. Obviously, persistence rewards, but the relationship between pyridoxine and epilepsy is complex.

The wide range of reactivity of vitamin B_6 with a number of drugs and other chemicals encountered in the environment must be considered in the diagnosis. These interactions involve a condensation between the xenobiotic and pyridoxal phosphate, and vitamin B_6 absorption, coenzymes, and specific vitamin B_6-dependent enzymes can also be affected. Isoniazide is probably the most extensively studied drug with respect to effects on vitamin B_6 metabolism. Other drugs reported to interact with vitamin B_6 include ampicillin, anticonvulsants, levodopa, oral contraceptives and ethanol. The mechanism of anticonvulsant drug and vitamin B_6 interaction is not well determined. One study showed that the vitamin was decreased only in males treated with anticonvulsants. Another showed that pyridoxine supplements resulted in lower plasma phenytoin and phenobarbital concentrations. An interaction between the vitamin and dyes added to medications during manufacture has also been demonstrated (Dubick MA. Interactions of vitamin B_6 (pyridoxine) and xenobibotics. In Nutritional Toxicology, Vol III, ed. JN Hathcock. New York, Academic Press, 1989 .)-Editor. *Ped Neur Briefs* Sept 1992.

OCCIPITAL LOBE SEIZURES AND CELIAC DISEASE

The electroclinical ictal findings of 4 epileptic patients with clinically asymptomatic celiac disease are reported from the University of Bologna, Italy. All patients had paroxysmal visual manifestations and EEG seizure discharges arising from the occipital lobe. CT in 2 patients showed occipital calcifications. A gluten-free diet was not beneficial and polytherapy with antiepileptic drugs aggravated the seizures in 3 cases. Epilepsy and evidence of steatorrhea and growth failure were present in early childhood. The diagnosis of celiac disease was made by tests for serum folate level, a d-zylose absorption test, anti-gliadin antibody test and jejunal biopsy which showed villous atrophy (Ambrosetto G et al. Occipital lobe seizures related to clinically asymptomatic celiac disease in adulthood. Epilepsia May/June 1992; 33:476-481). (Reprints: Professor G. Ambrosetto, Institute of Neurology, Via Ugo Foscolo 7, 40123, Bologna, Italy.)

COMMENT. The same authors had investigated 10 patients with epilepsy and occipital cerebral calcification and had found evidence of celiac disease in 6. All patients with epilepsy and posterior cerebral calcification should be investigated for possible celiac disease. (Gobbi G, Ambrosetto P et al. Celiac disease, posterior cerebral calcifications and epilepsy. Brain Dev Jan 1992; 14:23-29.)-Editor. *Ped Neur Briefs* Aug 1992.

CEREBROVASCULAR ABNORMALITIES AND CELIAC DISEASE

Cortical vascular abnormalities including pial angiomatosis and fibrosis of small veins are described in a 12 year old girl with celiac disease, occipital calcifications, and folate deficiency who underwent surgery for intractable complex partial seizures at the Montreal Neurological Institute, Canada. She was first diagnosed with Sturge-Weber syndrome without nevus flammeus. A right occipital resection was performed and was followed by seizure remission. Subsequently, low folic acid levels and iron deficiency anemia led to a diagnosis of celiac disease. Antigliadin antibodies were 182 arbitrary units (normal: < 25), and small bowel biopsy showed villous atrophy. A gluten-free diet with folate, vitamin E, and iron supplementation resulted in improved appetite and weight increase. (Bye AME et al. Cortical vascular abnormalities in thc syndrome of celiac disease, epilepsy, bilateral occipital calcifications, and folate deficiency. Ann Neurol Sept 1993;34:399-403). (Respond: Dr Anderman, Montreal Neurological Hospital, 3801 University St, Montreal, Quebec, Canada H3A 2B4).

COMMENT. The pathological abnormalities in this case were considered similar but not identical to those in Sturge-Weber syndrome. A syndromc of celiac disease, epilepsy, and cerebral calcifications, resembling Sturge-Weber syndrome, has been reported frequently, especially in Italy (Gobbi G et al. Lancet 1992;340:439; Tiacci C et al. Epilepsia 1993;34.528; Piattella L et al. Child's Nerv Syst 1993;9:172.).

Patients with occipital cerebral calcification of unknown cause and patients with celiac disease should receive an EEG, followed by an MRI if the EEG is abnormal. A new, rapid, noninvasive screening test for celiac disease, a strip-AGA (antigliadin antibody) test, performed on a drop of whole blood, is described from the Instituto per l'Infancia, Trieste, Italy (Not T et al. J Pediat Sept 1993;123:425-7).-Editor. *Ped Neur Briefs* Sept 1993.

KETOGENIC DIET FOR INTRACTABLE SEIZURES

The efficacy of the ketogenic diet in 58 children with multiple seizure types resistant to antiepileptic drugs has been evaluated at the Johns Hopkins University School of Medicine, Baltimore. All patients had severe neurologic handicaps: mental retardation (84%), cerebral palsy (45%), and microcephaly (15%). Mean age at diet initiation was 60 months (range 12-235 months). EEGs showed Lennox-Gastaut pattern (33%), hypsarrhythmia (19%), and focal activity (14%). Antiepileptic drugs, including valproate, showed no adverse interaction. Seizures were completely controlled in 29%, and reduced by half in 38%. Diet was continued for an average of 24 months in those controlled and for 4 months in the unimproved group. Dietary benefit was not determined by seizure type. Renal stones required withdrawal of the diet in 2 patients. (Kinsman SL et al. Efficacy of the ketogenic diet for intractable seizure disorders: Review of 58 cases. Epilepsia Nov/Dec 1992; 33:1132-1136). (Reprints: Dr SL Kinsman, Kennedy Krieger Institute, 707 N Broadway, Baltimore, MD 21205).

COMMENT. Despite further demonstration of its efficacy and relative safety, the ketogenic diet is not a popular method of therapy among neurologists generally. Apart from the Mayo Clinic and Johns Hopkins, the diet is not frequently promoted in the training of pediatric neurologists and dieticians. Furthermore, the bias against fat in the diet in today's society adds to the difficulty in convincing mothers to become enthusiastic partners in the treatment program. Millichap JG at the Mayo Clinic (Epilepsia 1964; 5: 239) and Schwartz RM at the John Radcliffe Hospital, Oxford (Dev Med Child Neurol 1989; 31: 145) studied the metabolic effects of the diet and were unable to document any significant changes in blood lipid profiles using the classical diet. For an account of the mechanism of action of the diet, see Millichap JG. Progress in Pediatric Neurology, Chicago, PNB Publ, 1991, p 87-88.-Editor. *Ped Neur Briefs* Jan 1993.

E COLI FOOD POISONING AND HEMOLYTIC-UREMIC ENCEPHALOPATHY

Twenty-seven children, ages 6 months - 13 years, with encephalopathy complicating hemolytic-uremic syndrome are reported from The University of British Columbia, Vancouver, Canada. Seventeen had seizures and 2 died. An increased risk for developing a neurological manifestation was correlated with the female sex, the prolonged use of an antimotility agent (e.g. codeine, anticholinergic drugs) and an increased hemoglobin (Cimolai N et al. Risk factors for the central nervous system manifestations of gastroenteritis-associated hemolytic-uremic syndrome. Pediatrics Oct 1992; 90:616-621. (Reprints: N. Cimolai, M.D., Department of Pathology, British Columbia's Children's Hospital, 4480 Oak St., Vancouver, British Columbia, Canada V6H 3V4.)

COMMENT. These authors have previously found an association between the prolonged use of antimotility drugs and the likelihood for progression of E coli enteritis to hemolytic-uremic syndrome. Systemically absorbed verotoxins are thought to be responsible for the multiple organ involvement. A food reservoir and improper handling are the most likely vehicles for transmission of the E coli.-Editor. *Ped Neur Briefs* Nov 1992.

E COLI HEMORRHAGIC COLITIS AND NEUROLOGIC SYMPTOMS

The neurological manifestations of hemorrhagic colitis in seven kindergarten children with *Escherichia coli* 0157:H7 infection are reported from the Saitama Children's Medical Center, Saitama, Japan. Generalized convulsions, occurring in 5 comatose patients, seizures were intractable in 3 and required toxic doses of anticonvulsants for their control. Two patients died after 5 and 7 days of illness. Transient symptoms, delayed in onset for 2 to 6 weeks and after consciousness improved, included phrenic nerve paralysis in 1 patient, neurogenic urinary incontinence in 3, gaze nystagmus in 3, action tremor and oral dyskinesia in 1, and vertigo in 1 patient. Pyrexia and hemolytic uremic syndrome were seen only in patients with neurologic complications. Diarrhea, bloody diarrhea, and abdominal pain were more frequent and severe in this group compared to 7 patients with no neurologic symptoms who were admitted to hospital. Contaminated well water was the source of infection, and verotoxin-I (Shiga-like toxin I) was the likely cause of neurological symptoms. (Hamano S et al. Neurological manifestations of hemorrhagic colitis in the outbreak of *Escherichia coli* 0157:H7 infection in Japan. Acta Paediatr May 1993; 82: 454-458). (Respond: S Hamano MD, Division of Neurology, S Children's Medical Center, 2100 Magome, Iwatsuki, Saitama 339, Japan).

COMMENT. Fever, high white blood cell count, young or old age, and prolonged antimotility drug use are risk factors for complications of this strain of E *coli* infection. For a comprehensive review of the neurologic and other complications of foodborne and waterborne infections, pollutants, and additives, see Environmental Poisons in Our Food, Millichap JG, Chicago, PNB Publishers, 1993.-Editor. *Ped Neur Briefs* June 1993.

AUTHOR INDEX

JOURNAL INDEX

A
Acta Paediatrica Scandinavica (Stockholm)
Acta Paediatrics Scandinavica Supplement
American Journal of Diseases of Children
American Journal of Human Genetics
American Journal of Medical Genetics
American Journal of Mental Retardation
American Journal of Neuroradiology
American Journal of Psychiatry
Anatomy & Embryology
Annals of Neurology
Annals of Nutrition and Metabolism
Annals of Pediatrics (Paris)
Archives of Disease in Childhood
Archives of General Psychiatry
Archives of Internal Medicine
Archives of Neurology
Archives of Neurology and Psychiatry

B
Biological Psychiatry
Brain
Brain & Development
British Medical Journal

C
Canadian Journal of Neurological Sciences
Cell
Cephalalgia
Child's Nervous System
Chinese Medical Journal
Clinical Electroencephalography
Clinical Neuropathology
Clinical Neuropharmacology
Clinical Pediatrics
Clinical Toxicology

D
Development
Developmental Biology
Developmental Brain Research
Developmental Medicine and Child Neurology
Developmental Review

E
Electroencephalography and Clinical Neurophysiology
Epilepsia
European Journal of Pediatrics
European Neurology
Exceptional Children

H
Headache

I
Intelligence
International Pediatrics (Miami)

J
Journal of the American Academy of Child and Adolescent Psychiatry
Journal of the American Medical Association
Journal of Child Neurology
Journal of Child Psychology and Psychiatry and Allied Disciplines
Journal of Clinical Neurophysiology
Journal of Clinical Psychiatry
Journal of Developmental Behavior and Pediatrics
Journal of Ethnopharmacology
Journal of Inherited Metabolic Disease
Journal of Laboratory and Clinical Medicine
Journal of Learning Disabilities
Journal of Medical Genetics
Journal of Nervous and Mental Disease
Journal of the Neurological Sciences
Journal of Neurology, Neurosurgery and Psychiatry
Journal of Neuropathology and Experimental Neurology
Journal of Pediatrics
Journal of Reproductive Medicine
Journal of the Royal Society of Medicine
Journal of Toxicology and Environmental Health

K
Klinische Padiatrie (Stuttgart)

L
Lancet

M
Mayo Clinic Proceedings

N
Nature
Neurology
Neuron
Neuropediatrics

Neuropsychologia
Neuroradiology
Neuroscience Letters
Neurotoxicology and Teratology
New England Journal of Medicine
Nutrition Reviews
Nutritional Toxicology

P
Pediatric Clinics of North America
Pediatric Infectious Disease Journal
Pediatrics
Pediatric Neurology
Pediatric Neurology Briefs
Pediatric Neurosurgery
Proceedings of the National Academy of Sciences (USA)
Progress in Pediatric Neurology
Psychological Medicine
Psychoneuroendocrinology

S
Scandinavian Journal of Educational Research
Science
Seminars in Neurology
Surgical Neurology

T
Transactions of the American Neurological Association

V
Visual Neuroscience

W
Weiner Medizinische Wochenschrift (Wien)